Communicable Disease Control and Health Protection Handbook

About the authors

Dr Jeremy Hawker has worked at local, regional and national levels in communicable disease control and health protection in the UK and has led work on evidence-based communicable disease control for the European Centre for Disease Prevention and Control (ECDC). He is currently Regional Epidemiologist for the Health Protection Agency in the West Midlands Region of England and is also the Registrar of the UK Faculty of Public Health, the standard setting body for specialist public health practice in the UK.

Dr Norman Begg is Chief Medical Officer of GlaxoSmithKline Biologicals, based at their global headquarters in Wavre, Belgium. He trained in public health and worked for many years as a consultant at the UK Public Health Laboratory Service (now Health Protection Agency) where he was head of the Immunisation Division. He has acted as a regular advisor to the World Health Organization. He has published extensively in the field of paediatric vaccines and is a former co-editor of *Immunisation Against Infectious Disease* (the *Green Book*).

Dr Iain Blair is an Associate Professor in the Department of Community Medicine at the Faculty of Medicine and Health Sciences of the United Arab Emirates University. As a GP, he worked in Canada and the Middle East before starting a career in public health. He has been a Consultant for Communicable Disease Control and a Regional Epidemiologist. In 2003 with the establishment of the UK Health Protection Agency he was Director of a Health Protection Unit before moving to the United Arab Emirates in 2008.

Professor Ralf Reintjes holds a full professorship for Epidemiology and Public Health Surveillance in Hamburg, Germany, and is Adjunct Professor for Infectious Disease Epidemiology in Tampere, Finland. He was a Fellow of the European Programme for Intervention Epidemiology Training at the National Institute of Public Health and the Environment in the Netherlands, head of the Department of Hygiene, Infectious Disease Epidemiology and Vaccinations at the Institute of Public Health of NRW, Germany, and head of the Emerging Risks Unit at the European Food Safety Authority in Parma, Italy. He has acted as consultant for the World Health Organization, the EU and other organisations in many European, African and Asian countries. He has published extensively in the field of Epidemiology, Surveillance, Health Systems and Policy Research.

Professor Julius Weinberg is Vice Chancellor at Kingston University London. He trained as an infectious disease physician, and then in public health. He was a consultant epidemiologist and head of Epidemiological Programmes at the PHLS/CDSC and has worked in Zimbabwe and Eastern Europe as well as the UK. He was involved in the development of European Infectious Disease Surveillance collaborations and the UK National Electronic Library for Infection; he was expert advisor to a House of Lords Select Committee inquiry into infectious disease.

Professor Karl Ekdahl is head of the Public Health Capacity and Communication Unit at the European Centre for Disease Prevention and Control (ECDC), where since 2005 he has held various positions including acting director. He is a specialist in infectious diseases, and prior to joining ECDC he was Deputy State Epidemiologist for Sweden. In 2007, he was appointed Adjunct Professor in Infectious Disease Epidemiology at the Karolinska Institutet in Stockholm. He is also the former editor-in-chief of the scientific journal *Eurosurveillance*.

Communicable Disease Control and Health Protection Handbook

Dr Jeremy Hawker *Regional Epidemiologist, Health Protection Agency, West Midlands; Registrar, UK Faculty of Public Health, UK*

Dr Norman Begg *Chief Medical Officer, GlaxoSmithKline Biologicals, Wavre, Belgium*

Dr Iain Blair *Associate Professor, Department of Community Medicine, Faculty of Medicine and Health Sciences, United Arab Emirates University, United Arab Emirates*

Professor Ralf Reintjes *Professor of Epidemiology and Public Health Surveillance, Hamburg, Germany; Adjunct Professor of Infectious Disease Epidemiology, Tampere, Finland*

Professor Julius Weinberg *Vice Chancellor, Kingston University, London, UK*

Professor Karl Ekdahl *Head of Public Health Capacity and Communication Unit, European Centre for Disease Prevention and Control (ECDC); Specialist in Infectious Diseases; Adjunct Professor in Infectious Disease Epidemiology, Karolinska Institutet, Stockholm, Sweden*

Third edition

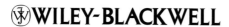

WILEY-BLACKWELL

A John Wiley & Sons, Ltd., Publication

Blackwell Publishing was acquired by John Wiley & Sons in February 2007. Blackwell's publishing program has been merged with Wiley's global Scientific, Technical and Medical business to form Wiley-Blackwell.

Registered office: John Wiley & Sons, Ltd, The Atrium, Southern Gate, Chichester, West Sussex, PO19 8SQ, UK

Editorial offices: 9600 Garsington Road, Oxford, OX4 2DQ, UK
The Atrium, Southern Gate, Chichester, West Sussex, PO19 8SQ, UK
111 River Street, Hoboken, NJ 07030-5774, USA

For details of our global editorial offices, for customer services and for information about how to apply for permission to reuse the copyright material in this book please see our website at www.wiley.com/wiley-blackwell

Library of Congress Cataloging-in-Publication Data

Communicable disease control and health protection handbook / Jeremy Hawker ... [et al.]. – 3rd ed.
    p. ; cm.
  Rev. ed. of: Communicable disease control handbook. 2nd ed. c2005.
  Includes index.
  ISBN 978-1-4443-3567-5 (pbk.)
    1. Communicable diseases–Handbooks, manuals, etc.   2. Communicable diseases–Prevention–Handbooks, manuals, etc.   I. Hawker, Jeremy.   II. Communicable disease control handbook.
    [DNLM: 1. Communicable Disease Control–Handbooks. WA 39]
    RC112.C626 2012
    616.9–dc23
                                                                                              2011018728

A catalogue record for this book is available from the British Library.

This book is published in the following electronic formats: ePDF [978-1-4443-4693-0]; Wiley Online Library [978-1-4443-4696-1]; ePub [978-1-4443-4694-7]; Mobi [978-1-4443-4695-4]

Typeset in 8/11pt Stoneserif by Aptara Inc., New Delhi, India
Printed in Singapore by Ho Printing Singapore Pte Ltd

First Impression 2012

Contents

Section 4: Services and organisations

Section 5: Communicable disease control in Europe

Appendices

Foreword

In the mid 1990s, EU-level co-operation against infectious diseases was a topic that interested no more than a few dozen experts in public health institutes across Europe. And the WHO's International Health Regulations were, in those days, regarded by most public health professionals as a rather obscure set of agreements of little practical relevance to their day-to-day work.

Fast forward to the year 2009, and co-operation within the EU system and under the WHO's revised International Health Regulations had a prominent role in the public health response to the first influenza pandemic of the twenty-first century. Subsequent evaluations of the EU and WHO responses to the 2009 influenza A (H1N1) pandemic indicated the value of this co-operation, while also pointing to areas where it needed to be strengthened.[1] Co-operation within the EU and internationally has now become part of the routine work of many public health professionals working on infectious diseases in Europe. This fact is recognised in the Third Edition of the *Communicable Disease Control and Health Protection Handbook*, which now contains two chapters on EU level and international public health structures for infectious disease control.

How did we reach this point? In his Foreword to the First Edition, Sir Donald Acheson wrote eloquently of the factors that drove communicable diseases up the national public health agenda during his time as Chief Medical Officer at the Department of Health in London. Sir Liam Donaldson, in his Foreword to the Second Edition, showed great insight in his analysis of the implications of the 2003 outbreak of severe acute respiratory syndrome (SARS) for international co-operation against infectious diseases. The issues identified by Sir Donald and Sir Liam have, if anything, increased in importance over the last few years.

Infectious diseases continue to matter in a relatively rich region such as the EU because, despite all of our medical technology, Europeans continue to die from these diseases. Even worse, significant outbreaks of infectious diseases can, and do, still occur in our societies. When this happens, they have the potential to cause great distress and disruption. Our citizens are not used to seeing previously healthy young and middle-aged people die from infections. Neither they, nor the health professionals who serve them, are willing to accept seeing a significant number of such deaths. National and EU level health authorities must therefore strive to provide their citizens with a high level of health protection.

Add to this the fact that the world, and particularly the EU, is ever more interconnected and the importance of co-operation across borders becomes clear. The influenza pandemics of the twentieth century took many months to spread around the world. In 2009, the first influenza pandemic of the twenty-first century reached over 100 countries within a matter of weeks of the new virus being identified.[2] To take another example, for the past decade or more a number

---

[1] See Report of the Review Committee on the functioning of the International Health Regulations (2005) and on Pandemic Influenza A (H1N1) 2009, WHO, Geneva, 2011 and Assessment Report on the EU-wide response to Pandemic (H1N1) 2009 (covering the period 24 April 2009–31 August 2009) and Assessment Report on EU-wide pandemic vaccine strategies both published by European Commission, Brussels, 2010.

---

[2] On 24 April 2009 the US Centers for Disease Control and Prevention (CDC) announced it had identified eight cases of infection with a new influenza A (H1N1) virus. On 24 June 2009, the ECDC published a situation report showing that a total of 56,129 cases of infection had been

of EU countries have been unable to achieve the 95% vaccine coverage needed to eliminate measles. In 2011 we are seeing large measles epidemics in these countries, with cases being exported across the EU. Individual EU countries cannot keep themselves measles free by national efforts alone. We need to achieve high vaccine coverage across the EU if we are going to keep our countries measles free.

One final example of the interconnectedness of health in the EU is the outbreak of enterohaemorrhagic *Escherichia coli* (EHEC) centred on northern Germany, which is taking place as I write. All of the infections in this outbreak are connected with a relatively limited region of northern Germany. But though the source of infection is localised, its impact has been international. At the time of writing, cases linked to this outbreak have been identified in 13 EU Member States as well the USA and Canada. The investigation, assessment and control of this outbreak has required collaboration between an array of regional and federal authorities in Germany: the ECDC, the European Commission, the European

Food Safety Authority and networks of public health and food safety experts across the EU. It is a good reminder that success in the fight against infectious diseases requires action and co-operation at all levels: local, regional, national and international.

The multilevel and multidisciplinary nature of communicable disease control in the modern world is complex. Finding your way through this maze is not always easy, especially when you face the acute pressures of a crisis situation. The modern disease control professional needs authoritative and easy to use information at his or her fingertips to point them rapidly in the right direction. This is what the *Communicable Disease Control and Health Protection Handbook* exists to give. I am sure you will find it an indispensible companion.

Marc Sprenger, MD PhD
Director
European Centre for Disease
Prevention and Control
Stockholm

---

identified by health authorities in a total of 109 countries and territories worldwide (see: http://ecdc.europa.eu/en/healthtopics/ Documents/090624_Influenza_AH1N1_ Situation_Report_1700hrs.pdf).

Abbreviations

ACDP	Advisory Committee on Dangerous Pathogens
AFB	Acid-fast bacilli
AIDS	Acquired immune deficiency syndrome
AMT	Antimicrobial management team
ART	Antiretroviral therapy
BBV	Blood-borne virus
BCG	Bacille Calmette–Guérin (vaccine against TB)
BSE	Bovine spongiform encephalopathy
CAP	Community-acquired pneumonia
CCDC	Consultant in Communicable Disease Control (local public health doctor with executive responsibilities for CDC)
CCHF	Congo–Crimean haemorrhagic fever
CDC	Communicable Disease Control
CDAD	*Clostridium difficile* associated disease
CDI	*Clostridium difficile* associated infection
CDP	Continuing professional development
CDR	Communicable Disease Report
CDT	Cytolethal distending toxin
CFT	Complement fixation test
CICN	Community infection control nurse
CIPC	Community infection prevention and control
CJD	Creutzfeldt–Jakob Disease
CMV	Cytomegalovirus
CNS	Central nervous system
COSHH	Control of Substances Hazardous to Health
CSF	Cerebrospinal fluid
D	Diarrhoea
DAEC	Diffuse-adherance *Escherichia coli*
DHEA	Diarrhoea-associated haemolytic *Escherichia coli*
DHF	Dengue haemorrhagic fever
DIC	Disseminated intravascular coagulation
	District Immunisation Committee
DIF	Direct immunofluorescence
DIPC	Director of Infection Prevention and Control
DNA	Deoxyribonucleic acid
DPH	Director of Public Health
DSN	Disease-specific surveillance network
DTP	Diphtheria, tetanus and pertussis (whole-cell)
EAAD	European Antibiotic Awareness Day
EAGA	Expert Advisory Group on AIDS
EAggEC	Enteroaggregative *Escherichia coli*
EARS-Net	European Antimicrobial Resistance Surveillance Network
EARSS	European Antimicrobial Resistance Surveillance System
EBV	Epstein–Barr virus
ECDC	European Centre for Disease Prevention and Control
EHEC	Enterohaemorrhagic *Escherichia coli*
EHO	Environmental Health Officer
EIA	Enzyme immunoassay
EIEC	Enteroinvasive *Escherichia coli*
ELISA	Enzyme-linked immunosorbent assay
EM	Electron microscopy
EPEC	Enteropathogenic *Escherichia coli*
EPP	Exposure-prone procedure
ERL	Emergency Reference Level
ETEC	Enterotoxigenic *Escherichia coli*
EU	European Union
EWRS	Early Warning and Response System
GBS	Group B streptococci
GP	General practitioner (primary care physician)
GRE	Glycopeptide-resistant emterococci
GUM	Genitourinary medicine

HA	Health authority	MLST	Multi-locus sequence typing
HACCP	Hazard Analysis Critical Control Point	MMR	Measles, mumps and rubella
		MMRV	Measles, mumps, rubella, varicella
HAI	Hospital-acquired infection	MRI	Magnetic resonance imaging
HAV	Hepatitis A virus	MRSA	Methicillin-resistant *Staphylococcus aureus*
HBeAg	Hepatitis B e antigen		
HBsAg	Hepatitis B surface antigen	MSM	Men who have sex with men
HBIG	Hepatitis B immunoglobulin	MSSA	Methicillin-sensitive *Staphylococcus aureus*
HBV	Hepatitis B virus		
HCAI	Healthcare-associated infection	NAAT	Nucleic acid amplification test
HCV	Hepatitis C virus	NPA	Nasopharyngeal aspirate
HCW	Healthcare worker	nvCT	New variant *Chlamydia trachomatis*
HELICS	Hospitals in Europe Link for Infection Control through Surveillance	OPV	Oral poliovirus vaccine
		PCR	Polymerase chain reaction
HEV	Hepatitis E virus	PCT	Primary care trust
HFMD	Hand, foot and mouth disease	PEP	Post-exposure prophylaxis
HFRS	Haemorrhagic fever with renal syndrome	PFGE	Pulsed field gel electrophoresis
		PHEIC	Public health emergency of international concern
HHV	Human herpesvirus		
Hib	*Haemophilus influenzae* type b	PPE	Personal protective equipment
HIV	Human immunodeficiency virus	PrP	Prion protein
HNIG	Human normal immunoglobulin	PMC	Pseudomembranous colitis
HP	Health Protection	PVL	Panton–Valentine leukocidin
HPA	Health Protection Agency	RCGP	Royal College of General Practitioners
HPAI	Highly pathogenic avian influenza		
HPS	Hantavirus pulmonary syndrome	RIDDOR	Reporting of Injuries, Diseases and Dangerous Occurrences
HPU	Health Protection Unit		
HPV	Human papillomavirus	RNA	Ribonucleic acid
HSV	Herpes simplex virus	RSV	Respiratory syncytial virus
HTLV	Human T-cell lymphotropic virus	RT-PCR	Reverse transcription polymerase chain reaction
HUS	Haemolytic uraemic syndrome		
ICC	Infection control committee	SARS	Severe acute respiratory syndrome
ICD	Infection control doctor (hospital)	SCID	Severe combined immunodeficiency
ICN	Infection control nurse		
ICT	Infection control team (hospital)	SFP	Staphylococcal food poisoning
ICU	Intensive care unit	SHEC	Shiga toxin producing *Escherichia coli*
ID$_{50}$	Median infective dose		
IDU	Injecting drug use/user	sp	Species
IFA	Indirect immunofluorescent antibody (test)	SSTI	Skin and soft tissues infection
		STI	Sexually transmitted infection
IgG	Immunoglobulin class G	SVR	Sustained virological response
IgM	Immunoglobulin class M	TB	Tuberculosis
IGRA	Interferon-gamma release assay	TBE	Tick-borne encephalitis
IHR	International Health Regulations	TSE	Transmissable spongiform encephalopathy
IPV	Inactivated poliovirus vaccine		
LA	Local authority	TTP	Thrombotic thrombocytopaenic purpura
LGV	Lymphogranuloma verereum		
LHPT	Local health protection team	TWAR	Taiwan acute respiratory agent
MDG	Millennium Development Goals	UK	United Kingdom of Great Britain and Northern Ireland
MIF	Microfluorescence		

vCJD	Variant Creutzfeldt–Jakob disease
VHF	Viral haemorrhagic fever
VRE	Vancomycin resistant *Enterococcus*
VTEC	Verocytotoxin-producing *Escherichia coli*
VZIG	Varicella-zoster immunoglobulin
VZV	Varicella-zoster virus
WHO	World Health Organization (OMS)
WNV	West Nile virus

Vaccine abbreviations (used in section 5)

D	Diphtheria vaccine (normal dose)*
d	Low dose diphtheria vaccine (booster dose)*
T	Tetanus vaccine (normal dose)*
t	Low dose tetanus vaccine (booster dose)*
aP	Acellular pertussis vaccine (normal dose)*
ap	Low dose acellular pertussis vaccine (booster dose)*
wP	Whole cell pertussis vaccine*
HiB	Haemophilus influenzae type b vaccine
OPV	Live oral polio vaccine
IPV	Inactivated polio vaccine
Var	Varicella vaccine
HepB	Hepatitis B vaccine
MenC	Meningococcal meningitis C conjugate vaccine
MMR	Measles, mumps and rubella vaccine
R	Rubella vaccine
RV	Rotavirus vaccine
BCG	Bacillus Calmette–Guérin vaccine
PCV	Pneumococcal conjugate vaccine
PPV	Pneumococcal polysaccharide vaccine
HPV	Human papilloma virus vaccine

*Given as part of DTaP, DTwP, DT, dT, dTaP or dtap.

Section 1
Introduction

1.1 How to use this book

This book is for those working in the field of communicable disease control (CDC) and health protection. It provides practical advice for specific situations and important background knowledge that underlies CDC activities; therefore it will be of interest to all these working in this broad field, including (but not exclusively) public health physicians, epidemiologists, general practitioners, public health nurses, infection control nurses, environmental health officers, microbiologists and policy makers at all levels, as well as students in medical, public health and related fields.

Since the publication of the second edition, there have been many important changes in CDC and health protection. The world has faced its first pandemic of influenza for many decades and other new or re-emerging threats have been identified. There have been successes, such as new vaccine programmes, improvements in knowledge, new evidence reviews, updating of consensus guidelines and new laboratory tests, particularly in relation to molecular epidemiology. The combination of these with administrative changes in the European Union, the accession of new member states, the increasing role and outputs of the European Centre for Disease Prevention and Control (ECDC) and new administrative changes in countries like the UK has led to major revisions in the content of this Handbook.

The structure of the book is as follows:

Section 1 contains important background material. Chapter1.2 runs through the basic principles of transmission and control, which underlie later chapters. **Chapter 1.3** is aimed primarily at those who undertake on-call duties but do not practice in mainstream CDC or health protection and those undertaking health protection response duties for the first time.

Section 2 addresses topics in the way they often present to CDC staff in the field, i.e. as syndrome-related topics rather than organism-based, such as an outbreak of gastroenteritis of (as yet) undetermined cause, or a needlestick injury. In these chapters, we discuss the differential diagnosis (infectious and non-infectious), including how to decide the most likely cause based on relative incidence, clinical and epidemiological differences and laboratory tests. We also give general advice on prevention and control, including how to respond to a case or cluster when the organism responsible is not yet known. A new chapter in this section addresses measures that can be taken by individuals to reduce the risk of infection. When the organism becomes known, Section 3 should be consulted.

Section 3 addresses CDC in a more traditional way, by disease/organism. We have continued to make these chapters more European, using EU wide data and policies where these exist. We have used England and Wales (or the UK if appropriate) as an example in other instances: for differences relating to surveillance and control in other countries, the relevant country specific chapter in Section 5 should be consulted (e.g. those working in Germany should consult Chapter 5.13).

The chapters in Section 3 conform to a standard pattern, which we hope will make instant reference easier. Most chapters are ordered as follows:

1 A short introduction mentioning the syndrome(s) common synonyms and the main public health implications of the organism.

2 A box of *suggested on-call action*. This relates only to what needs to be done if cases are reported outside of normal office hours. Further action may be needed during the next working day, which will be identified in 'response to a case'.

Communicable Disease Control and Health Protection Handbook, Third Edition. Jeremy Hawker, Norman Begg, Iain Blair, Ralf Reintjes, Julius Weinberg and Karl Ekdahl.

3 *Epidemiology* will give the relevant points on burden of disease, important differences by age/sex/season/year/risk group are given and important differences within Europe are noted.

4 Two sections deal with diagnosis of the infection: *clinical features* and *laboratory confirmation*. Both sections highlight the important points to practising CDC professionals. They are not meant as a substitute for clinical and microbiological textbooks.

5 *Transmission* details the main sources, reservoirs, vehicles and routes of spread of the organism. The main aim of this section is to give the investigator clues as to how a case or outbreak may have arisen to aid identification and control.

6 *Acquisition* deals with the incubation period, infectious period (if communicable), infective dose (if known) and any important factors affecting immunity or susceptibility.

7 The final five sections relate to control of infection. These are based on current available guidance and evidence: where this is unclear, they are based on practice in the UK (supplemented by our own views) although the principles will be equally relevant to European readers. These sections are:

- actions likely to be effective in the *prevention* of infection;
- *surveillance* activities relevant to the organism;
- suggested public health actions to be taken in *response to a case;* and
- suggested approach to an *investigation of a cluster* of cases of that organism, and suggested actions to help *control of an outbreak*, including a *suggested case-definition* for use in an epidemiological study.

New chapters have been added on *Burkholderia* and chickungunya. Diseases that are generally less of a public health issue in Europe are summarised in the tables that follow Section 3.

Section 4 refers to the organisation of CDC/health protection services and could be titled 'how to run a CDC service'. For the authors who have worked as consultants in CDC, this is the textbook that we wished we'd had on appointment! It deals with the

services that a CDC department is expected to provide, including the non-communicable disease functions that have been attached to the health protection role in some countries. Some of those chapters are UK focused, although this has been reduced and most (e.g. surveillance, outbreak management, hospital infection, clinical governance) will be of equal use to European colleagues. New chapters on antimicrobial resistance, pandemic preparedness and global health have been added to this section.

Section 5 gives a brief overview of structures for infectious disease notification and Public Health action internationally (consisting of two new chapters) and in the 27 EU Member States (including new chapters on the new members states), plus Norway, Switzerland and a new chapter on Iceland. The objective of this section is to allow an orientation on Public Health structures relevant for infectious disease control in various European countries and to offer a starting point for further information on individual countries. Lengthy descriptions have been avoided, but Internet addresses for contact points in the countries and for further information, reports and data have been given.

Finally, the two appendices and two lists of useful websites detail further sources of information and advice for those undertaking CDC functions routinely or on-call.

In updating the evidence base for this edition, we have often referred to the systematic review of 57 infections that was undertaken on behalf of ECDC by a combined team from the Health Protection Agency and the Royal College of Paediatrics and Child Health (which was led by JH) and we gratefully acknowledge this help. We are indebted to a number of individuals who have helped us in commenting on parts of the book, including Andrew Kibble, Amal Rushdy and numerous advisors for the country-specific chapters, including Reinhild Strauss and Franz Allerberger (Austria), René Snacken, Carl Suetens and Emmanuel Robesyn (Belgium), Angel Kunchev (Bulgaria), Chrystalla Chadjianastassiou (Cyprus), Jozef Dlhý (Czech Republic), Kåre Mølbak (Denmark), Kuulo

Kutsar and Jevgenia Epštein (Estonia), Petri Ruutu and Leino Tuija (Finland), Jean-Claude Desenclos (France), Gérard Krause and Andreas Gilsdorf (Germany), Sotirios Tsiodras (Greece), Ágnes Csohan (Hungary), Haraldur Briem (Iceland), Darina O'Flannagan (Ireland), Stefania Salmaso (Italy), Irina Lucenko (Latvia), Loreta Ašoklienė (Lithuania), Robert Hemmer (Luxembourg), Tanya Melillo Fenech (Malta), Roel Coutinho and George Haringhuizen (The Netherlands), Preben Aavitsland (Norway), Andrzej Zielinski (Poland), Ana Maria Correia (Portugal), Florin Popovici (Romania), Mária Avdičová (Slovakia), Irena Klavs and Eva Grilc (Slovenia), Karoline Fernández de la Hoz (Spain), Daniel Koch (Switzerland), Meirion Evans, Brian Smyth and Martyn Donaghy (UK) and Guénaël Rodier (WHO). Linda Parr and Leanne Baker's administrative skills were essential as was the help of Jennifer Seward at Wiley. Finally, we are grateful to our families and work colleagues for their patience and support whilst we were preoccupied with this project.

1.2 Basic concepts in the epidemiology and control of infectious disease

The epidemiological framework

Identification

Infections can be identified by their clinical features, epidemiology and the use of appropriate laboratory procedures.

Infectious agent

The traditional model of infectious disease causation is the epidemiological triangle. It has three components: an external agent, a susceptible host and environmental factors that bring the host and the agent together.

The agent is the organism (virus, rickettsia, bacterium, fungus, etc.) that produces the

infection. Host factors influence an individual's exposure, susceptibility or response to a causative agent. Age, sex, socio-economic status, ethnicity and lifestyle factors such as smoking, sexual behaviour and diet are among the host factors that affect a person's likelihood of exposure, while age, genetic makeup, nutritional and immunological status, other disease states and psychological makeup influence susceptibility and response to an agent. Environmental factors are extrinsic factors that affect the agent and the opportunity for exposure. These include geology, climate, physical surroundings, biological factors (such as insect vectors), socioeconomic factors such as crowding and sanitation and the availability of health services.

Occurrence

The occurrence or amount of an infectious disease will vary with place and time. A persistent low or moderate level of disease is referred to as *endemic* and a higher persistent level is called *hyper-endemic*. An irregular pattern with occasional cases occurring at irregular intervals is called *sporadic*. When the occurrence of an infection exceeds the expected level for a given time period, it is called *epidemic*. The term outbreak or cluster is also used. When an epidemic spreads over a wide geographical area, such as a continent or continents, it is called *pandemic*. Epidemics vary in size and duration. An *epidemic curve,* a frequency histogram of number of cases against time or date of onset (see Figures 4.2.1–4.2.3), should be plotted. If exposure to the infectious agent takes place over a relatively brief period, a *point source* outbreak occurs. Intermittent or continuous exposure broadens the peaks of the epidemic curve, and so an irregular pattern is observed. An outbreak that spreads from person to person is called a *propagated* outbreak. In theory, the epidemic curve of a propagated outbreak would have a series of peaks at intervals approximating to the incubation period. Usually, the epidemic wanes after a few generations because the number of susceptible people falls below a critical level. Some epidemic curves have both common source epidemic and propagated epidemic features because of secondary person-to-person spread. These are called *mixed epidemics*.

Two rates are commonly used to describe the occurrence of infectious diseases:

$$\text{Incidence} = \frac{\text{New cases over a given time period}}{\text{Persons at risk}}$$

$$\text{Prevalence} = \frac{\text{Existing cases at a given point in time}}{\text{Persons at risk}}$$

The chain of infection

Transmission occurs when the agent leaves its *reservoir* or host through a *portal of exit* and is conveyed by a mode of *transmission* and enters through an appropriate *portal of entry* to infect a susceptible host. This is the *chain of infection*.

Reservoir

The reservoir of an infectious agent is any person, animal, arthropod, plant, soil or substance (or combination of these) in which the infectious agent normally lives and multiplies. The reservoir may be different from the *source* or *vehicle* of infection. This is the person, animal, object or substance from which an infectious agent actually passes to a host. Many of the common infectious diseases have human reservoirs which include clinical cases, those who are incubating the disease and convalescent carriers. *Colonisation* is the presence of a micro-organism in or on a host, with growth and multiplication, but without evidence of infection. Shedding of an organism from a colonised host may be intermittent. Infectious diseases that are transmissible from animals to humans are called *zoonoses*. The *portal of exit* is the path by which an agent leaves the source host, which usually corresponds with the site at which the agent is localised, for example respiratory tract, genitourinary system, gastrointestinal system, skin or blood. The *portal of entry* is the route by which an agent enters a susceptible host.

For any given infection, understanding the chain of infection allows appropriate control measure to be recommended.

Mode of transmission

This is the mechanism by which an infectious agent is spread from a source or reservoir to a susceptible person. The mechanisms are detailed in Table 1.2.1.

Natural history of disease

This refers to the progress of a disease in an individual over time without intervention. Following exposure to an infectious agent there is a period of subclinical or inapparent pathological changes, which ends with the onset of symptoms. This period is known as the *incubation period*. For a given infectious disease, the incubation period has a range and a mean value. For hepatitis A the range is 2–6 weeks with a mean of 3 weeks. During the incubation period, pathological changes may be detectable with laboratory or other tests. Most screening programmes attempt to identify the disease process during this early phase of its natural history, since early intervention may be more effective than treatment at a later stage. The onset of symptoms marks the transition from the subclinical to the clinical phase. Most diagnoses are made during this stage. In some people the disease may never progress to a clinically apparent illness. In others the disease process may result in a wide spectrum of clinical illness, ranging from mild to severe or fatal.

Infectious period

This is the time during which an infectious agent may be transmitted directly or indirectly from an infected person to another person. Some diseases are more communicable during the incubation period than during the actual illness. In others such as tuberculosis, syphilis and *Salmonella* infection the communicable period may be lengthy and intermittent. The communicable period may be shortened by antibiotic treatment (though in some

Table 1.2.1 Modes of transmission of infectious agents

Types of transmission	Examples
Direct transmission Transmission by direct contact such as touching, biting, kissing, sexual intercourse or by droplet spread on to the mucous membranes of the eye, nose or mouth during sneezing, coughing, spitting or talking. Droplet spread is usually limited to a distance of one metre or less.	**Direct route** Infections of the skin, mouth and eye may be spread by touching an infected area on another person's body or indirectly through a contaminated object. Examples are scabies, head lice, ringworm and impetigo. Sexually transmitted infections are also spread by the direct route. **Respiratory route** Sneezing, coughing, singing and even talking may spread respiratory droplets from an infected person to someone close by. Examples are the common cold, influenza, whooping cough and meningococcal infection. **Faecal-oral route** Gastrointestinal infections can spread when faeces are transferred directly to the mouth of a susceptible host.
Indirect transmission This may be *vehicle-borne* involving inanimate materials or objects (*fomites*) such as toys, soiled clothes, bedding, cooking or eating utensils, surgical instruments or dressings; or water, food, milk or biological products such as blood. The agent may or may not multiply or develop in or on the vehicle before transmission. It may be *vector-borne*. This in turn may be *mechanical* and includes simple carriage by a crawling or flying insect as a result of soiling of its feet or proboscis or by passage of organisms through its gastrointestinal tract. This does not require multiplication or development of the organism. It may be *biological* when some form of multiplication or development of the organism is required before the arthropod can transmit the infected form of the agent to human when biting.	**Faecal-oral route** Faeces contaminate food or objects like toys or toilet flush handles. Animal vectors such as cockroaches, flies and other pests may transfer faeces. Environmental surfaces may be contaminated. This is particularly important in viral gastroenteritis when vomiting occurs because the vomit contains large numbers of infectious viral particles. Examples of infections spread in this way are food poisoning and hepatitis A. **The blood-borne route** There is transfer of blood or body fluids from an infected person to another person through a break in the skin such as a bite wound or open cut or through inoculation, injection or transfusion. Blood-borne infections include infection with HIV, and hepatitis B and C infections. Spread can also occur during sexual intercourse **Respiratory route** Droplets from the mouth and nose may also contaminate hands, cups, toys or other items and spread infection to others who may use or touch those items.
Air-borne spread *Air-borne* spread is the dissemination of a microbial aerosol to a suitable port of entry, usually the respiratory tract. Microbial aerosols are suspensions of particles that may remain suspended in the air for long periods of time. Particles in the range 1–5 µm are easily drawn into the alveoli and may be retained there. Droplets and other larger particles that tend to settle out of the air are not considered air-borne. Microbial aerosols are either droplet nuclei or dust.	Examples are infection with *Legionella*, *Coxiella* and in some circumstances TB.

Box 1.2.1 Terms used to describe the outcomes of exposure to an infectious agent

- *Infectivity*: the proportion of exposed persons who become infected, also known as the *attack rate*.
- *Pathogenicity*: the proportion of infected persons who develop clinical disease.
- *Virulence:* the proportion of persons with clinical disease who become severely ill or die (*case fatality rate*).

---

infections antibiotics may prolong carriage and hence the communicable period).

Susceptibility and resistance

This describes the various biological mechanisms that present barriers to the invasion and multiplication of infectious agents and to damage by their toxic products. There may be inherent resistance in addition to immunity as a result of previous infection or immunisation.

Hepatitis A in children has low pathogenicity and low virulence (Box 1.2.1). Measles has high pathogenicity but low virulence, whereas rabies is both highly pathogenic and highly virulent. The *infectious dose* is the number of organisms that are necessary to produce infection in the host. The infectious dose varies with the route of transmission and host susceptibility factors. Because of the clinical spectrum of disease, cases actually diagnosed by clinicians or in the laboratory often represent only the tip of the iceberg. Many additional cases may remain asymptomatic. People with subclinical disease are nevertheless infectious and are called carriers.

Preventing spread of infection

Standard precautions

It is not always possible to identify people who may spread infection to others, therefore standard precautions to prevent the spread of infection must be followed at all times (Box 1.2.2). In addition, for patients with respiratory infections, droplet precautions may be recommended (Box 1.2.3) and in those

---

Box 1.2.2 Standard precautions to prevent the spread of infection

- Hand hygiene: handwashing with soap and water or use of an alcohol hand rub or gel. Cover wounds or skin lesions with waterproof dressings.
- Appropriate use of gloves, gowns and aprons and facial protection (eyes, nose, and mouth).
- Prevention and management of needlestick injuries, injuries from other sharp instruments and blood splash incidents.
- Respiratory hygiene and cough etiquette.
- Safe disposal of contaminated waste.
- Managing spillages of blood and body fluids.
- Safe collection and transport of specimens.
- Decontaminating equipment including cleaning, disinfection and sterilisation.
- Maintaining a clean clinical environment.
- Safe management of used linen.
- Place patients with infections in appropriate accommodation.

World Health Organization (2007). Standard precautions in health care. Geneva: World Health Organization. http://www.who.int/csr/resources/publications/EPR_AM2_E7.pdf [Accessed March 2010].

Box 1.2.3 Droplet precautions when managing respiratory infections

- Wear a medical mask if working within approximately 1 m of the patient or upon entering the room/cubicle of a patient.
- When performing aerosol-generating procedures (chest physiotherapy, nebulisation) wear a particulate respirator, perform procedures in an adequately ventilated room and limit other persons in the room only to those required for the patient's care.

---

with diarrhoea and/or vomiting enteric precautions should be followed (Box 1.2.4).

Handwashing

Handwashing is the single most important part of infection control. The technique illustrated in Figure 1.2.1 should be used when washing soiled hands with soap and water. At other times an alcohol gel or rub can be used. Hands should be washed before contact with patients, after any activity that contaminates the hands (removal of protective clothing and gloves, using the toilet) and before handling food. Nails should be kept short, rings should not be worn, artificial nails should be avoided and cuts and abrasions should be covered with a waterproof dressing. Adequate handwashing facilities must be available in all patient areas. Liquid soap dispensers, paper hand towels and foot-operated waste bins should be provided.

Box 1.2.4 Enteric precautions when managing diarrhoea and vomiting

- Patients should normally use a flush toilet for the disposal of excretions and soiled materials. Attendants should wear disposable plastic gloves and wash hands thoroughly.
- Faecal material on soiled clothing and bed linen should be flushed into the toilet bowl. Linen should then be washed in washing machine on a 'hot' cycle. Soaking in disinfectant before washing is not necessary.
- Use of disinfectants is important in schools, nursery schools and residential institutions. Toilet seats, flush handles, wash-hand basin taps and toilet door handles should be cleaned daily and after use with a bleach-based household cleaner, diluted according to manufacturer's instructions. Alcohol-based wipes may be used on seats and other hard surfaces. Bedpans and urinals should be emptied into the toilet bowl, washed with a disinfectant and rinsed.
- Patients and carers should be advised about personal hygiene and the hygienic preparation and serving of food. Children and adults in jobs likely to spread infection should stay away from work or school for 48 h after the diarrhoea has stopped.

WASH HANDS WHEN VISIBLY SOILED! OTHERWISE, USE HANDRUB

Duration of the entire procedure: **40-60 seconds**

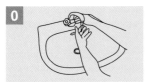

Wet hands with water;

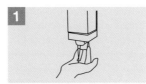

Apply enough soap to cover all hand surfaces;

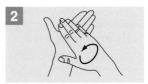

Rub hands palm to palm;

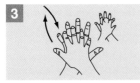

Right palm over left dorsum with interlaced fingers and vice versa;

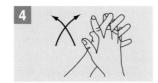

Palm to palm with fingers interlaced;

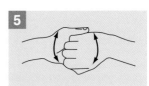

Backs of fingers to opposing palms with fingers interlocked;

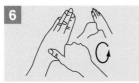

Rotational rubbing of left thumb clasped in right palm and vice versa;

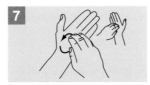

Rotational rubbing, backwards and forwards with clasped fingers of right hand in left palm and vice versa;

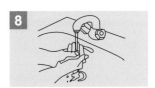

Rinse hands with water;

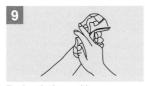

Dry hands thoroughly with a single use towel;

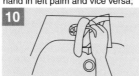

Use towel to turn off faucet;

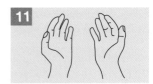

Your hands are now safe.

Fig. 1.2.1 How to wash hands correctly and reduce infection. (From World Health Organization (2009). WHO Guidelines on Hand Hygiene in Health Care. Geneva: World Health Organization. http://whqlibdoc.who.int/publications/2009/9789241597906_eng.pdf [Accessed March 2011].)

1.3 Health protection on-call

During office hours health protection activity is usually undertaken by individuals who are expert in their field and have access to a full range of supporting services. Outside of office hours, this is not always the case, for example in the UK health protection on-call at a local level may be integrated with general public health rotas and laboratories also offer a much reduced service.

Requirements for on-call staff

Undertaking health protection on-call should present few problems for those adequately trained in public health, as the skills applied are the same as those used in everyday public health practice, i.e.
- defining the problem;
- collecting the necessary information;
- undertaking a risk assessment;
- identifying good practice;
- implementing the response; and
- evaluating the outcome.

In addition to these generic public health skills, basic specialist health protection knowledge and experience is needed for safe out-of-hours health protection practice. A suggested list of the competences required is given in Box 1.3.1. These competencies need to be maintained by incorporating them into the continuous professional development plan for each individual, for example by attending an on-call updating course and participating in simulations and exercises.

Access to knowledge on-call is important and is available from:
- this handbook: on-call actions and underlying theory are given for all the most common pathogens;
- a local on-call pack, detailing local policies, procedures, plans and contact details;
- national guidance documents (see Appendix 2);

- websites, including those of the national communicable disease control or health protection organisation (see inside covers); and
- local, regional and national specialist on-call, for example the local acute hospital will usually have a consultant medical microbiologist on-call and the national health protection organisation will usually provide access to a communicable disease epidemiologist.

Public health response to a case of infection

The two key questions in dealing with a case of communicable disease are:
- *Where did the case get it from?* This is important because there may be a continuing source which needs to be controlled and because there may be others who have also been exposed and need advice and/or treatment. Others exposed may be known to the case (e.g. household or fellow tourists), but this is not always the case (e.g. a *Legionella* source in the environment).
- *Is the case likely to pass it on?* This may be to close contacts (e.g. household or sexual contacts) that need to be protected by advice to the case and perhaps prophylaxis for the contacts (e.g. hepatitis B), or it may be via the patient's occupation (e.g. a food handler who has a gastrointestinal infection).

Syndromes and diseases

At the time that health protection issues emerge, the causative agent may not yet be clear, for example an outbreak of diarrhoea and vomiting in a hospital or an outbreak of respiratory disease at a nursing home. This may be especially true out-of-hours. Section 2 of this book looks at problems from this angle. The important issues to consider are as follows:
- What investigations are needed to identify the agent (e.g. *Salmonella*), the cause of the incident (e.g. poor hygiene practices) and, if relevant, the vehicle of infection (e.g. a particular food served to guests)? Such investigations

Box 1.3.1 Suggested competences required to undertake consultant level health protection on-call duties

1 Familiarity with the principles and practice of being on-call, including:
- professional obligations;
- legal issues; and
- professional responsibility to ensure appropriate public health action taken in response to all incidents.

2 Ability to perform a risk assessment of a problem, decide whether public health action is necessary and decide appropriately whether action is required out of hours.

3 Ability to effectively exercise the local on-call procedures, including:
- administration of urgent prophylaxis; and
- handover before and after on-call.

4 Experience of practicalities of working with others out of hours, particularly:
- local and national health protection agency;
- microbiology laboratory; and
- environmental health department.

5 Up-to-date knowledge of relevant aspects of natural history, epidemiology, clinical presentation, laboratory diagnosis and methods of transmission and control of common hazards that may require public health intervention out of hours, including:
- meningococcal disease and meningitis;
- gastrointestinal infections, including *E. coli* O157;
- respiratory infection, including *Legionella* and TB;
- blood-borne viruses (hepatitis B, hepatitis C, HIV);
- infections requiring prophylaxis/advice (e.g. pertussis, hepatitis A, measles);
- most common chemical/environmental hazards (asbestos, CO, smoke, mercury, ammonia, chlorine); and
- other hazards with increased local/regional occurrence.

6 Ability to interpret national guidelines and local policies for the most common scenarios that present on-call and to coordinate public health action effectively. Includes single cases of infections listed in Section 5.

7 Awareness of the basic principles of control and sources of advice and support (particularly out of hours) for serious, less common public health problems that may present out of hours, including:
- imported infections (e.g. viral haemorrhagic fever, diphtheria, rabies exposure, possible SARS/avian flu);
- exposure of particularly vulnerable groups (e.g. chickenpox in immunosuppressed/ neonates; rubella in pregnancy);
- exposure to blood-borne viruses or TB in community or healthcare settings (including needlestick injuries and potential lookback exercises);
- potential public health emergencies (e.g. food-borne botulism);
- potential deliberate release (e.g. 'white powder' exposures);
- exposure to contaminated water;
- acute exposure to chemical hazards;
- urgent travel health enquiries;
- major emergencies (e.g. floods, explosions); and
- recently emerged diseases/hazards.

8 Understanding of the principles and practice of management of outbreaks and incidents.

> **Box 1.3.1 (*Continued*)**
>
> **9** Ability to effectively coordinate the public health investigation and control of common local outbreaks and incidents out of hours, including:
>   • potentially linked cases of meningococcal disease;
>   • potential community outbreaks of gastrointestinal illness; and
>   • chemical incidents.
> **10** Ability to contribute effectively to the control of:
>   • hospital outbreaks/incidents;
>   • radiological incidents;
>   • major emergencies; and
>   • deliberate release incidents.
> **11** Ability to communicate effectively on public health issues, including:
>   • preparing appropriate press releases out of hours;
>   • giving effective media interviews; and
>   • communicating directly with public.
>
> Source: UK Faculty of Public Health, 2006.

usually have microbiological, environmental and epidemiological components.

• What generic control measures can be applied to limit morbidity, whilst awaiting confirmation (e.g. enhanced handwashing, environmental cleaning and excluding ill food handlers in outbreaks of gastrointestinal illness)?

Public health action on-call

There are two key questions that define what action is taken on-call:
• Is public health action necessary?
• Does it need to be done now?

The factors in deciding whether public health action is necessary are a combination of the following:
• Is the index case at risk of a poor outcome? A death from meningitis or any case of a viral haemorrhagic fever are examples that lead to public anxiety and media interest.
• Is the index case likely to pass infection on to others? If so, action may be required to limit onward transmission from the index case and any infected contacts.
• Is there likely to be an ongoing source that needs controlling? Some stages in investigat-

ing possible sources take considerable time, so the earlier they are started, the sooner the result.
• Do contacts or others exposed to the same source need to be traced? This will be important if their outcome can be improved by an intervention or if it will help limit onward transmission.
• Do the public need information or reassurance? This is often affected by the 'scariness' of the disease, whether particularly vulnerable groups are exposed (e.g. children) and issues of 'blame'.

If public health action is necessary, it does not automatically follow that it should occur out-of-hours. Issues that affect timing include the following:
• The seriousness of the disease. Some infections such as viral haemorrhagic fevers, diphtheria or *Escherichia coli* O157 may require prompt action to prevent even one more additional case in vulnerable groups, whereas others such as norovirus or mumps are less of a threat to most individuals.
• How transmissible is the infection? Not only are some infections more transmissible than others, but some cases of the same infection can transmit more easily than others (e.g. e-antigen positive hepatitis B or smear positive TB).

• How long is the incubation period? Secondary (or co-primary) cases of meningococcal infection may present very quickly, but the incubation period for TB is weeks or months.
• How vulnerable are the people that may have been exposed? Some pathogens are particularly likely to lead to infection or a poor outcome in particular groups e.g. *E. coli* O157 in young children and the frail elderly or chickenpox in immunosuppressed patients. This will heavily influence speed of response.
• What is the public, media or political reaction? Even if not a health protection priority to react on-call (e.g. an HIV positive healthcare worker), action may be required if information becomes public.
• What is 'expected' or good practice?
• When will normal service be resumed? The risk of delaying until normal office hours is obviously proportional to the length of time until a 'normal' response can be activated. Thus, action is more likely on a Saturday morning before a national holiday Monday than on a Sunday night before a normal working Monday.

Collection of baseline data

Collecting information and recording it in a systematic way is important in order to:
• aid management of the incident: the information will be useful to you and to others who take over management later in the incident;
• be available for later scrutiny, either for professional purposes (audit, lessons learnt) or legal purposes (public inquiries or civil actions).
    A good basic minimum dataset is usually required, preferably by completion of a standard form/dataset, covering the following:
• Administrative details for those providing information (name, organisation/position, contact details) and cases and contacts (name, address, phone, GP, hospital).
• Epidemiological information on cases in relation to person (age, sex, occupation), place (residence, travel, institution) and time (onset).

• Diagnosis, consisting of clinical and laboratory information.
• Record of advice given.

Risk assessment

The next stage is usually to undertake a risk assessment, which includes the principles identified above (see 'Public health action on-call'), but often also includes an assessment of whether contacts have been put at significant risk. The three general questions that are asked in assessing the likelihood of transmission are:
• How infectious is the source (or case)?
• How close is the contact?
• How susceptible are those exposed?
An example of how this is applied for a particular disease is given in Box 3.80.2.

Possible interventions

If it is decided that action is required, possible interventions include the following:
• Action to improve outcome for cases by ensuring appropriate care is provided. This may include provision of immunoglobulins (rabies), antitoxins (diphtheria), antidotes (chemicals) or different antibiotics from usual (e.g. *Legionella*).
• Action to trace others exposed to source or cases in order to provide advice, antibiotics or vaccines (e.g. in contacts of meningococcal disease, all three may be provided).
• Action to prevent others being exposed to cases or contacts, for example by rendering them non-infectious by use of antibiotics and/or isolation (e.g. diphtheria or TB); by provision of hygiene advice and/or exclusion from work or school (e.g. gastrointestinal illness); or by closure of premises associated with incident (e.g. cooling tower or food premises).
• Action to identify a possible source so that control measures can be implemented and monitored.

Communications

Communication is vital in public health incidents. Communication needs can be considered from a number of perspectives:
• Who needs to know for public health purposes? Some may need to be contacted on-call (may include the case (or parents), contacts or clinicians) and some can wait until the next working day (e.g. school).
• Who needs to know before the press? This may include officers of local public health organisations (press officer, chief executive, Director of Public Health) and regional or national organisations (e.g. the national health protection agency and the Department of Health may sometimes need to be told).
• Who can offer advice or help in management of the incident? Such individuals may be able to contribute from a microbiological, epidemiological or environmental health aspect.
• Is there any advantage in wider dissemination of information or advice? This may be to primary or secondary healthcare services (e.g. identification and treatment of cases) or the public and press (e.g. to allay anxiety).

Governance issues

Ensuring an appropriate quality of response on-call can be considered as a mixture of preparation and follow up.

Preparation for on-call includes the following:
• Access to an up-to-date on-call pack.
• Access to up-to-date local policies and contingency plans.
• Undertaking appropriate training and updating.
• Exercising contingency plans and multiagency response.
• Ensuring effective authorisation for use of legal powers.
• Ensuring access to required support, including surge capacity.

Follow-up issue include:
• debrief to review individual cases with local health protection team as learning exercise;
• systematic audit;
• adverse incident reporting;
• written reports, including any lessons learnt; and
• review of policies and plans.

Section 2
Common topics

2.1 Meningitis and meningism

Meningitis is inflammation of the meninges. Meningism is the group of signs and symptoms that accompanies the inflammation. The symptoms of meningism are headache, neck stiffness, nausea or vomiting and photophobia. The classical physical sign of meningism is a positive Kernig's test; however, this may be negative in mild cases. Typical features of meningism are uncommon in infants and young children, who are usually simply floppy and pale with fever and vomiting. A bulging fontanelle may be present in a young infant.

Meningitis is a notifiable disease in many countries. However, this is a rather unhelpful term for communicable disease control purposes, as bacterial meningitis (particularly due to *Neisseria meningitidis*), can present as septicaemia without any features of meningitis, and many types of meningitis require no public health action. Meningococcal septicaemia presents with a typical haemorrhagic rash, which may be accompanied by shock, circulatory collapse, and confusion or coma. Many patients with meningococcal disease will have features of both meningitis and septicaemia (see Chapter 3.50).

Infectious and other causes

Meningitis is the most common cause of meningism; however, meningism can occur in the absence of meningitis (Table 2.1.1). It may accompany upper lobe pneumonia, urinary tract infection and other febrile conditions. Cerebrospinal fluid (CSF) examination is normal in these conditions. Meningism without fever can also occur in non-infectious conditions, the most important of which is subarachnoid haemorrhage; malignancy affecting the meninges can also present as meningism.

Clinical and epidemiological differences

Many infectious agents can cause meningitis. Acute meningitis is nearly always either viral or bacterial; fungal and protozoal infections occasionally occur, mainly in the immunosuppressed patient.

The overall incidence is relatively stable across Europe, having declined by half during the past decade. The decline was due to both the introduction of meningococcal group C vaccine and a general reduction in serogroup B infections. *Haemophilus influenzae* type b (Hib) meningitis is well controlled as all countries in Europe routinely vaccinate in infancy; progressively vaccination with pneumococcal conjugate vaccines is also having an impact.

Viral meningitis

Viral meningitis is common; however, most cases are mild or inapparent. Notifications are an unreliable estimate of incidence as only the more severe cases are investigated.

The most common cause is an enterovirus infection (either an echovirus or coxsackievirus) (Box 2.1.1). In enterovirus meningitis there is sometimes a history of a sore throat or diarrhoea for a few days before the onset of headache, fever and nausea or vomiting. The headache is severe; however, there is no alteration of neurological function. Meningism is usually present to a greater or lesser degree. Recovery is usually complete and rapid (within a week). The CSF is clear, with 40–250 cells, all lymphocytes, elevated protein and normal glucose. An enterovirus infection can

Communicable Disease Control and Health Protection Handbook, Third Edition. Jeremy Hawker, Norman Begg, Iain Blair, Ralf Reintjes, Julius Weinberg and Karl Ekdahl.
© 2012 Jeremy Hawker, Norman Begg, Iain Blair, Ralf Reintjes, Julius Weinberg and Karl Ekdahl.
Published 2012 by Blackwell Publishing Ltd.

Table 2.1.1 Differential diagnosis of meningism

Cause	Distinguishing features
Viral meningitis	Fever, clear CSF with a lymphocytosis and raised protein
Bacterial meningitis	Fever, purulent CSF with a neutrophil pleiocytosis, raised protein and lowered glucose. In TB, the CSF is not purulent and the fever may be absent or low grade
Other febrile conditions	Fever. Normal CSF
Subarachnoid haemorrhage	No fever. Abrupt onset, rapid deterioration. Blood-stained CSF
Meningeal malignancies	No fever. Insidious onset. Variable CSF features

CSF, cerebrospinal fluid.

be confirmed by detection of virus in a faecal sample or by serology. Enterovirus meningitis occurs mainly in later summer. It affects all age groups, although it is most common in preschool children.

Mumps can cause meningitis, although it is now rare in countries where MMR vaccine is used. It is easily recognized by the accompanying parotitis. The diagnosis can be confirmed by detection of specific immunoglobulin class M (IgM) in blood or saliva, or by serology.

In herpes simplex meningitis, the illness is more severe and may persist for weeks. It is associated with primary genital herpes.

Non-paralytic poliomyelitis can present as meningitis, indistinguishable clinically from other causes of enteroviral meningitis. Poliovirus is detectable in faeces or CSF.

Box 2.1.1 Causes of viral meningitis

Common
- Echovirus
- Coxsackievirus

Rare
- Poliovirus
- Mumps virus
- Herpes simplex type 2
- Herpes zoster
- Influenza types A or B
- Arbovirus
- Rubella
- Epstein–Barr virus

Bacterial meningitis

Bacterial meningitis is a medical emergency. The clinical presentation depends on the age of the patient, and the infecting organism (Table 2.1.2). In the neonate, the presentation is non-specific, with features of bacteraemia. The infant is febrile, listless, floppy and does not feed. There may also be vomiting, drowsiness, convulsions or an abnormal high-pitched cry. In this age group, the most common causes are *E. coli* and group B streptococci.

Signs and symptoms in older infants and young children are also non-specific. Meningococcal infection is the most common cause at this age and is often accompanied by a haemorrhagic rash (see Chapter 3.50).

In older children and adults the symptoms are more specific. Fever, malaise and increasing headache are accompanied by nausea and often vomiting. Photophobia may be extreme. Meningism is usually present. Meningococcal infection is also the most common cause in this group and the typical rash of meningococcal septicaemia may be present. Patients with rapidly advancing meningococcal disease may, over the course of a few hours, develop hypotension, circulatory collapse, pulmonary oedema, confusion and coma.

Other causes of acute bacterial meningitis in older children and adults are uncommon. *Haemophilus influenzae* meningitis occasionally occurs in unvaccinated children or adults; it has a slower onset than

Table 2.1.2 Causes of bacterial meningitis

Neonate	Infant/preschool child	Older child/adult
Common		
E. coli	N. meningitidis	N. meningitidis
Group B streptococci		S. pneumoniae
Uncommon		
L. monocytogenes	H. influenzae	L. monocytogenes
N. meningitidis	S. pneumoniae	Staphylococci
Staphylococci		H. influenzae
		M. tuberculosis

meningococcal meningitis and a rash is rare. Pneumococcal meningitis also has a more insidious onset and the symptoms are less specific than meningococcal meningitis. It usually occurs in adults with an underlying risk factor such as dura mater defect due to trauma or surgery, chronic intracranial infection, asplenia, terminal complement deficiency or alcoholism. *Listeria* meningitis presents either as a neonatal infection following intrapartum exposure or as a food-borne illness in older children and young adults, often in the immunosuppressed.

Tuberculous meningitis is a manifestation of primary tuberculosis, which occurs mainly in children and young adults. It has an insidious onset; meningism is usually mild and other features (except fever) are often absent.

Laboratory diagnosis

With the exception of TB, bacterial meningitis causes neutrophil pleiocytosis in the CSF, with raised protein and lowered glucose. A Gram's stain will often demonstrate the typical appearance of the infecting organism, allowing a definitive diagnosis to be made.

Conventional culture of CSF and blood should always be carried out; however, these may be negative, particularly if the patient has been given antibiotics before hospital admission. In addition, a CSF specimen may not be available, as clinicians are often reluctant to undertake a lumbar puncture.

Polymerase chain reaction (PCR) diagnosis for meningococcal disease (see Box 3.50.1

for suggested investigations) and serology are available. Other useful investigations include throat swab and microscopic examination of a rash aspirate, if present.

General prevention and control measures

• *Hygiene.* Enteroviral meningitis usually spreads as result of environmental contamination, particularly under conditions of crowding and poor hygiene. General hygiene measures such as handwashing will help prevent spread. This is particularly important in hospitals.
• *Pregnancy.* Group B streptococcal meningitis in neonates can be prevented by intrapartum antibiotic treatment of colonised women (see Chapter 3.74).
• *Immunisation.* Childhood immunisation schedules in Europe ensure protection against meningitis caused by mumps, polio and Hib. In some countries, *Neisseria meningitidis* group C and TB are also in the schedule. Quadrivalent vaccines for *N. meningitidis* serogroups A, C, Y and W135 have recently become available. The 7, 10 and 13 valent conjugate pneumococcal vaccines are licenced in Europe and have been implemented in several countries.
• *Chemoprophylaxis* is indicated for close contacts of meningococcal and Hib disease (see Chapters 3.50 and 3.38) and investigation for close contacts of TB (see Chapter 3.80). It is not necessary for contacts of pneumococcal or viral meningitis.

• *Food safety*. *Listeria* meningitis is preventable by avoiding high-risk foods such as soft cheese, paté and cook-chill foods, particularly for the immunosuppressed and in pregnancy.
• *Optimising case management*. In cases of suspected meningococcal disease, benzyl penicillin should be given urgently (see Chapter 3.50).

Response to a case or cluster

The first priority when a case is notified is to establish the diagnosis. This requires close liaison with clinicians and microbiologists to ensure that appropriate investigations are carried out. If the initial diagnosis is viral meningitis, then no further action is needed at this stage, although it may be necessary to provide information to GPs and parents if the case appears to be linked with others.

If bacterial meningitis is suspected, then further measures will depend on the cause. Again, optimum investigation is essential as the nature of the public health response differs for each organism. Typing of the organism is needed to determine whether cases are linked. Chemoprophylaxis, and sometimes also vaccination, is indicated for cases due to *N. meningitidis* or *H. influenzae* (see Chapters 3.50 and 3.38). With the introduction of Hib vaccine, meningococcal infection is by far the most likely diagnosis in a patient with acute bacterial meningitis and it may sometimes be appropriate to initiate control measures before laboratory confirmation.

In the UK, useful information leaflets on meningitis are available from the National Meningitis Trust and the Meningitis Research Foundation (see Appendix 1).

2.2 Gastrointestinal infection

Every year in the UK, approximately 1 in 30 people attend their GP with an acute gastroenteritis (usually diarrhoea and/or vomiting) and many more suffer such an illness without contacting the health service. Although an infectious cause is not always demonstrated, there is strong epidemiological evidence to suggest that most of these illnesses are caused by infections. A wide variety of bacteria, viruses and parasites may cause gastrointestinal infection: commonly identified ones in the EU are listed in Table 2.2.1. Less common but highly pathogenic infections may be imported from abroad including amoebic or bacillary dysentery, cholera, typhoid and paratyphoid fevers. Other infectious causes of gastroenteritis include other *Escherichia coli*, *Bacillus subtilis*, *Clostridium difficile*, *Vibrio parahaemolyticus*, *Yersinia enterocolitica* and viruses as adenovirus, astrovirus, calicivirus and coronavirus. Non-infectious causes of acute gastroenteritis include toxins from shellfish, vegetables (e.g. red kidney beans) and fungi (such as wild mushrooms), and chemical contamination of food and water.

Laboratory investigation

Identification of the causative organism is dependent upon laboratory investigation, usually of faecal samples. It is important that such samples are taken as soon after the onset of illness as possible, as the likelihood of isolating some pathogens (e.g. viruses) decreases substantially within a few days of onset. Collecting at least 2 mL of faeces and including the liquid part of the stool will increase the chances of a positive result. Delay in transport to the laboratory, particularly in warm weather, should be minimised. If delay is likely, samples should be refrigerated or stored in a suitable transport medium. A local policy on sampling and transport should be agreed with the local microbiology laboratory. Samples of vomit may sometimes be helpful. In both cases, the patient should receive instructions on the collection and storage or transport of the specimen. Serum samples may be helpful, particularly if some cases become jaundiced. It is often difficult to distinguish between bacterial and chemical food-borne gastroenteritis on clinical grounds, although some toxins cause an unpleasant taste and/or burning in the mouth or throat. If a chemical cause is suspected, advice on sampling should be obtained from a toxicologist (e.g. public analyst).

A suitable list of organisms to test for in all community outbreaks of gastroenteritis is as follows:
• Salmonellae;
• *Campylobacter* species;
• *Shigella* species;
• *E. coli* O157;
• Norovirus; and
• Protozoa (*Cryptosporidium* and *Giardia*).
Plus, if food poisoning is suspected or if clinical features suggest (Table 2.2.1):
• *Bacillus* species;
• *Clostridium perfringens*; and
• *Staphylococcus aureus*.
Also consider if clinical or epidemiological features suggest or if first list above is negative:
• Rotavirus;
• *Vibrio* species;
• *Yersinia* species;
• *Clostridium difficile*;
• Other *E. coli;*
• Other viruses; and
• Toxins or poisons.
In hospitals, the most common causes of outbreaks are:
• Norovirus;
• *Clostridium difficile;*
• Salmonellae; and
• Rotavirus;

Prevention and control

Vaccines are not yet available against most of the major causes of gastrointestinal infection and so public health efforts concentrate on reducing exposure to the organisms responsible. Most gastrointestinal infections are either food-borne or spread person to person. The role of the consumer in demanding safe food via pressure on government and food retailers is underdeveloped in many countries.

At the local level, prevention of gastrointestinal or food-borne infection is achieved by the following measures.
• Working with food businesses and staff to reduce the likelihood of contamination of food (from the environment, food handlers or cross-contamination), inadequate cooking and storage at inadequate temperatures. The hazard analysis critical control point (HACCP) system is used by the food industry in identifying and assessing hazards in food, and establishing control measures needed to maintain a cost-effective food safety programme. Important features are that HACCP is predictive, cheap, on-site and involves local staff in the control of risk. In the UK, this approach is reinforced by inspection of premises by the Environmental Health Department of the Local Authority and other enforcement agencies.
• Use of statutory powers: UK Local Authorities can exclude cases or carriers of infection from work or school and compensate them for any loss of earnings. Other powers include seizure of food and closure of premises that present an 'imminent risk to Public Health'. Officers of the Environmental Health Department usually exercise these powers. The Meat Hygiene Service (part of the Food Standards Agency) is the enforcing authority for licensed fresh meat/poultry premises in Great Britain.
• Advising the public on safe food handling and the reduction of faeco-oral spread. This includes the importance of handwashing immediately after going to the toilet and before handling or eating food. This is of vital importance, as approximately 80% of people with gastrointestinal infection do not consult the health service when ill.
• Adequate infection control policies in all institutions including hospitals, nursing and residential homes, schools and nurseries, including use of enteric precautions (see Table 1.2.2) for cases of diarrhoea or vomiting.
• Regular surveillance to detect outbreaks and respond to individual cases. Food poisoning (proven or suspected and including waterborne infection), dysentery and viral hepatitis are all statutorily notifiable, as are cholera,

Table 2.2.1 Differential diagnosis of common gastrointestinal infection

| Organism | Laboratory confirmed cases from EU member states in 2007** | | Incubation period (approx.) | | Clinical clues in outbreaks | | |
	Cases (No.)	Notification rate per 100,000 population	Usual	Range	Symptoms*	Severity	Other features
Campylobacter	200,779	46.6	2–5 days	1–10 days	D often with blood. Abdominal pain ± fever	Usually lasts 2–7 days	Peaks in early summer
Giardiasis	172,735	62.7	5–16 days	1–28 days	D, malaise, flatulence smelly stools; cramps, bloating	Often prolonged. May be malabsorption and weight loss	Often travel associated. Possibility of water-borne outbreak
Salmonella	153,823	34.3	12–48 hours	4 hours–5 days	D often with fever. May be myalgia, abdominal pain, headache	Can be severe. Lasts several days to 3 weeks	Peaks in late summer
Hepatitis A	13,921	2.8	Mean 28 days	15–50 days	Fever, nausea, malaise. Jaundice fairly specific but not sensitive	Worse in adults. Lasts up to 4 weeks	Children may be asymptomatic
Shigellosis	7929	2.1	24–72 hours	12–96 hours. Possibly up to 1 week for Shigella dysenteriae	Shigella sonnei: Often watery D; May be mucus. Other shigellae: D, mucus, blood, fever and colic common	S. sonnei: Self-limiting in 3–5 days. Other shigellae: Lasts average of 7 days, often severe	S. sonnei: Often children or institutions: secondary spread common. Other shigellae: Often imported, secondary spread common
Cryptosporidium	6253	2.4	4–7 days	1–28 days	D, bloating and abdominal pain common	Self-limiting but lasts up to 4 weeks	Severe in immunocompromised. Increase in spring and autumn

			Incubation	Duration	Symptoms	Severity/duration	Comments
E. coli O157	2906	0.6	2–4 days	6 hours–10 days	D, blood not uncommon	Variable, may be very severe (e.g. HUS, TTP)	Consider in all cases of bloody D
Rotavirus	n/a	n/a	2–4 days	1–4 days	Watery D, fever vomiting ± respiratory symptoms	Usually lasts a few days, but occasionally severe	Usually children, common in winter
Norovirus	n/a	n/a	15–50 hours	6–72 hours	Nausea/vomiting common. Cramps, mild D may occur	Usually mild lasts 1–2 days	Secondary spread common More common in winter
Clostridium perfringens	n/a	n/a	8–18 hours	5–24 hours	D, abdominal pain common (vomiting and fever are rare)	Usually mild and short-lived lasts approx. 1 day	Usually failure of temperature control post cooking
Bacillus cereus	n/a	n/a	1–24 hours	Usually mild and short-lived, lasts approx. 1 day	Syndrome of nausea, vomiting + abdominal pain Syndrome of D, abdominal pain	Usually mild and short-lived lasts approx. 1 day	Often from rice or pasta High attack rate
Staphylococcus aureus	n/a	n/a	2–4 hours	0.5–8 hours	Vomiting, abdominal pain (D rare). Often abrupt onset	May be very acute	Food handler may have skin infection

HUS, haemolytic uraemic syndrome; TTP, thrombotic thrombocytopaenic purpura.

* D, diarrhoea, which can be defined as three or more loose stools in 24 hours.

** ECDC, Annual epidemiological report on communicable diseases in Europe, 2009.

paratyphoid and typhoid fever in almost all European countries. However, there are no generally accepted clinical case-definitions for these notifiable infections in some countries including the UK and there may often be no laboratory confirmation of the organism responsible. It is therefore often necessary to initiate action before the causative organism is known. Arrangements should also be in place for reporting of isolates of gastrointestinal pathogens from local microbiology laboratories (see Chapter 4.1). However, around 90% of cases seen by GPs are not identified by either of these systems: obtaining surveillance data from computerised primary care providers may help address this.

Response to an individual case

It is not usually possible to identify the organism causing gastroenteritis on clinical grounds in individual cases. The public health priorities in such cases are as follow:
• To limit secondary spread from identified cases by provision of general hygiene advice to all and by specific exclusion from work/school/nursery of those at increased risk of transmitting the infection (Box 2.2.1).

• To collect a minimum dataset to compare with other cases to detect common exposures or potential outbreaks. It is best to collect such data on standardised forms and a subset should be entered on a computerised database for both weekly and annual analysis. A possible dataset is given in Box 2.2.2.
• Ideally, a faecal sample would be collected from all clinical notifications of food poisoning or dysentery to detect clusters by organism/type, to detect potentially serious pathogens requiring increased intervention and to monitor trends.

A local policy to address these priorities should be agreed with local Environmental Health Officers (EHOs), microbiologists and clinicians. The role of the GP in public health surveillance and in preventing secondary spread is of particular importance and needs to be emphasised regularly (e.g. via a GP newsletter).

Response to a cluster

The most common setting for a cluster of clinical cases of gastroenteritis is in an already defined cohort, for example a nursing home or amongst attendees at a wedding. Such a

---

Box 2.2.1 Groups that pose an increased risk of spreading gastrointestinal infection

1 Food handlers whose work involves touching unwrapped foods to be consumed raw or without further cooking.
2 Staff of healthcare facilities with direct contact, or with contact through serving food, with susceptible patients or persons in whom an intestinal infection would have particularly serious consequences.
3 Children aged less than 5 years who attend nurseries, nursery schools, playgroups or other similar groups.
4 Older children and adults who may find it difficult to implement good standards of personal hygiene (e.g. those with learning disabilities or special needs); and in circumstances where hygienic arrangements may be unreliable (e.g. temporary camps housing displaced persons). Under exceptional circumstances (e.g. *E. coli* O157 infection) children in infant schools may be considered to fall into this group.

  Guidelines for the exclusion of cases in risk groups 3 and 4 assume that, once cases have recovered and passed normal stools, they can subsequently practice good hygiene under supervision. If that is not the case, individual circumstances must be assessed.

Source: PHLS Salmonella Committee, 1995

Box 2.2.2 Possible district dataset for investigation of cases of gastrointestinal infection

---

Administrative details (name, address, telephone, Date of birth, GP, unique number*)

Formally notified?   Yes/No

Descriptive variables (age*, sex*, postcode*)

Date* and time of onset

Symptoms

Diarrhoea	Yes/No
Nausea	Yes/No
Vomiting	Yes/No
Fever	Yes/No
Abdominal pain	Yes/No
Blood in stool	Yes/No
Malaise	Yes/No
Headache	Yes/No
Jaundice	Yes/No

Others (specify): _____

Duration of illness

Stool sample taken? (source, date, laboratory)

Microbiological result (organism details*, laboratory, specimen date)

Food history: functions, restaurants, takeaways

Food consumed in last 5 days (for unknown microbial cause)

Raw water consumed outside the home in previous 14 days

Other cases in household?

Travel abroad?

Animal contact?

Occupation, place of work/school/nursery

Advised not to work?

Formally excluded?

Part of outbreak?*

   Organism-specific questions may be added if microbiological investigation reveals an organism of particular public health importance (e.g. *E. coli* O157, *Cryptosporidium*, *Salmonella typhi*, *Salmonella paratyphi*).

* Minimum dataset to be recorded in computerised database.

---

situation is slightly different from investigating a laboratory-identified cluster.

It is important to discover the microbiological agent. Following discussion with the relevant microbiologist, stool specimens should be obtained without delay from 6–10 of the patients with the most recent onset of illness and submitted to the laboratory for testing for all relevant organisms (see list above: the laboratory may not test for all these unless requested). The identity of the agent will dictate the urgency of the investigation (e.g.

to prevent further exposure to a source of *E. coli* O157), the control measures to be introduced (e.g. to limit person-to-person spread of norovirus in institutions) and provide valuable clues as to how the outbreak may have happened (e.g. inadequate temperature control in a *Bacillus cereus* outbreak).

As microbiological results will not be available for a number of days, clinical details should be collected from all reported cases so that the incubation period, symptom profile, severity and duration of illness can be used

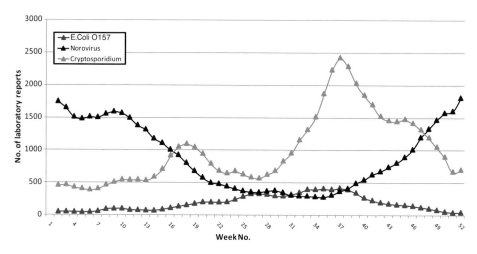

Fig. 2.2.1 Seasonal distribution of gastrointestinal pathogens, 1999–2009, England, Wales and Northern Ireland (3-week rolling averages).

to predict which organism(s) are most likely to be the cause (Table 2.2.1). The likelihood of different microbiological causes also varies by season (Figures 2.2.1 and 2.2.2). There may also be clues as to whether the illness is likely to be food-borne or spread person to person (Box 2.2.3). In many such outbreaks a formal hypothesis-generating study is not necessary, and it is often possible to progress to an analytical study to investigate possible food vehicles early in the investigation (see Chapter 4.2).

The environmental component of the investigation is often illuminating as to why the outbreak happened (i.e. how did an infectious dose of the organism occur in the identified food vehicle). This investigation will look at the following:

1 Food sources, storage, food preparation, cooking procedures, temperature control after cooking and reheating.

2 Symptoms of gastrointestinal or skin disease, or testing for faecal carriage in food handlers.

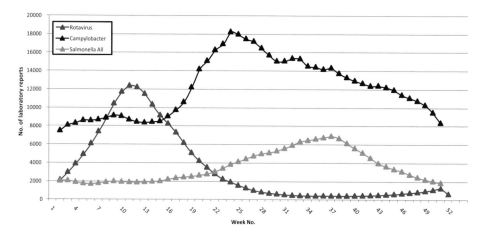

Fig. 2.2.2 Seasonal distribution of gastrointestinal pathogens, 1999–2009, England, Wales and Northern Ireland (3-week rolling averages).

Box 2.2.3 Clues as to whether an outbreak of gastroenteritis could be food-borne or spread person to person

May suggest food-borne	May suggest person to person
Dates of onset (epidemic curve) clustered indicating a point source outbreak	Dates and times of onset do not cluster but occur in waves coinciding with the incubation period of the responsible pathogen
All wards, classes, buildings or units supplied by the kitchens or food supplier are affected	Patients and staff in a single ward, class, building or unit are affected
Food handlers and catering staff are affected	People in the households of staff-members or pupils are also affected
Clinical features and laboratory tests indicate an organism predominantly spread via food and water rather than person to person (e.g. *C. perfringens*, *B. cereus*)	Clinical features and laboratory tests suggest organism predominantly spread person to person (e.g. rotavirus, *Shigella*)
Environmental investigation reveals poor food handling practices or premises	Environmental investigation reveals poor infection control practice or hygiene facilities

Warnings

These are not invariable rules, assess each outbreak on its own merits, for example:
- some food-borne outbreaks may be prolonged by person-to-person spread
- food-borne outbreaks may be due to a continuing source
- some outbreaks may be augmented by environmental contamination

3 General state of knowledge of the staff and condition of the premises.

4 Examination of records of key controls, such as temperatures and pest controls.

5 Whether samples of food are available for examination/analysis and whether environmental swabbing or water sampling is appropriate.

General control measures to prevent spread from those affected can be instituted early, as can addressing important problems identified in the environmental investigation. This includes the exclusion from work of infected food handlers and measures to avoid secondary spread from cases. More specific measures can be instituted when the organism and vehicle are identified (see appropriate chapter in Section 3). In institutions, such as hospitals and nursing homes, institute measures to reduce risk of person-to-person spread (see Chapter 3.55 for details).

2.3 Community-acquired pneumonia

Respiratory tract infections are the most common infectious disease in developed countries and pneumonia remains one of the most common causes of death. Community (as opposed to hospital) acquired pneumonia (CAP) affects all ages, although its incidence increases dramatically beyond 50 years of age.

Table 2.3.1 Differential diagnosis of community-acquired pneumonia

Organism	Percentage of cases[1]	Incubation period	Clinical clues[2]	Epidemiological clues
Streptococcus pneumoniae	29	1–3 days (exogenous)	Acute. Rusty sputum, fever, chest pain. Prominent physical signs	More common in infants, elderly, unvaccinated and in winter
Mycoplasma pneumoniae	9	6–32 days (median = 14 days)	Gradual onset, scanty sputum, headache, malaise, sore throat	May be 4-yearly epidemics. Often affects younger patients or military
Influenza A	8	0–3 days (median = 1.4 days)	Headache, myalgia, coryza, fever, sore throat	May be seasonal community epidemic. Particularly affects the unvaccinated
Chlamydophila pneumoniae	6	Unclear: 10–30 days?	Hoarseness, sore throat, prolonged cough, scanty sputum, sinus tenderness. Insidious onset	Often affects young adults. No obvious seasonality
Gram-negative bacteria	6	Variable	Severe. Acute onset. Redcurrent jelly sputum	Particularly common in nursing homes. More likely if chronic respiratory disease, diabetes, alcohol
Haemophilus influenzae	5	Unclear: 2–4 days?	Purulent sputum. Onset may be insidious	Often associated with chronic lung disease and elderly
Legionella pneumophila	4	2–10 days (median = 6 days)	Anorexia, malaise, myalgia, headache, fever. Some with diarrhoea, confusion and high fever. Upper respiratory symptoms rare. Often severe	May be associated with aerosol source. More common in summer and autumn. Mostly over 30 years; male excess
Staphylococcus aureus	4	1–4 days (exogenous)	Often serious. May be ring shadows on X-ray	May complicate influenza infection. More common in nursing homes

Parainfluenza	2	1–6 days (median = 2.6 days)	Croup wheezing or hoarseness. Ear or upper respiratory infection	Mostly affects children and immunocompromised. Para 1 and 2 more common in autumn or early winter (but para 3 endemic)
Chlamydophila psittaci	2	4–28 days (median = 10 days)	Fever, headache, unproductive cough, myalgia. May be rash. Often severe	Possible link to birds. May be severe. Mostly adults, more often male
Influenza B	1	0–2 days (median = 0.6 days)	Headache, myalgia, coryza fever, sore throat	May be seasonal community epidemic. Affects the unvaccinated
Coxiella burnetii	1	9–33 days (median = 20 days)	Fever, headache, myalgia, cough. May be fatigue, chills, anorexia, arthralgia, nausea. Possibly neurological symptoms or hepatitis	Possible link to sheep, other animals or animal products. May be increase in April–June. Male excess, rare in children
RSV	1	3–7 days (median = 4.4 days)	Wheezing, rhinitis, fever	May be more common in spring. Peaks every November to January. Causes outbreaks in nursing homes
Adenovirus	0.7	4–8 days (median = 5.6 days)	Fever, sore throat, runny nose	Usually children or young adults (e.g. military recruits). Highest in January–April

[1] Average from a number of prospective studies of patients admitted to hospital (Farr and Mandell, 1988). Will vary according to epidemic cycles.
[2] Clinical picture is not a reliable indicator of organism in individual cases.

Other risk factors include chronic respiratory disease, smoking, immunosuppression (including HIV/AIDS) and residence in an institution. Approximately 20% of cases require hospitalisation, of which 5–10% die.

In general, the symptoms of CAP are fever, cough, sputum production, chest pain and shortness of breath, with accompanying chest X-ray changes. The most common causes of CAP are listed in Table 2.3.1. Although the clinical picture cannot be used to diagnose individual cases, clues may be obtained to help identify the causes of outbreaks. Some organisms may be more likely to cause 'typical' pneumonia (e.g. pneumococcus, *Haemophilus*, *Moraxella*, *Klebsiella*) and others 'atypical' with significant non-pulmonary features (e.g. *Mycoplasma*, *Chlamydophila*, *Legionella*, *Coxiella*).

Rare causes of pneumonia for which there may be an environmental cause (most likely abroad, but perhaps due to deliberate aerosol release) include anthrax, brucellosis, hantavirus, histoplasmosis, leptospirosis, tularaemia, Q fever and plague. Respiratory infection may also be caused by rare or emerging organisms, such as severe acute respiratory syndrome (SARS) coronavirus, avian influenza, metapneumovirus and *Moraxella catarrhalis*, or, in immunosuppressed individuals, opportunistic pathogens such as *Pneumocystis carinii*. Similar symptoms may also be seen in exacerbations of chronic respiratory disease and non-infective respiratory conditions, for example pulmonary oedema, pulmonary infarction, alveolitis (may follow exposure to inorganic particles) and eosinophilic pneumonias (may be associated with drugs or parasites).

Laboratory investigation

Microscopy and culture of sputum was traditionally the mainstay of diagnosis. However, about one-third of pneumonia cases do not produce sputum, culture is only moderately sensitive and contamination with oropharyngeal flora is not an uncommon event. Blood culture is highly specific but relatively insensitive.

Serology was the mainstay of diagnosis for viral and 'atypical' causes, but this is often not diagnostic until 2–6 weeks into the illness, although *Mycoplasma*-specific IgM may be apparent earlier. PCR tests on respiratory samples can now be carried out for viruses, *Mycoplasma*, *Chlamydophila* and *Legionella* (lower respiratory samples preferred). Influenza and respiratory syncytial virus (RSV) may be cultured from nasopharyngeal swabs or aspirates, and viral antigen may also be detected from these specimens. Antigen tests are available for *Legionella pneumophila* (serogroup 1 only) in urine and pneumococcus in urine, sputum or serum, even if antibiotics have already been given.

A proportion of cases may be infected with more than one pathogen.

Prevention and control

• Immunisation of elderly and those with chronic disease and immunocompromised with influenza and pneumococcal vaccines.
• Immunisation of children with conjugated vaccines against *Haemophilus influenzae* type b and pneumococcus.
• Reduction of smoking.
• Promotion of breastfeeding.
• Avoiding overcrowding, especially in institutions.
• Good infection control in institutions.
• Environmental measures to reduce *Legionella* exposure.
• Surveillance of CAP, especially for influenza, *Mycoplasma*, *Legionella*, *Coxiella* and *Chlamydophila psittaci*. Surveillance of antibiotic-resistant pneumococci.
• Reporting of outbreaks in institutions to public health authorities.

Response to a case

• If resident or attender at institution, or if severely ill, investigate to obtain microbiological cause.

• Follow up individual cases of legionellosis, psittacosis and Q fever for source of organism.
• Advise personal hygiene, particularly hand-washing, coughing and disposal of secretions.
• Limit contact with infants, frail elderly and immunocompromised individuals.

Response to a cluster

• Discuss investigation with microbiological colleagues. A suitable set of investigations could be as follows:
  (a) take nasopharyngeal aspirates or nose and throat swabs from most recently infected cases for virus culture, PCR and antigen testing;
  (b) take serum samples from recovered cases or those with date of onset 10 days or more ago;
  (c) send sputum samples for microbiological culture and possibly pneumococcal antigen;
  (d) send blood cultures from febrile cases; and
  (e) send urine for *Legionella* and pneumococcal antigen.
• If an institutional cluster, isolate or cohort cases until cause known. Stop new admissions. Avoid discharges to institutions containing elderly, frail or immunocompromised individuals. Measures should aim to limit transmission by large droplets, droplet nuclei, respiratory secretions and direct contact. In RSV season, also consider transmission via inanimate objects.
• Collect data on immunisation history (influenza, pneumococcus), travel, exposure to water and aerosols, animals, birds and other potential sources of *Legionella*, Q fever, *Chlamydophila psittaci*, brucellosis.
• Advise community cases on hygiene measures (e.g. handwashing, coughing, discharges) and to avoid individuals susceptible to severe disease (e.g. elderly, chronically ill).
• Specific interventions as appropriate to identified organism (see organism-specific chapter).
• During influenza season, may wish to give anti-influenza prophylaxis to contacts in res-

idential care institutions for elderly, whilst awaiting diagnosis (see Chapter 3.40).
• A cluster of CAP could arise as a result of a deliberate release of an aerosol of a serious or rare infection such as anthrax or plague (see Chapter 4.15).

2.4 Rash in pregnancy

Infections and other causes

There are many possible causes of a rash in a pregnant woman. Most causes are non-infectious and include drug reactions and allergies. There are also a number of unusual non-infectious causes of rash that occur in pregnancy, which may require specialist referral (polymorphic eruption of pregnancy, papular dermatitis of pregnancy, prurigo gestationis, pemphigoid gestationis and impetigo herpetiformis). The important differentiating feature from an infectious cause is the absence of fever. Infectious causes are relatively uncommon, but important because of the potential harm to the developing fetus. Rubella, parvovirus B19, varicella and syphilis can all cause severe congenital disease or intrauterine death.

Clinical and epidemiological differences

Viral infections in pregnancy are often mild or inapparent with variable or absent fever. The exceptions are varicella, which presents with a characteristic rash, and measles. Bacterial infections are more severe and usually accompanied by a high fever (with the exception of syphilis). The clinical presentation of each of the infections in Box 2.4.1 is described in more detail in the relevant chapters.

The most common infections in pregnancy are parvovirus B19 (1 in 400 pregnancies), varicella (1 in 500 pregnancies) and the enteroviruses. Rubella and measles are now both rare as a result of successful immunisation

---

Box 2.4.1 Infections that may present with a rash in pregnancy

Viral
- Rubella
- Parvovirus B19
- Varicella-zoster
- Measles
- Enterovirus
- Infectious mononucleosis

Bacterial
- Streptococcal
- Meningococcal
- Syphilis

---

programmes. Enterovirus infections and measles during pregnancy do not carry a specific risk for the fetus although they may result in abortion (enteroviruses) or intrauterine death and pre-term delivery (measles). Infectious mononucleosis sometimes presents with a rash, but poses no risk to the fetus. Bacterial causes of rash in pregnancy are very uncommon.

Laboratory investigation

The laboratory investigation of suspected meningococcal and streptococcal disease and syphilis is described in Chapters 3.50, 3.74 and 3.28, respectively.

Where a viral infection is suspected, it is important to exclude varicella, parvovirus B19 and rubella. Varicella can usually be diagnosed on the basis of the typical vesicular rash, but where there is doubt, serology should be performed. Rubella and parvovirus B19 can both be diagnosed by detection of IgM in or rising IgG in saliva or serum. PCR testing is also available. Testing should be carried out irrespective of previous testing or vaccination.

The investigation of a pregnant woman who has been in contact with someone with a rash illness is more complex. The aim of investigation is to determine whether the contact case has varicella, rubella or parvovirus

B19, and whether the pregnant patient is susceptible to these three infections. A significant contact is defined as being in the same room for over 15 minutes, or face to face contact. Testing algorithms have been published by the UK Health Protection Agency (Communicable Disease and Public Health 2002, 5 (1) 59–71, available at www.hpa.org.uk).

Prevention and control

Rubella infection in pregnancy can be prevented both directly, by vaccination of susceptible women of childbearing age, and indirectly, by universal childhood immunisation (which reduces circulation of wild virus and thus prevents exposure). All pregnant women should be screened for rubella in each pregnancy and vaccinated postpartum. Rubella vaccine (usually given as MMR) is a live vaccine and should not be given during pregnancy, although the risk to the fetus is theoretical and immunisation in pregnancy is no longer an indication for termination of pregnancy.

Varicella vaccine is licensed in most countries in Europe, including the UK, and can be used for both direct prevention of varicella in pregnancy (by vaccination of susceptible women) and indirect prevention (universal childhood immunisation). A specific varicella-zoster immunoglobulin (VZIG) is also available for post-exposure prophylaxis of susceptible women exposed in pregnancy (see Chapter 3.8).

No specific measures are available for prevention of parvovirus B19 in pregnancy, although pregnant women may wish to avoid outbreak situations, and healthcare workers who have been in contact with B19 infection should avoid contact with pregnant women for 15 days from the last contact or until a rash appears (see Chapter 3.57).

Response to a case

Laboratory investigations should be undertaken as described above. Pregnant women with varicella, rubella or parvovirus B19 should be counselled regarding the risks to the fetus and managed accordingly. Oral aciclovir should be considered for pregnant women who present within 24 hours of onset of varicella. The risk to the fetus of rubella in the first 16 weeks is substantial; rubella prior to estimated date of conception or after 20 weeks carries no documented risk and rubella between 16 and 20 weeks gestation carries a minimal risk of deafness only. Parvovirus B19 in the first 20 weeks of pregnancy can lead to intrauterine death and hydrops fetalis, so regular ultrasound screening is recommended for such cases. The public health management of the close contacts is the same as for non-pregnant cases (see Chapters 3.8, 3.67 and 3.57).

Response to a cluster

As for response to a case, but consider community-wide vaccination programme for clusters of rubella or measles.

2.5 Rash and fever in children

Rashes in children are common and result from various causes (Box 2.5.1). Where fever is present, this usually means the cause is infectious (although rash and fever can be an early sign of an unusual inflammatory disease in childhood, such as juvenile rheumatoid arthritis). In the absence of fever, a non-infectious cause (e.g. allergy or drug reaction) is the most likely cause, although in some infections (e.g. enterovirus infections) the fever may be mild or absent.

Clinical and epidemiological differences

In addition to fever, other features that suggest an infectious cause are the presence of swollen lymph nodes, general malaise and a history of recent contact with another infectious case. A full vaccination history should always be obtained from a child with a rash.

There are four main types of rash: vesicular, maculopapular, punctate and haemorrhagic. Vesicular rashes have a blister-like appearance and sometimes contain fluid. Maculopapular rashes are flat or slightly raised and there is sometimes joining together of areas of the rash. Punctate rashes have small, discrete pinpoint lesions. Haemorrhagic rashes look like bruising. The main causes of each type are shown in Table 2.5.1.

Laboratory investigation

General investigations that are useful in differentiating infectious from non-infectious causes are a full blood count, erythrocyte sedimentation rate, blood culture, specimens for viral culture and an acute serum sample for serology. Other investigations will depend on the possible differential diagnoses. A saliva test should be obtained if measles or rubella is suspected.

Prevention and control

General hygiene measures such as handwashing may help limit the spread of some infectious causes of rashes. Transmission of measles, rubella, meningococcal disease (serogroups A, C, W135 and Y) and

---

Box 2.5.1 Causes of rash in children

Common
- Infection
- Drug reaction
- Allergy

Rare
- Inherited bleeding disorder
- Leukaemia
- Purpura

Table 2.5.1 Types of rash

	Prodrome	Fever	General malaise	Distribution of rash	Pruritus	Special features
Vesicular rashes						
Chickenpox	None or short Coryzal	Mild to moderate	Mild	Mostly truncal	Yes	Contact with sufferers is common; crops
Dermatitis herpetiformis	Nil	Nil	Nil	Trunk	Yes	Sporadic cases eventually leave depigmentation
Eczema herpeticum	Nil	Moderate to high	Moderate	In areas of eczema	Yes	May be seriously ill
Hand, foot and mouth disease	Nil	Minimal	Minimal	Palms, soles and inside mouth	No	Often occurs as minor epidemics
Herpes simplex gingivostomatis	Nil	Moderate to high	Moderate (may be dehydrated)	Mouth and lips	Yes (at onset)	Frequent history of contact with cold sores
Impetigo	Nil	Nil	Nil	Face and hands	Yes	Vesicles often replaced by yellow crusting
Insect bites	Nil	Nil	Rare	Variable	Yes	Usually isolated lesions
Molluscum contagiosum	Nil	Nil	Nil	Variable	Yes	Characteristic pearly vesicles with central dimples
Maculopapular and punctate rashes						
Enteroviral infections	Short	Mild	Mild	General	No	Rash often pleomorphic
Fifth disease	Uncommon; mild fever and respiratory symptoms	Mild, if any	Minimal	Face ('slapped cheeks') trunk and limbs	No	Rash may come and go. Heat brings it out. Can have a reticular pattern
Glandular fever	Malaise, mild fever and sore throat	Moderate	Common	General	No	Exudate in throat especially marked swollen glands and spleen
Kawasaki disease	Mild fever, malaise and sore throat	Moderate to high and persistent	Mild to moderate	General	No	Palms and soles, lips and conjunctivae affected
Measles	Rising fever, cough and conjunctivitis	Moderate to high	Substantial	Around ears, then face, then trunk Confluent	No	Koplik's spots in mouth before rash on 4th day of illness

Disease	Prodrome			Distribution	Itch	Features
Meningococcal disease	None or short with coryza or fever	Variable	Profound	Variable	No	Petechial rash may be preceded by maculopapular rash. Evolves rapidly
Pityriasis rosea	Nil	Nil	Nil	Trunk	Initially	Usually in older children; herald patch at onset
Roseola infantum (exanthem subitum)	High fever and irritability	Moderate	Moderate	Trunk then face	No	Dramatic improvement in child when rash appears on 4th or 5th day
Rubella	Short, mild fever and malaise	Mild	Mild or absent	Face then trunk and limbs	No	Posterior occipital lymphadenopathy
Scarlet fever	Fever and sore throat	Moderate to high	Moderate	Face, then rapidly generalised	No	Remains blanched for several seconds after pressure; strawberry tongue and perioral pallor
Haemorrhagic rashes						
Acute lymphoblastic leukaemia	Mild, non-specific	Absent or mild/moderate	Moderate	Anywhere, including mucous membranes	Nil	Pallor, lymphadenopathy and hepatosplenomegaly may be present
Henoch–Schönlein purpura	Mild, sometimes symptoms of upper respiratory tract infection	Mild or moderate	Moderate	Mainly limbs, especially legs and buttocks	No	Rash is urticarial initially. Arthralgia, joint swelling and abdominal pain may be present
Idiopathic thrombocytopaenic purpura	Nil to mild	Nil	Nil	Anywhere, including mucous membranes	Nil	Child is usually well, apart from effects of bleeding
Inherited bleeding disorder	Nil	Nil	Nil	Anywhere, including mucous membranes	Nil	Spontaneous bruises. Family history may be present
Meningococcal disease	None or short with coryza or fever	Variable	Severe	Variable	No	Petechial rash may be preceded by maculopapular rash

From E.G. Davies et al. Manual of Childhood infections, second edition. Royal College of Paediatrics and Child Health, 2001 with permission.

chickenpox are all preventable by vaccination (see Chapters 3.49, 3.67, 3.50 and 3.8, respectively).

Response to a case

• Obtain clinical details, especially whether fever present.
• Check vaccination status.
• Obtain history of contact with other case(s).
• Most childhood rashes are mild and do not warrant any specific public health action.
• Exclusion from school is indicated for the vaccine-preventable diseases (see above) and for scarlet fever (see Chapter 3.74).
• Exclusion of contacts of a case of fifth disease who are non-immune healthcare workers may be indicated (see Chapter 3.57).
• If meningococcal infection is suspected ensure rapid admission to hospital and administration of pre-admission benzyl penicillin and chemoprophylaxis for close contacts (see Chapter 3.50).

Response to a cluster

As for a case, although it may be important to give out information to parents and GPs to allay anxiety and to increase disease awareness.

2.6 Illness in returning travellers

In 2008, the World Tourism Organization recorded 922 million international arrivals of which half were for leisure and recreation. Travel abroad by UK residents numbered 69 million people in 2008 (UK International Passenger Survey). Compared with 2007 this represented a slight fall due to a decline in business travel but visits to friends and relatives and for holidays increased. Of the visits, 1.5 million were to India, Pakistan or Sri Lanka, 1.2 million were to Africa and 660,000 were to Egypt. Prospective studies of over-seas travellers have shown that 10% may report an illness, often an infection, and 2% may experience an injury. Risk factors for illness include young age, pre-existing medical conditions, duration of travel over 4 weeks and travel to low-income countries. Persons travelling abroad should be therefore be prepared for infection risks. Before they depart they should obtain health advice (including advice about immunisation) and if they are ill when they return they should seek appropriate medical attention. Their medical attendants should be aware of the infections that may affect the returning traveller (see also Chapter 4.10).

Travel-related infections

The likelihood of a travel-related infection will depend on the presence of risk factors and these should be assessed by a careful travel history including the following:
• Countries and areas that were visited (rural, urban);
• Duration of stay;
• Exact times and dates (in relation to incubation periods);
• Accommodation (luxury hotels, hostel, camping);
• Activities (hiking, walking, work, contact with local population, contact with animals, looking after ill persons or animals);
• Health status;
• Vaccinations;
• Protection against insect bites;
• Malaria prophylaxis;
• Incidents (animal bites, healthcare, sexual contact, injections, consumption of exotic foodstuffs);
• Exposure to healthcare activities/facilities.

It may be helpful to make enquiries about the local epidemiology of infections and any unusual infections or outbreaks that have been reported in the area. There are several websites that may help with this. The common presentations of travel-related infections are fever, diarrhoea and skin rash, and all of these may be due to conditions common in non-travellers such as pneumonia, urinary

Table 2.6.1 Presentations of travel-related infections

Fever	Malaria (see Chapter 3.48)
	Dengue (see Chapter 3.21)
	Enteric fever (see Chapters 3.56 and 3.82)
	Legionnaires' disease (see Chapter 3.43)
	Rickettsial infections spotted fever (see Chapter 3.83)
	Epidemic typhus (see Chapter 3.83)
	Chikungunya virus (see Chapter 3.9)
	Viral haemorrhagic fever (see Chapter 3.85)
	Influenza (see Chapter 3.40)
	SARS (see Chapter 3.69)
Diarrhoea	Toxigenic *Escherichia coli* (travellers' diarrhoea) (Table 3.26.1)
	Salmonella (see Chapter 3.68)
	Campylobacter (see Chapter 3.7)
	Shigella (see Chapter 3.71)
	Cryptosporidium species (see Chapter 3.18)
	Giardia (see Chapter 3.27)
	Entamoeba histolytica (see Chapter 3.1)
	Cyclospora (see Chapter 3.19)
	Vibrios (see Chapters 3.13 and 3.84)
Jaundice	Hepatitis A, B, C and E (see Chapters 3.32–3.36)
Rash	Rickettsial infections (see Chapter 3.83)
Pharyngitis	Diphtheria (see Chapter 3.22)
Skin lesions	Diphtheria (see Chapter 3.22)
	Leishmaniasis (see Chapter 3.91.2)
Other	Intestinal helminths (see Chapter 3.91.1)
	Schistosomiasis (see Chapter 3.91.1)

tract infection or neoplasia. The travel-related causes of these presentations is summarised in Table 2.6.1. In 2007 the majority of cases of typhoid and paratyphoid reported in the UK were cases acquired in India, Pakistan and Bangladesh while most malaria cases were acquired in Ghana, Nigeria and Uganda.

Response to a case

• From the detailed travel history, assess risk and determine possible exposures.
• Exclude malaria.
• Follow relevant algorithms (where available) to ensure that diagnostic tests and infection control measures are appropriate.
• Manage contacts, carers and health staff appropriately
• In the case of viral haemorrhagic fever (VHF), severe acute respiratory syndrome (SARS) or other serious imported infections

ensure that the relevant public health authorities and specialist secure infectious disease unit are alerted.
• Inform national surveillance unit so that incidents that may potentially be a 'public health emergency of international concern' can be notified to the World Health Organization (WHO) as required by the International Health Regulations.

Investigation of a cluster

In Europe, due to good sanitary conditions and the absence of appropriate biological vectors, onward transmission is unusual for most imported infections and secondary cases are therefore uncommon. If a cluster does occur urgent investigation is required to determine whether it is the result of primary exposure abroad or secondary transmission in the home country.

Surveillance

Surveillance of travel-related infection is largely unsystematic and there are few good estimates of the risks of acquiring an infection when visiting a particular location. Laboratory surveillance systems rarely capture accurate travel data and when these data are available they are subject to reporting bias. Infections that are typically imported may be made the subject of enhanced surveillance (e.g. typhoid surveillance in the UK). Single cases of unusual infections and clusters of cases should be reported to the public health authorities and may be publicised on dedicated websites such as *ProMED-mail* (http://www.promedmail.org/pls/apex/f?p=2400:1000, accessed September 2010).

2.7 Sexually transmitted infections

Sexually transmitted infections (STIs) are infections that are spread by direct sexual contact. Table 2.7.1 lists the common infectious agents that cause STIs, their clinical features, diagnosis and common sequelae. STIs are an important cause of ill health and may lead to long-term complications such as infertility, ectopic pregnancy and genital cancers. These complications disproportionately affect women. The health service costs of diagnosing and treating STIs and their complications are considerable. STIs such as gonorrhoea in men can be an indicator of

Table 2.7.1 Clinical features and laboratory confirmation of acute sexually transmitted infections (STIs)

Infection and infectious agent	Clinical features and sequelae	Diagnosis
Genital chlamydial infection, *Chlamydia trachomatis*	80% of cases in women and 50% cases in men are asymptomatic. In women there is cervicitis and urethritis which may be complicated by pelvic inflammatory disease, tubal damage, infertility and ectopic pregnancy. In men there is urethritis and possibly epididymitis. Incubation period 7–21 days	NAATs have improved the diagnosis of genital chlamydial infection. NAATs are highly sensitive and specific and allow the use of non-invasive specimens such as urine and self-taken vaginal swabs. Diagnoses of chlamydial infection can now be made outside the GUM clinic setting
Bacterial vaginosis, *Gardnerella vaginalis*, other anaerobes	Presents with vaginal discharge and itching. There is debate about the importance of sexual transmission	Wet mount of the discharge reveals vaginal epithelial cells studded with *clue cells*
Chancroid, *Haemophilus ducreyi*	A painful ulcerating genital papule appears 4–10 days after exposure. If untreated, suppurating lymphadenopathy follows	Diagnosis is confirmed by a Gram-stained smear or culture on special media
Genital candidiasis, *Candida albicans*	Presents with vaginitis with irritation and discharge. *C. albicans* is a vaginal commensal and infection is often endogenous although sexual spread may occur. In males, infection is often asymptomatic but irritation and a rash on the glans penis may occur	The organism can be identified in a Gram stain, wet mount or by culture

Table 2.7.1 (*Continued*)

Infection and infectious agent	Clinical features and sequelae	Diagnosis
Genital HSV. Usually HSV-2 but HSV-1 causes 20% of cases	Primary infection produces painful vesicles or ulcers on the penis, labia, cervix and adjacent genital areas. There may be fever and malaise. Incubation period is 2–10 days. Healing occurs within 17 days. In the majority of cases, recurrent secondary episodes, usually less severe, occur as often as once a month due to HSV latency in local nerve ganglia. Precipitating factors include menstruation, sexual intercourse and stress Subclinical attacks are common and are important in transmission. Serious HSV infection of the neonate may be acquired during delivery	Genital herpes may have an atypical appearance so diagnosis should be confirmed by demonstrating HSV in the genital lesions. This can be done by culture or PCR
Genital warts, HPV	Sessile warts are 1–2 mm in diameter and affect dry areas of skin. Condylomata acuminata are large fleshy soft growths and occur particularly when cellular immunity is depressed. Genital warts are often multiple and may occur anywhere on the external genitalia and within the vagina. Subclinical HPV infections of the genitalia are common. Certain HPV types are associated with genital tract neoplasia. Possible sequelae are carcinoma of anus, cervix, penis and vulva. Incubation period is from 1 month to several months	HPV cannot be cultured. Diagnosis may be made histologically on examining cervical cytology specimens. PCR-based assays are now available that are capable of distinguishing between the 40 different HPV types that affect the genital tract
Gonorrhoea, *Neisseria gonorrhoeae*	Cause cervicitis in females and urethritis in males, with purulent discharge. Anorectal and oropharyngeal infection can occur. Incubation period is 2–5 days. Subclinical infection is common and an important source of transmission. Salpingitis is a complication in 10–15% of females but local complications in males are uncommon	Urethral or cervical swabs should be requested. Gram-negative diplococci may be seen on microscopy *N. gonorrhoea* may be cultured. NAATs are more sensitive than culture and can be used as diagnostic/screening tests on non-invasively collected specimens (urine and self-taken vaginal swabs)

(*Continued on p. 42*)

Table 2.7.1 (*Continued*)

Infection and infectious agent	Clinical features and sequelae	Diagnosis
Non-chlamydial, non-gonococcal urethritis	*Ureaplasma urealyticum* and *Mycoplasma hominis* are causes of urethritis and pelvic inflammatory disease. Possible sequelae are infertility and ectopic pregnancy	Specific diagnostic tests for these organisms are not usually clinically indicated
Granuloma inguinale *Calymmatobacterium granulomatis*, a Gram-negative coccobacillus	Destructive ulcerating genital papules appear 1–12 weeks after exposure. Possible sequelae are genital lymphoedema, urethral stricture	Biopsy of the edge of the ulcer shows Donovan bodies on appropriate staining
HTLV	Leukaemia, lymphoma, tropical spastic paraparesis	Tests for HTLV-specific antibodies are available
Lymphogranuloma venereum Types L-1, L-2 and L-3 of *Chlamydia trachomatis* distinct from those that cause trachoma and oculogenital infection	Starts with a painless penile vesicle 1–4 weeks after exposure. This heals but is followed 1–2 weeks later by fever and regional lymphadenopathy, which leads to suppuration and fibrosis	Diagnosis is made by serology, culture of aspirates or direct fluorescence of smears
Syphilis, *Treponema pallidum*	The clinical manifestations of syphilis are varied. The primary and secondary stages are characterised by mucocutaneous lesions. The primary chancre occurs on average 21 days after exposure. A variable secondary rash follows after 6–8 weeks, often with fever and malaise. Gummata (tertiary lesions) appear after several years. Almost any organ of the body can be affected. Transplacental spread of *T. pallidum* may result in fetal death, prematurity or congenital syphilis. Possible sequelae are fetal and neonatal infection, neurological and cardiovascular disease	The diagnosis of syphilis is based upon clinical examination and demonstration of *T. pallidum* in early infectious lesions by dark ground microscopy. Serological tests, particularly EIA for anti-treponemal IgM and PCR are available
Trichomoniasis, *Trichomonas vaginalis*, a flagellated protozoan	Vaginitis with offensive discharge. Asymptomatic urethral infection or colonization common in males. Incubation period is 5–21 days	Motile organisms may be seen on unstained wet preparation

EIA, enzyme immunoassay; GUM, genitourinary medicine; HPV, human papillomavirus; HSV, herpes simplex virus; HTLV, human T-cell lymphotropic virus; NAAT, nucleic acid amplification test; PCR, polymerase chain reaction.

sexual behaviour, which may carry a risk of transmission of HIV infection. STIs, which result in genital ulceration, may enhance HIV transmission. Interventions that reduce STI incidence have great potential for health gain.

Surveillance

As with any infectious disease, control of STIs depends on good surveillance. The main UK sources of surveillance data are summarised in Table 2.7.2. Most European countries have

Table 2.7.2 UK STI surveillance

Surveillance type	Comment
KC60 mandatory, quarterly return	Aggregate data on the total number of episodes of STIs or sexual health services provided by 232 GUM clinics in England, Wales and Northern Ireland. GUM clinics are open access clinics that offer free, confidential sexual health services, including diagnosis and treatment of STIs. Data is aggregated by diagnosis, sex, age group and homosexual acquisition (for selected infections in males)
Genitourinary Medicine Clinic Activity Dataset (GUMCAD)	GUMCAD has replaced the KC60 return. The dataset is collected electronically and comprises patient level disaggregated data on area of residence, age, sexual orientation, ethnic group and country of birth in addition to clinical and risk factor data. The data are more timely and have the potential to identify outbreaks of STI
Routine laboratory reporting of STIs to HPA	Voluntary laboratory reports of gonorrhoea, genital *Chlamydia* and genital herpes from healthcare settings by sex and age group
National Chlamydia Screening Programme (NCSP) returns, England	The NCSP offers opportunistic chlamydia screening to those aged 15–24 years attending a variety of non-GUM clinic settings, includes index cases and partners/contacts
Gonococcal Resistance to Antimicrobial Surveillance Programme (GRASP)	All gonococcal isolates during July, August and September of each year at 24 collaborating laboratories in England and Wales are submitted to HPA. Clinicians are asked to provide detailed demographic and behavioural data including age group, sex, ethnic group, sexual orientation, previous infection, sexual lifestyle, antimicrobial susceptibility
Enhanced surveillance for syphilis	Following laboratory identification, in England and Wales, of cases of syphilis clinicians are asked to provide enhanced patient data including gender, age, ethnic background, sexual orientation, stage of infection, HIV status, location where infection was likely to have been acquired and connection with sexual networks such as saunas and bars
Enhanced surveillance for LGV	Following laboratory confirmation, cases are followed up to collect demographic, clinical and behavioural information from clinicians throughout the UK
HPV surveillance	It is proposed to test for type-specific HPV DNA on a representative sample of normal and abnormal cervical smears and on genital samples from females in vaccine cohorts undergoing opportunistic chlamydia screening

HPA, Health Protection Agency; HPV, human papillomavirus; LGV, lymphogranuloma venereum.
Outputs from these surveillance sources are published regularly by the Health Protection Agency on its website http://www.hpa.org.uk/Topics/InfectiousDiseases/InfectionsAZ/STIs/ [accessed September 2010]. European surveillance data can be accessed at http://www.ecdc.europa.eu/en/publications/Publications/0910_SUR_Annual_Epidemiological_Report_on_Communicable_Diseases_in_Europe.pdf [accessed September 2010]. Variations in surveillance makes comparisons between EU countries difficult.

STI surveillance systems but there are major variations in terms of coverage, completeness and representativeness, and this prevents useful international comparisons.

The most recent UK STI surveillance data (2009) suggest that the upward trend in STI incidence apparent over the past 10 years is continuing. Between 2008 and 2009 annual STI diagnoses rose by 3% to 482,000. This rise is mainly due to increased diagnoses of genital *Chlamydia* (7%), gonorrhoea (6%) and genital herpes (5%). New diagnoses of genital warts were relatively unchanged while diagnoses of syphilis and non-specific genital infection fell slightly. The increase in diagnoses is due in part to increased transmission as a result of unsafe sexual behaviour but increasing use of newer molecular tests for gonorrhoea and genital herpes and the availability of community-based *Chlamydia* screening will also have contributed to the increase. The greatest burden of STIs continues to fall on young people aged 16–24 years who comprise only 12% or the population but account for more than half of new STI diagnoses. Homosexual and bisexual men and those of black ethnic origin are also disproportionately affected and there are geographical variations in incidence influenced by sexual behaviour and access to services.

Although total STI diagnoses remain higher than 10 years ago, STI surveillance data are susceptible to ascertainment factors including use of new diagnostic tests so the increased transmission of bacterial STIs seen recently in the UK may be due to improved availability and uptake of sexual health screening. The recent epidemiology of the main STIs is summarised in Table 3.28.1.

Prevention and control

The source of STIs is controlled by early diagnosis of cases of infection and prompt effective treatment. Contacts are actively followed up and offered diagnostic testing and prophylactic antibiotics if appropriate. All pregnant women are screened for syphilis by serology and increasingly there is opportunistic screening for genital *Chlamydia* infection.

In the UK, genitourinary medicine (GUM) clinics are open access clinics that offer free, confidential services and treatment for all STIs including HIV infection. A national network of GUM clinics was created as a result of the Venereal Disease Regulations 1916.

Transmission of STIs is controlled by promoting safer sexual behaviour including condom use through education and information. Vaccines are not available for the major STIs but susceptible individuals and populations may be offered immunisation against hepatitis A, hepatitis B and human papillomavirus (HPV).

2.8 Jaundice

Differential diagnosis

The differential diagnosis of jaundice includes many infectious and non-infectious causes (Boxes 2.8.1 and 2.8.2). In a previously well patient with acute onset of jaundice, the most likely cause is viral hepatitis.

Box 2.8.1 Non-infectious causes of jaundice

- Drug reaction (paracetamol, phenothiazines, alcohol)
- Recent anaesthetic
- Haemolysis (e.g. due to G6PD deficiency, sickle cell disease)
- Physiological (in the neonate)
- Toxin causing liver damage
- Primary biliary cirrhosis
- Gallstones
- Biliary or pancreatic cancer
- Genetic disorders (e.g. Gilbert's disease. NB mild forms may first become apparent due to the stress of an infection)

Box 2.8.2 Infectious causes of jaundice

Common
- Viral hepatitis
- Malaria

Uncommon
- Acute infections of the biliary system (cholecystitis, cholangitis, pancreatitis)
- Leptospirosis
- Epstein–Barr virus infection
- Cytomegalovirus
- Yellow fever

Viral hepatitis can be clinically distinguished from other causes of jaundice by the presence of a prodrome of fever, anorexia, nausea and abdominal discomfort. The liver is often enlarged and tender. There may be a history of travel to endemic areas, contact with a case or high-risk behaviour. Bilirubin is present in the urine, and serum transaminase levels (ALT, AST) are markedly elevated.

In viral hepatitis, the fever usually subsides once jaundice has developed. If the fever persists, other liver infections should be considered, such as Epstein–Barr virus or leptospirosis.

Laboratory investigations to distinguish between the different types of viral hepatitis and other liver infections are covered in the relevant chapters.

Prevention and control

General measures for the prevention of gastrointestinal infection (see Chapter 2.2) and blood-borne virus infection (see Chapter 2.10) will help prevent jaundice due to viral hepatitis. Malaria prophylaxis is covered in Chapter 3.48. Vaccines are available for hepatitis A (see Chapter 3.32), hepatitis B (see Chapter 3.33) and yellow fever (see Chapter 3.89).

Response to a case

Determine whether infectious or non-infectious cause. No specific public health measures are needed for non-infectious causes. For infectious causes, specific measures will usually be indicated, depending upon the causal agent. Assume blood, body fluids and (until 1 week after start of jaundice) stools are infectious until the cause is known.

Investigation of a cluster and response to an outbreak

Investigate to determine whether infectious or non-infectious cases. For non-infectious cases, consider common toxic exposure. For infectious cases, the response will depend upon the causal agent.

2.9 Infection in the immunocompromised

Impaired immunity is common; it may be congenital or acquired (ageing, treatments, underlying disease). Infection should be considered in an unwell immunocompromised person (and immunocompromise in unusual or recurrent infection). Infection may present in unusual ways in unusual sites, both common and unusual pathogens may be found.

Particular infections may be associated with specific immune defects (e.g. invasive aspergillosis with neutropenia and intracellular organisms with T-cell defects); knowledge of the immune defect may guide preventative measures, investigation and therapy. The risk of infection rises as the neutrophil count falls.

Infections with common organisms usually respond to routine treatment. Immunocompromised patients are often exposed to healthcare facilities, and to courses of antimicrobials, and are at increased risk of infection with resistant organisms.

Treating infection in the immunocompromised is highly specialised. This chapter concentrates upon issues of concern to a health protection specialist whose major role is ensuring systems are in place to minimise the risk of infection in the immunocompromised.

Specific causes and health protection issues

Groups at increased risk include the following:
• Extremes of age;
• Impaired anatomical barriers: burns, catheters, intubation; and
• Impaired host defence: genetic or acquired, underlying malignancy, chronic infection, immunosuppressive drugs, HIV.

Specific syndromes

HIV

HIV-positive patients are particularly at risk when they associate with other immunocompromised patients in healthcare surroundings. Services should be organised to minimise transmission of likely pathogens, in particular TB. Outbreaks of resistant TB associated with healthcare have occurred. Associated infections include *Pneumocystis*, TB, *Cryptosporidium*, cytomegalovirus.

Post-splenectomy

Post-splenectomy or as a consequence of hyposplenism, patients are at risk of infection from capsulate bacteria, particularly *Streptococcus pneumoniae*, *Neisseria meningitidis* and *Haemophilus influenzae*. Asplenic children under 5 years, especially those with sickle cell anaemia or splenectomised for trauma, have an infection rate of over 10%. Most infections occur within 2 years following splenectomy; however, the increased risk of dying of serious infection is probably lifelong. Hyposplenic patients should receive the following:

• Pneumococcal immunization;
• *Haemophilus influenzae* type b vaccine (if not already immune);
• Conjugate meningococcal group C immunization;
• Influenza immunization;
• Prophylactic antibiotics, probably lifelong (oral phenoxy-methylpenicillin or an alternative);
• Advice on prevention of malaria: hyposplenic patients are at risk of severe malaria; and
• An alert card to carry.

Laboratory diagnosis

A search for infection, including blood and urine cultures and a chest X-ray, will be necessary as soon as an immunocompromised patient spikes a fever. Opportunistic organisms that do not cause disease in the immunocompetent must be sought but it should be remembered that immunocompromised patients are most often infected by common pathogens.

Prevention and control

Immunization

The following infections can be prevented through immunisation of the immunocompromised patient:
• Pneumococcus;
• *H. influenzae* (Hib);
• Influenza; and
• Meningcococcus (group C).

Varicella risk can be reduced by vaccine for close non-immune contacts of immunocompromised where unavoidable continuing contact (e.g. sibling of a child with leukaemia).

Live vaccines are contraindicated in many immunocompromised patients. Avoid giving live vaccines (except MMR and BCG) to siblings of immunocompromised patients. Immunocompromised children should avoid close physical contact with children vaccinated with oral poliovirus vaccine (OPV) for 4–6 weeks following administration (this does not require school withdrawal).

Prophylaxis

The following chemoprophylaxis is available to reduce risk of infection in appropriate cases:
• Pneumocystis (oral co-trimoxazole) in HIV/AIDS;
• Malaria chemoprophylaxis;
• Penicillin in hyposplenism.

Managing the environment

Patients with T-cell deficiency are advised to boil their drinking water. This group includes the following:
• HIV-positive patients with a low T-cell count;
• Children with severe combined immunodeficiency (SCID); and
• Others with specific T-cell deficiencies.

Travel advice

Immunocompromised patients are at increased risk of travel-related infection. Asplenic patients are at risk of severe malaria and patients with AIDS are at risk from gastrointestinal parasites. The advice given will be dependent upon the epidemiology of disease in the area to be visited and the cause of immunosuppression.

Organisation of clinical services

• Treatment of TB and HIV-positive: examining the geographical layout of services so that infected and at-risk patients do not come into contact.
• Avoid healthcare staff who are zoster-susceptible working with immunocompromised individuals, or vaccinate non-immune healthcare workers.

Fungal infection and building work

Outbreaks of fungal infection have been associated with building work occurring close to healthcare areas that immunocompromised patients have frequented. Consider relocating services if major building work is undertaken.

Surveillance

All units treating significant numbers of immunocompromised patients should have ongoing surveillance of infection and be aware of the risk of outbreaks in the patient population.

Investigation of a cluster

Clusters of infection in the immunocompromised should be investigated with urgency. A cluster suggests a group of vulnerable people exposed to a common source.

Control of an outbreak

Rapid removal of any source. If necessary, closure of a ward if environmental contamination is feared.

2.10 Blood-borne viral infections

Human immunodeficiency virus (HIV), hepatitis B and hepatitis C are the main blood-borne viruses (BBV) of public health importance. These viruses persist in the blood and body fluids of affected persons and can be transmitted to others by various routes, often in an occupational setting (Table 2.10.1). Although immunisation and post-exposure prophylaxis may be available, the key to minimising the public health impact of these infections is prevention of exposure by careful management of contact with blood, body fluids and tissues. Exposure to BBV can be minimised by limiting exposure to blood and tissues (Table 2.10.2).

Management of blood exposure incidents

Following a needlestick or other sharps injury (from an infected patient) the risk of

Table 2.10.1 Routes of transmission of blood-borne viruses (BBVs)

Common	Less common
1 Sexual intercourse **2** Sharing injecting equipment **3** Skin puncture with sharp objects contaminated with blood of infected person **4** Vertical transmission from mother to infant before or during birth or by breastfeeding **5** Transfusion of infected blood or blood products when screening for BBVs has not been carried out	**1** Open wound contaminated with blood of infected person during sporting activities **2** Skin lesions (e.g. eczema) contaminated with blood of infected person **3** Splashes of the mucous membranes of eye, nose or mouth with blood of infected person **4** Human bites (which break skin) by infected person

Table 2.10.2 Minimising exposure to blood-borne viruses (BBV)

Prevention of exposure and use of PPE	Avoid contact with blood or body fluids. Cover cuts and abrasions with waterproof dressings. Control environmental contamination by blood and body fluids Protect skin, eyes, mouth and nose from blood splashes by using PPE including gloves, plastic aprons, impermeable gowns, rubber boots or overshoes, protective eye wear and masks
Avoid sharps injury, stay 'sharp safe'	Avoid using needles and sharp instruments if possible. Where available use innovative products that reduce the risk of sharps injuries Dispose of sharps into a container (UN Standard 3291, British Standard 7320) immediately after use and at the point of use. Do not re-sheath. Do not overfill the container
Dispose of waste safely	Healthcare staff have a duty to dispose of waste properly. In the UK, the safe disposal of waste is regulated by the 2005 Hazardous Waste regulations made under the Environmental Protection Act. Guidance on implementing these regulations is available: *Safe management of health care waste*, UK Royal College of Nursing. http://www.rcn.org.uk/__data/assets/pdf_file/0013/111082/003205.pdf [accessed September 2010] Healthcare waste is classified as infectious clinical waste, medicinal waste or offensive/hygiene waste. Waste should be classified and segregated in colour-coded and labelled receptacles before collection, transport and disposal. BBV-contaminated waste will usually be classified as infectious clinical waste and will require incineration
Managing blood and body fluids: spillages	Spills of blood and body fluids are a source of potential infection for others and should therefore be made safe as soon as possible. Local procedures should be followed which may specify use of spill kits and disinfectants
Collection and transport of specimens	Only staff who have been trained should collect and handle specimens. Local procedures should be followed. A guidance document *Transport of Infectious Substances* is available from: http://webarchive.nationalarchives.gov.uk/+/http://www.dft.gov.uk/pgr/freight/dgt1/publications/otherpublications/guidanceontransportofinfecti3186
Decontamination	HIV, HBV and HCV can all survive outside the human body for several weeks and so blood-contaminated surfaces, equipment and clothing that have not been decontaminated may lead to transmission. Decontamination is a combination of processes that removes contamination so that BBVs cannot reach a susceptible site in sufficient quantities to produce infection. Decontamination may include cleaning, disinfection and sterilisation Wherever possible single-use disposable devices should be used. Re-usable medical devices should be decontaminated in a sterile services department (SSD)

Table 2.10.2 (*Continued*)

	Best practice advice on decontamination of medical equipment is available on the Medicines and Healthcare Products Regulatory Agency (MHRA) website (http://www.mhra.gov.uk) and the decontamination section of the NHS website (http://www.dh.gov.uk/en/Managingyourorganisation/Workforce/Leadership/Healthcareenvironment/NHSDecontaminationProgramme/DH_077611
	Household bleach is usually supplied at a strength of 100,000 parts per million (ppm) free chlorine. Adding one part bleach to nine parts cold water gives a solution for disinfecting blood and body fluids (10,000 ppm). For general use, such as disinfecting work surfaces, a 1000 ppm solution of bleach is adequate (i.e. 1 in 100 dilution of household bleach). Undiluted Milton is equivalent to a strength of 10,000 ppm. All dilutions become ineffective with time and should be freshly made up every day
Linen	Blood-stained linen should not be sorted but should be placed in a water-soluble primary bag. This in turn should be placed within a secondary bag for storage and transport. The washing programme should include a disinfection cycle. Guidelines are available (HSG (95)18: Hospital laundry arrangements for used and infected linen. Department of Health 1995).
	http://www.dh.gov.uk/prod_consum_dh/groups/dh_digitalassets/@dh/@en/documents/digitalasset/dh_4012310.pdf

HBV, hepatitis B virus; HCV, hepatitis C virus; PPE, personal protective equipment.

HIV infection is 0.3%, the risk of hepatitis C virus (HCV) infection is 3% and the risk of hepatitis B virus (HBV) infection is 30%. The risk of acquiring HIV infection from a mucous membrane exposure is less than 0.1%. There should be a written policy detailing the local arrangements for risk assessment, advice, the provision of post-exposure prophylaxis and follow up. The policy should designate one or more doctors to whom exposed persons may be referred urgently for advice and should ensure that adequate 24-hour cover is available. Primary responsibility usually rests with the occupational health service, with out-of-hours cover provided by accident and emergency departments. These arrangements should be included in the programme of mandatory staff training.

Following an exposure, the wound should be washed liberally with soap and water and free bleeding should be encouraged. Exposed mucous membranes including conjunctivae should be irrigated and contact lenses should be removed. The injury should be reported promptly.

The designated doctor should assess the risk of transmission of HIV, HBV and HCV infection and the need for post-exposure management. The risk assessment is based on the type of body fluid involved and the route and severity of the exposure.

As a routine, the designated doctor or member of the clinical team (not the exposed worker) should approach the source patient (if known) and obtain informed consent, after pre-test discussion, to test for anti-HIV, hepatitis B surface antigen (HBsAg), anti-HCV and HCV RNA. Testing of the source patients should be completed within 8–24 hours.

If there is an HIV risk, post-exposure prophylaxis (PEP) should be started ideally within 1 hour. Subsequently, PEP may be discontinued if it is established that the source patient is HIV negative. Various PEP regimens have been recommended. In the UK, on the basis of acceptability and shelf life, the following PEP starter packs are used:

• One Truvada tablet (245 mg tenofovir and 200 mg emtricitabine (FTC)) once a day

   plus

• Two Kaletra film-coated tablets (200 mg lopinavir and 50 mg ritonavir) twice a day.

PEP should be started within 1 hour and certainly within 48–72 hours of exposure and continued for at least 28 days. The healthcare worker should be followed up weekly during the period of PEP, to monitor treatment side effects and ensure compliance.

The HBV immunity status of the healthcare worker should be assessed and if necessary blood should be taken for urgent anti-HBs testing. An accelerated course of vaccine, a booster dose of vaccine and/or hepatitis B immunoglobulin (HBIG) may be given. For HCV no immunisation or prophylaxis is available.

A baseline blood sample should be obtained from the exposed worker and stored for 2 years. If the source is HIV infected, the worker should be tested for anti-HIV at least 12 weeks after the exposure or after HIV PEP was stopped, whichever is the later. Testing for anti-HIV at 6 weeks and 6 months is no longer recommended. If the source is HCV infected, the worker should be tested for HCV RNA at 6 and 12 weeks and for anti-HCV at 12 and 24 weeks.

In the absence of seroconversion, modification of working practices is not necessary but infection control measures, safer sex practices and avoiding blood donation should be observed during the follow-up period. Generally, management of workers exposed to a potential BBV source whose status is unknown or a source that is unavailable for testing will depend upon a risk assessment and a discussion of the benefits of intervention.

Healthcare providers should follow local policies on reporting occupational exposures. In the UK, exposures to known BBV positive sources should be reported to the Health Protection Agency. Some types of occupational exposure are required to be reported under the Reporting of Injuries, Diseases and Dangerous Occurrences (RIDDOR) legislation.

Employment policies

In the UK, guidelines for healthcare workers with BBV infections who carry out exposure-prone procedures (EPP) have been published (*Health clearance for tuberculosis, hepatitis B, hepatitis C and HIV: New healthcare workers*. London: Department of Health. http://www. dh.gov.uk/prod_consum_dh/groups/dh_digi talassets/@dh/@en/documents/digitalasset/ dh_074981.pdf [accessed September 2010]).

EPPs are those in which there is a risk that injury to the healthcare worker could result in exposure of the patient's open tissues to the blood of the healthcare worker. Such procedures occur mainly in surgery, obstetrics and gynaecology, dentistry and midwifery. Healthcare workers who will perform EPPs should be HIV antibody negative, HBsAg negative (or, if positive, e-antigen negative with a viral load of 10^3 genome equivalents/mL or less) and hepatitis C antibody negative (or, if positive, negative for hepatitis C RNA).

In the UK, employers are required by the Control of Substances Hazardous to Health Regulations (COSHH) to assess the risk to their staff from exposure to BBVs and implement any protective measures. There are no vaccines available against HCV or HIV but routine pre-exposure HBV immunisation is recommended for healthcare workers, laboratory staff, staff of residential and other accommodation for those with learning difficulties, morticians and embalmers and prison service staff. Other occupational groups such as police and fire and rescue services, tattooists and needle exchange service staff may also be at risk and for these groups of staff an assessment of the frequency of likely BBV exposure should be carried out prior to immunisation. Generally, those who receive HBV immunisation because they are at occupational risk should have their immunity confirmed by post-immunisation testing for anti-HBs.

Advice for people living with blood-borne viral infections

All persons found to be infected with a BBV should be considered potentially infectious and should be counselled concerning infectivity. The following advice should be given:
• Keep cuts or grazes covered with a waterproof plaster until the skin has healed.
• Avoid sharing your razor or toothbrush (or anything that might cut the skin or damage the gums and cause bleeding). Use your own towel and face cloth.

- If you cut yourself, wipe up any blood with paper tissues and flush these down the toilet. Wipe any surfaces where blood has been spilt with household bleach diluted in cold water (1 part bleach to 10 parts water). Do not use this on your skin or on any fabrics. In these circumstances wash thoroughly with soap and water.
- Tell any helpers that you are a carrier of a BBV and that blood precautions should be taken. If available they should wear plastic gloves. Otherwise, they can use a towel or cloth to prevent them from getting blood on to their skin.
- If your clothing is soiled with blood or other body fluids, wash them using a pre-wash and hot washing machine cycle.
- Dispose of used tampons straight away by flushing down the toilet. Dispose of sanitary towels in your rubbish after first sealing inside a plastic bag.

- If you go for medical or dental treatment, tell your doctor or dentist you have a BBV infection.
- Do not donate blood or carry an organ donor card.
- Do not have acupuncture, tattooing, ear piercing or electrolysis.
- If you are an injecting drug user do not share your works and dispose of used needles and syringes safely by putting them in a rigid container with a lid. If possible use a local needle exchange scheme. Return used works to the scheme in the special plastic sharps bin.
- If you have HCV infection you should limit weekly alcohol consumption to less than 21 units for women and 28 units for men. BBV infections are not infectious under normal school or work conditions. There is no need to stay away from school or work.
- Sexual intercourse, pregnancy and birth advice is given in Table 2.10.3.

Table 2.10.3 Sexual intercourse, pregnancy and birth: advice to patients

	HCV	HBV	HIV
Sexual intercourse	If you are in a stable relationship with one partner you may not feel the need to start using condoms; however, it is advisable to avoid sexual intercourse during a menstrual period Otherwise, condom use should be encouraged and safe sex should continue to be promoted for the prevention of HIV and other sexually transmitted infections	Condom use recommended until sexual partners are immunised against HBV and have had immunity confirmed	Condom use recommended
Pregnancy and birth	The risk of transmission from mother to child appears to be very low. At the present time there is no need to advise against pregnancy based on HCV status alone Mothers who are viraemic should not breastfeed	All babies of HBsAg positive mothers should receive hepatitis B vaccine. Those whose mothers are e-antigen positive, HBsAg positive without e-markers (or where e-marker status has not been determined) or had acute hepatitis during pregnancy also require HBIG	The risk of transmission from mother to child can be reduced by anti-viral treatment in pregnancy, caesarean section and avoiding breastfeeding

HBsAg, hepatitis B surface antigen; HBV, hepatitis B virus; HBC, hepatitis C virus; HBIG, hepatitis B immunoglobulin.

2.11 Vaccine queries

Vaccine queries are very common and can generate significant work for the public health practitioner. Those who administer vaccines often receive little or no training on the subject and may rely heavily on the local public health team for support. The questions in this chapter are a selection of those commonly encountered in public health practice.

Schedule

One of my patients had the first two doses of the primary schedule as a baby and has now turned up 3 years later for the third dose – do I need to restart the course?

An interrupted immunisation course should be treated as normal – there is no need to restart the course.

A baby in my practice was born at 27 weeks' gestation – should I delay his/her immunisations?

It has been shown in several studies that even very premature babies mount an adequate immune response when they are vaccinated starting at 2 months. There is no need to delay.

I've got a 14-year-old patient who has never had any immunisations – is it too late to start now?

It is never too late. Your patient needs a full course of immunisation against all antigens in the national schedule (except for pertussis, which can be omitted in older children). No-one should be unprotected.

I've got a family of asylum seekers in my practice and they have no medical records. What vaccinations do they need?

Assume they are unimmunised and give a full course of immunisations according to the national schedule

I've given the first dose of DTP-IPV-Hib vaccine to a 7-week old baby by mistake – what should I do?

Although the response may not be optimal, DTP-containing vaccines provide adequate protection from 6 weeks of age. Complete the course at the recommended ages, no extra dose is needed.

A 6-month-old baby was born in Italy and had two injections there – what should I do to complete the course?

The immunisation schedule is different in every country. Current vaccination schedules in Europe can be found at www.euvacc/net. DTP, polio and Hib vaccines are given in all EU countries; most countries (including Italy) also vaccinate against hepatitis B. Meningococcal vaccine and pneumococcal vaccines are only given in some countries. Vaccination of children moving between countries needs to be adapted to the local schedule. In the example given, a baby moving from Italy to the UK would need meningococcal C and pneumococcal vaccines (two doses) and a further dose of DTPa-IPV-Hib. This could be given as DTPa-IPV-Hib-Hep B, available from the manufacturer, which would complete the hepatitis B course.

Contraindications

A 6-month-old child, who has not yet started vaccination, has had meningococcal meningitis. Does that mean I can skip the MenC vaccine?

Previous history of disease is not a contraindication to vaccination. Natural disease does not always confer immunity and there is no specific risk of vaccinating an individual with pre-existing immunity. Additionally, in the example given, the meningitis could have been caused by a non-group C strain.

Which vaccines can be given in pregnancy?

There is a theoretical risk that vaccination in pregnancy with live vaccines may infect the fetus. However, there is no evidence to date that any live vaccine causes birth defects but because of the theoretical risk of fetal infection, live vaccines should generally be delayed until after delivery. There is no theoretical risk of fetal infection with inactivated vaccines; however, unless protection is required without delay (e.g. during an influenza pandemic), vaccination should be delayed until after delivery.

I've got a patient who is highly allergic to eggs – are there any vaccines he/she can't have?

Non-anaphylactic allergic reactions are not a contraindication to any vaccine. Yellow fever and influenza vaccines should not be given to people with egg anaphylaxis but there is now evidence that MMR can be given to children with severe egg allergy, including anaphylaxis.

Safety and other concerns

I've given an adult dose of hepatitis A vaccine to a child – what should I do?

The risk of a vaccine reaction is normally not dose-related, so continue the vaccine course as normal and reassure. In the UK, the incident should be reported to the Committee on Safety of Medicines via a yellow card.

I've heard the MMR vaccines contain pork – what should I tell my Muslim patients?

Porcine material is used in the manufacturing process of some MMR vaccines, but is undetectable in the final product. Muslim leaders are aware of this and support the use of MMR vaccine.

Will giving so many vaccines to a young baby overload the immune system?

From birth, humans are exposed to countless foreign antigens and infectious agents in the environment; this is part of the process by which the immune system matures. Responding to the very small number of antigens contained in vaccines requires only a tiny proportion of the capacity of an infant's immune system. Studies have shown that vaccines do not increase susceptibility to serious infections.

One of my patients developed a rash and a temperature after the first dose of MMR vaccine. Is it safe to give the second dose?

Yes – a mild version of measles is a common side effect of MMR and usually resolves spontaneously. Reactions are less common after the second dose as most children will have developed antibodies that neutralise the vaccine virus.

I've given a vaccine which is out of date – do I need to repeat the dose?

There is usually some margin of error (up to a month) for out-of-date vaccine administration – consult the manufacturer. If in doubt repeat the dose.

Which vaccines contain thiomersal?

Some influenza and hepatitis B vaccines contain traces of thiomersal used in the manufacturing process. There is no evidence that the levels of thiomersal in vaccines (which are below levels found in natural sources) pose a safety risk.

Travel

One of my patients is off to India tomorrow – is it too late to give any vaccines?

Most vaccines will provide reasonable protection within 2 weeks even after a single dose. Give vaccines as appropriate but advise that protection will not be optimal.

I've got an HIV positive patient who is going on a trip to Africa and Asia – are there any vaccines he can't have?

Yellow fever and BCG vaccines should not be given; a letter of exemption from yellow fever may be required. Give IPV instead of OPV. All other vaccines can be given.

Occupational

I've given two complete courses of hepatitis B vaccine to a nurse but she still hasn't got any antibodies – what should I do?

Some adults are non-responders. Check for HBsAg carriage (if positive, may need to exclude from undertaking exposure-prone procedures). Consider giving a higher dose vaccine (specifically licensed for haemodialysis patients). May need HBIG if a needlestick injury is sustained.

A student nurse had a chickenpox vaccine last week, and now has a vesicular rash – does she need to be off work?

If the rash is localised and a vaccine reaction suspected, the rash should be covered and the nurse can continue to work, unless in contact with high-risk patients (risk assessment needed). If the rash is generalised the nurse should avoid patient contact until all the lesions have crusted.

Storage and administration errors

I came into the surgery this morning and found the cleaner had unplugged the fridge – are the vaccines still OK?

Vaccines are able to survive temperatures outside normal fridge limits for a limited period of time (up to 1 week). The manufacturer should be able to provide more advice on a specific vaccine. If in doubt it is better to discard the vaccines and order replacements.

Someone turned the fridge up and the vaccines are now frozen – are they still OK?

No – freezing causes irreversible deterioration of the vaccine. Discard and order more.

2.12 Individual measures against infections

General measures

A healthy lifestyle

Lifestyle has an important role in the transmission, acquisition, reactivation and response to infectious disease. The role of lifestyle in transmission of disease associated with drug misuse or sexual activity is well recognised. Activity such as outdoor pursuits is a risk factor in many tick-borne infections. Stress is associated with the reactivation of herpes simplex infection. Attention to general health, sufficient sleep (large interindividual variations), moderate intake of alcohol and reasonable levels of psychosocial stress decrease the risk of infection.

Hand hygiene

The human hand may be the most important of all disease transmitters. Our hands are in constant contact with the surrounding environment, and various pathogens can, via the hands, reach the mucous membranes in the mouth, nose, eyes and genitals and thus introduce an infection. Food can be contaminated via the hands, and auto-infection with *Enterobius vermicularis* sustained.

Proper hand hygiene is therefore the basis for all personal measures against infection. The hands should always be washed with soap and water before and after meals, after visits to the toilet and after direct contact with wounds, blood, nasal discharge and other body fluids (own and others), after direct contact with animals and after spending time in crowded conditions – especially during seasons with much respiratory tract or gastrointestinal infections.

Liquid soap is preferable. Thorough handwashing with liquid soap and water reduces the bacterial load on the hands by more than 90%, alcohol reduces the bacterial load a further 5%. Rings and jewellery should be removed before handwashing. It may be more practical to carry a small bottle of alcohol disinfectant than finding a place for handwashing when outdoors.

Exposure to low temperature

The effect of temperature on infections is much debated. The term 'common cold' refers to a general belief that low temperature increases the risk for upper respiratory tract infections. Experimental studies have not been able to prove such a relationship. However, exposure to low temperature is a risk factor for other infections such as pneumococcal pneumonia.

Prevention of food-borne infection

Food handling

In our globalised world we can find food from all parts of the world in our local grocery store, potentially exposing us to a global variety of pathogens. Changed eating habits, such as eating exotic food, fast food, microwave-heated food and less processed food, as well as changes in food preparation add variety if carried out correctly, but proper hygiene knowledge is necessary to avoid infections.

- It is important that groceries are transported home as quickly as possible. Do not let the grocery bags stay in the cars for hours. If it is not possible to return home immediately, use a cool box.
- Always check the 'best before' date to avoid buying food with high bacterial levels. It is important to note that food contaminated with pathogenic bacteria does not necessarily smell bad or look un-fresh. Many bacteria, such as *Yersinia enterocolitica*, *Listeria monocytogenes* and *Clostridium botulinum*, can grow well in low temperatures if stored in the refrigerator too long.
- When preparing large amounts of food it is important to chill the food as quickly as possible. During northern European winters with low temperatures, the food could be placed outdoors if well-covered. Alternatively, the food could be chilled in small containers placed in cold water.
- No raw food is free from micro-organisms. Always wash your hands before, during and after preparing food to prevent contamination and cross-contamination. Never cook for others when you have diarrhoea or an infected wound on the hands.
- Rinse vegetables, fresh herbs and fruit thoroughly before use – it is not possible to get rid of all bacteria, but the numbers could be substantially reduced.
- Cook meat thoroughly. This is especially important for chicken, which often contains *Campylobacter* or *Salmonella*.
- To avoid cross-contamination use different cutting boards for meat, vegetables and prepared food. Plastic cutting boards can be washed in a dishwasher. Change dishcloths often or boil them in water. Let them dry thoroughly between use.
- When barbequing, never put the meat back on plates that were used for the raw meat.

Risky food

Handling food to be eaten without being heated requires proper hygiene measures to ensure that it does not contain pathogenic microbes. Some food is associated with a higher risk of infection:

- Unpasteurised milk and milk products should be avoided, especially for small children, as verocytotoxin-producing *Escherichia coli* (VTEC) and *Campylobacter* are not uncommon, even in milk from healthy cows.
- Oysters and mussels filter large amounts of water, and micro-organisms (especially norovirus and hepatitis A virus) could be concentrated in the molluscs if they have been grown in contaminated water.
- Many large *Salmonella* outbreaks have been caused by contaminated bean sprouts. The sprouts are best stored in refrigerator.
- Fresh vegetable and herbs should always be rinsed, regardless of what is stated on the package.
- Raw or soft-boiled eggs may contain *Salmonella*. Risk for infection is highest if eggs are used in products that are not heated properly (e.g. custard on cakes).
- Frozen raspberries have caused several international norovirus outbreaks.
- Mycotoxins are produced by several moulds. Aflatoxin is highly carcinogenic, and may appear in peanuts and nuts.
- Because of the risk of poisoning it is important to have sufficient knowledge when picking mushrooms.

Measures against respiratory tract infections

Most respiratory tract infections have an airborne mode of transmission or are spread through droplets. An alternative important mode of transmission is through a direct contact between hands and mucous membranes. Especially during the flu season it is advisable to avoid crowded settings, avoid touching the face with the hands and wash the hands regularly.

Other effective measure to avoid respiratory tract infections include stopping smoking, immunization against respiratory tract pathogens as appropriate (depending on age and risk group) and using a face mask when being exposed for specific pathogens such as *Aspergillus* (renovations of cellars and attics), Puumala virus (environment soiled by urine from the bank vole *Clethrionomys glareolus*).

Measures against sexually transmitted infections

Sexually transmitted infections (STIs) require close person-to-person contact for transmission. It should therefore be noted that most other infectious diseases (e.g. gastrointestinal and respiratory tract infections) also easily transmit during sexual contact.

All forms of vaginal, oral and anal intercourse are associated with a risk of STI transmission even if condoms are used. It is therefore more appropriate to talk about 'safer sex' than 'safe sex'. Condoms should be used throughout intercourse. Even if they are generally durable, they may be torn by sharp nails or rupture during anal intercourse without lubrication. Lubrication should be water or silicon based, as oil-based lubricants such as Vaseline and skin creams may dissolve the condom.

Measures against blood-borne infections

Hepatitis B, hepatitis C and HIV are the three major viral infections transmitted via blood.

Intravenous drug use

The most important risk factor for blood-borne infections outside medical care settings is intravenous drug use. The infection is mainly transmitted through the use of non-sterile needles and syringes. A lesser-known route of infection, even among drug addicts, is the transmission through the cup or saucer in which the drugs are dissolved before being drawn into the syringe. Viruses can be killed through boiling the syringes and needles (for several minutes), alternatively by cleaning them in chlorine. To affect the hepatitis B viruses, which are hardier than HIV, the needles and syringes must be in contact with chlorine for at least 2 minutes.

Both these methods are effective, but not completely safe. The only safe way is never to share injection equipment. As a harm-reduction measure, most European countries organise needle-exchange programmes.

Tattoos

Becoming tattooed with a non-sterile needle carries the risk of blood-borne infection. It is therefore important to ensure that the tattoo is done by a reputable craftsman. In many countries there are associations of professional tattoo artists. If uncertain, it is advisable to consult the local public health department.

Tattooing abroad should be avoided as the prevalence of blood-infected persons may be high, and the regulation of tattoo artists is inadequate in many parts of the world.

Other blood exposure

Exposure to blood occasionally happens outside healthcare environments, for example in relation to accidents. The basic rule for all contact with blood is to consider it as infected. It is especially important to avoid getting blood splashes in the eyes, mouth or nose.

Blood-borne infection cannot occur through intact skin, but a broken skin barrier is not unusual (e.g. around the cuticles, or areas with eczema). Broken glass on the scene of an accident should never be picked up directly with the fingers. Blood on the skin should be immediately washed with soap and water. Blood spill, even minimal amounts, should be dried as soon as possible. Chlorine solution (1 part bleach to 9 parts water) effectively destroys the virus on blood-soaked surfaces or objects. Bleach solution should not be used directly on skin or on textiles. Blood-stained clothes should be washed with pre-wash and then at the highest possible temperature. Plastic or latex gloves and disposable plastic aprons should be included in car and home first aid kits. A nozzle with a check valve for mouth-to-mouth resuscitation is a valuable part of a first aid kit.

The risk of blood contamination increases with cuts and puncture wounds. If the skin is penetrated by contaminated needles, scalpels or similar, the risk of hepatitis B infection is about 30%, hepatitis C infection about 3% and HIV 0.3%. The injured area should be bled and the area should be washed thoroughly with soap and water. After any exposure that might have a risk of blood contamination a doctor should be immediately contacted.

Protection against insect-borne infections

Protection against tick bites

Several infections (e.g. tick-borne encephalitis (TBE), borreliosis, ehrlichiosis and tularaemia) are transmitted by *Ixodes* ticks. Ticks are widespread throughout large parts of northern and central Europe, and thrive in damp and shaded terrain with half-high grass. The tick season usually lasts from early spring to autumn.

The best protection against tick bites is to avoid the typical tick-infested terrains. In gardens, the number of ticks could be reduced by keeping the grass short and clearing away shady bushes and trees. Full dress, with trousers stacked in boots, is an effective protection. Furthermore, it is advisable to inspect the skin regularly, as the ticks often take some time before biting. Mosquito repellent has some effect even against ticks.

Ticks prefer to bite through thin skin. Most common areas in adults are the legs, while in children the bite is usually higher up on the body, often in the groins. Transfer of TBE virus is instantaneous after the bite, while the risk of infection with *Borrelia* and *Ehrlichia* increases with the time the tick is attached. Ticks are best removed with tweezers (preferably special tick tweezers which can be bought in pharmacies in tick-infested regions). A gentle, twisting motion increases the chance that the entire tick is removed and reduces the risk of bacterial transmission. Margarine or cooking oil should not be used. The wound is washed with soap and water. Any remaining tick parts give rise to an inflammatory reaction and can be removed after a few days. These do not increase the risk of infection. Doctors should be contacted if an erythema occurs around the bite site.

Protection against mosquito bites

Worldwide, mosquitoes are an extremely important vector for various infectious diseases such as malaria, dengue, yellow fever, chikungunya and Japanese encephalitis. In Europe, mosquito-borne diseases are less common, but nevertheless exist as seen in recent outbreaks of chikungunya fever, dengue fever and West Nile fever in areas of southern Europe, and endemic mosquito-borne transmission of tularaemia in areas of northern Europe.

The most common mosquito repellents for personal use contain diethyltoluamide (DEET) or icaridin (picaridine) and are very effective against mosquito bites. Used together with permethrin-treated clothes the reduction in the number of mosquito bites is around 85–95%. In order to achieve full protection DEET should be applied every fourth hour (more often if you sweat). Almost 10% of applied DEET can be absorbed through the skin, but despite this there are only a few reports of toxic side effects. Caution is urged in repeated application on small children.

Using permethrin and/or deltamitrin impregnated mosquito nets is recommended in tropical areas where malaria, dengue fever, Japanese encephalitis and other mosquito-transmitted diseases are endemic. The best effect is against mosquito species that have a preference to bite indoors at night. *Aedes* species that transmit dengue, chikungunya and yellow fever are primarily daytime biters, while the malaria-spreading *Anopheles* mosquitoes are most active at night and dawn. In air-conditioned rooms, mosquito nets can often be omitted.

Section 3
Diseases

3.1 Amoebic dysentery

Entamoeba histolytica is a cause of intestinal infection, which may include dysentery.

Suggested on-call action

- Exclude cases in high-risk groups for transmission of gastrointestinal infections (Table 2.2.1).
- If other non-travel-related cases known to you or reporting laboratory/clinician, consult local outbreak plan.

Epidemiology

Although much more common in tropical countries, amoebiasis does occur in Europe. Approximately 100 cases a year are reported in the UK, where infection is most common in young adults and unusual in pre-school children. Most cases occur in travellers to developing countries.

Clinical features

Intestinal infection may be asymptomatic; an intermittent diarrhoea with abdominal pain; amoebic colitis presenting as bloody diarrhoea; and a fulminant colitis with significant mortality in the malnourished, pregnant, immunosuppressed or very young. Extra-intestinal disease includes liver, lung and brain abscesses.

Laboratory confirmation

The diagnosis is confirmed by demonstrating either the trophozoites or cysts of *E. histolytica* on microscopy of very fresh stool samples. Three specimens are required to exclude amoebiasis. Many cysts are non-pathogenic (e.g. *Entamoeba dispar* and *Entamoeba moshkovskii*) but morphologically indistinguishable from *E. histolytica*: specific antigen detection and polymerase chain reaction (PCR) tests can differentiate between these organisms. Invasive disease may be diagnosed by serology.

Transmission

Entamoeba histolytica is predominantly spread by environmentally resistant cysts excreted in human faeces. Transmission may occur via contaminated water or food, or direct faeco-oral contact. Cysts resist standard water chlorination. Acute cases pose only limited risk.

Acquisition

The incubation period is usually 2–4 weeks but a range of a few days to years has been reported. The infectious period depends upon the excretion of cysts in the stool and may last several years. In acute dysentery only trophozoites are passed in the stool; these die within minutes in the environment. Almost all recovered patients appear to be immune to re-infection.

Prevention

- Avoidance of faecal contamination of water supplies, combined with adequate water treatment (e.g. filtration).
- Good personal, toilet and food hygiene.
- Care with food and water for travellers in developing countries.
- Sterilisation of re-usable colonic or rectal equipment (e.g. colonic irrigation or medical investigation).

Communicable Disease Control and Health Protection Handbook, Third Edition. Jeremy Hawker, Norman Begg, Iain Blair, Ralf Reintjes, Julius Weinberg and Karl Ekdahl.
© 2012 Jeremy Hawker, Norman Begg, Iain Blair, Ralf Reintjes, Julius Weinberg and Karl Ekdahl.
Published 2012 by Blackwell Publishing Ltd.

Surveillance

Cases of dysentery should be reported to the local public health department and confirmed *E. histolytica* to local and national surveillance systems.

Response to a case

• Exclude cases in groups at increased risk of spreading infection (Table 2.2.1) until 48 hours after first normal stool.
• If no history of travel abroad, then obtain detailed food history for the period 2–4 weeks before onset, including drinking water.
• Enteric precautions. Hygiene advice to case and household.
• Screen household or institutional contacts. Discuss with microbiologist further investigation of positives. Consider treatment for those with prolonged excretion of pathogenic cysts, especially if in risk group for spreading infection.

Investigation of a cluster

• Check to ensure that infection is not due to travelling abroad: inform relevant national centre if associated with particular country.
• Organise further testing to ensure that reported cases have infection with pathogenic *E. histolytica*.
• For symptomatic cases, obtain detailed food and water consumption history for period 2–4 weeks before onset of symptoms. Check home/work/travel against water supply areas (water-borne outbreaks have occurred rarely in Europe).
• Look for links with institutions with potential for faeco-oral spread (e.g. young adults with learning difficulties or camps with poor hygiene facilities).
• Consider transmission between men who have sex with men.

Control of an outbreak

• Rarely a problem in developed countries. Response will depend upon source identified.

• Enteric precautions for cases and carriers. Exclusion of those in risk groups (Table 2.2.1). Consider treatment if confirmed as *E. histolytica*. Ensure that treatment includes an agent that eliminates cysts (e.g. diloxanide).
• Sanitary disposal of faeces, handwashing, food hygiene and regular cleaning of toilet and kitchen areas.

Suggested case-definition for an outbreak

Diarrhoea with demonstration of trophozoites or cysts (speciation preferable).

3.2 Anthrax

Anthrax is a potentially serious infection caused by *Bacillus anthracis*, an organism that forms spores that may survive for many years. It is a potential agent of bioterrorism.

Suggested on-call action

• Ensure case admitted and treated.
• Identify likely source of exposure and other individuals who may have been exposed.
• Ensure exposed individuals are clinically assessed.

Epidemiology

Anthrax is a zoonosis, acquired from contact with infected herbivores or their products. It is endemic in the Middle East, Africa and in countries of the former Soviet Union, where it is usually a disease of rural herdsmen. In most of Europe it has been eliminated from livestock and is therefore rare, as are imported infections. In 2007, six cases were reported in Europe (four were confirmed: two in Romania, one in Spain and one in Bulgaria).

The sporadic cases reported in Europe usually result from occupational exposure to animal products, carcasses, hides, hair and wool. Fatal cases in 2009–2010 have been associated with the injection of contaminated heroin. Other than drug-related cases, concern is occasionally raised about renovating old buildings where animal hair was used in the construction; these have not been associated with cases.

Clinical features

The clinical features depend upon the route of infection:

Cutaneous anthrax (over 90% of cases): infection is through the skin. Over a few days a sore, which begins as a pimple, grows, ulcerates and forms a black scab, around which are purplish vesicles. There may be associated oedema. Systemic symptoms include rigors, headache and vomiting. The sore is usually diagnostic; 20% of cases are fatal.

Inhalation/pulmonary anthrax: spores are inhaled, with subsequent invasion of mediastinal lymph nodes. An abrupt onset of flu-like illness, rigors, dyspnoea and cyanosis is followed by shock and usually death over the next 2–6 days.

Intestinal anthrax occurs following ingestion of spores, with severe gut disease, nausea, vomiting, anorexia, fever and then septicaemia. Pulmonary and intestinal diseases are usually recognised late and have worse outcomes.

Laboratory confirmation

Swabs from cutaneous lesions, nasal swabs (if inhalational anthrax suspected), blood cultures, lymph node or spleen aspirates, or cerebrospinal fluid (CSF) (if meningitic) show characteristic bacilli on staining with polychrome methylene blue. Colonies may be grown overnight. The definitive test for *B. anthracis* is polymerase chain reaction (PCR).

Transmission

Transmission is usually from contact with contaminated animal products. Spores can remain viable in the soil for many years. Transmission may be by direct contact, inhalation or ingestion (e.g. of spores in meat). There is no recorded person-to-person spread via the inhalational route.

Acquisition

The incubation period varies between 1 and 7 days, inhalation anthrax usually within 48 hours, cutaneous anthrax rarely up to 7 weeks. Secretions from cutaneous lesions may be infectious. Environmental spores may be infectious for decades.

Prevention

• Pre-treatment of animal products and good occupational health cover are the mainstays of control.
• Animals believed to have died of anthrax should be disposed of under supervision. Mass vaccination of animals may reduce disease spread.
• Non-cellular vaccines for human use are available for individuals at risk from occupational exposure, such as veterinarians working in endemic areas, zoos, etc. Workers handling potentially infectious raw material should be aware of the risks. In the event of a deliberate release, individual risk would be assessed on a case-by-case basis. Post-exposure prophylaxis with antibiotics can be very effective in preventing disease if given early enough.

Surveillance

In most countries anthrax is a notifiable disease. Cases should be reported on clinical suspicion as a matter of urgency.

A suspected case includes any previously healthy person with the following:
• Rapid onset of severe, unexplained febrile illness or febrile death;
• Rapid onset of severe sepsis not due to a predisposing illness, or respiratory failure with a widened mediastinum; or
• Severe sepsis with Gram-positive rods or *Bacillus* species identified in the blood or CSF and assessed not to be a contaminant.
Cases should be immediately reported to the local Public Health authorities and to national authorities.

Response to a case

• Set up an incident team.
• Remove potentially contaminated clothes to reduce the possibility of secondary cutaneous cases. Instruct exposed persons to shower thoroughly. Use standard universal precautions for care.
• Investigate source: search for history of potentially infected animals or animal products and trace to place of origin. Liaise with veterinary officers. Particularly enquire as to travel and occupational exposure – include exposure to mail.
• Consider bioterrorism if:
  (a) single confirmed case of inhalational anthrax;
  (b) single confirmed case of cutaneous anthrax in individual with no contact with animals or animal hides; or
  (c) two or more suspected cases linked in time and place.
• Initial therapy of inhalational anthrax should be with ciprofloxacin 400 mg iv every 12 hours or doxycycline 100 mg every 12 hours plus additional antibiotics (rifampicin, vancomycin, chloramphenicol, penicillin, amoxicillin, imipenem, clindamycin, clarithromycin). Benzyl penicillin or amoxicillin should not be used alone.
• Other possible contacts of the source should be identified and placed under clinical surveillance for 7 days since last exposure.
• Contacts of cases are not at risk.

Investigation of a cluster

Check for history of exposure in endemic countries. If none:
• Undertake full hypothesis-generating study, using semi-structured interviews of all cases and re-interviewing as potential sources identified by other cases. Include full occupational history.
• Institute case-finding, both locally and nationally.
• Consider bioterrorism.

Control of an outbreak

• Trace exposure as a matter of urgency.
• Remove source.

Response to a deliberate release

• Report to local and national public health authorities.
• Define exposed zone and identify individuals exposed within it (some may have left scene).
• Cordon off exposed zone.
• Decontaminate those exposed: remove clothing and possessions, then shower with soap and water.
• Chemoprophylaxis (currently ciprofloxacin) as soon as possible for those exposed.
• Record contact details for all those exposed.
• Some health and emergency workers may also need prophylaxis.
• Police may take environmental samples.
For more general information see Chapter 4.15.

Suggested case-definition for an outbreak
Suspected   • Rapid onset of severe, unexplained febrile illness or febrile death.

• Rapid onset of severe sepsis not due to a predisposing illness, or respiratory failure with a widened mediastinum.
• Severe sepsis with Gram-positive rods or *Bacillus* species identified in the blood or CSF and assessed not to be a contaminant.
Confirmed case
• A case that clinically fits the criteria for suspected anthrax and, in addition, definitive positive results are obtained on one or more pathological specimens by the reference laboratory.

3.3 *Bacillus cereus*

Bacillus cereus is a rare cause of food poisoning that manifests as one of two mild gastrointestinal syndromes. It is not spread from person to person.

Suggested on-call action

If you or the reporting clinician/ microbiologist knows of associated cases, consult the Outbreak Control Plan.

Epidemiology

Bacillus cereus food poisoning occurs worldwide, accounting for around 0.2% of sporadic gastroenteritis cases presenting to GPs in the UK. A much higher incidence has been reported from Hungary, the Netherlands and Finland. Reported outbreaks are usually linked to institutions, including restaurants, schools and hospitals.

Clinical features

Two clinical syndromes may occur, caused by different toxins:

1 A short incubation illness consisting of vomiting accompanied by nausea, abdominal pain and, occasionally, diarrhoea later. This is usually a mild illness, which lasts less than 12 hours and is difficult to distinguish from staphylococcal food poisoning.
2 A short–medium incubation illness consisting of diarrhoea usually accompanied by abdominal pain and perhaps tenesmus, nausea or vomiting. Diarrhoea may be profuse and watery and lasts around 24 hours. It is difficult to distinguish clinically from *Clostridium perfringens* food poisoning.

Bacillus cereus may also cause local and systemic infections – these may be severe in the immunocompromised and intravenous drug users.

Laboratory confirmation

Bacillus cereus may be cultured from stool or vomit samples but is also found in a small number of healthy controls. It may be cultured from suspect foods; however, large numbers (e.g. $>10^5$/g) are necessary to prove that food was the source of infection. Serotyping is available to compare strains from different cases or with food isolates: however, more than one strain can be associated with an individual outbreak. Phage-typing may also be available. Reference laboratories can test the potential of the isolate for toxin production.

Transmission

Bacillus cereus is widespread in the environment and is found at low levels in many foodstuffs. Contamination of food may easily occur prior to cooking and spores can survive normal cooking (optimum temperature for spore activation is 65–75°C) and they are resistant to drying. Cell growth usually occurs between 10°C and 50°C (optimum 28–35°C) and so storage of food at ambient temperature after cooking allows multiplication of the organism. *B. cereus* produces two toxins: a heat-stable emetic toxin associated with the short incubation vomiting illness and a heat-labile enterotoxin associated with the longer incubation diarrhoeal illness. Both toxins occur preformed in food, but the latter may also be produced in the gut after digestion.

Many outbreaks of *B. cereus* vomiting have been linked to the method of making fried rice employed in Chinese restaurants. The rice is boiled, allowed to drain at room temperature (to avoid clumping), stored and then flash-fried at insufficient temperature to destroy preformed heat-stable emetic toxin. Attack rates of near 100% have been reported from such outbreaks.

Other reported food vehicles include pasta dishes, vanilla sauce, cream, meatballs, boiled beef, barbecue chicken and turkey loaf. Attack rates of 50–75% are reported for these outbreaks.

Nosocomial infection and cases in intravenous drug users have also been reported.

Acquisition

The incubation period is approximately 2–3 hours (range 1–6 hours) for the vomiting illness and 8–12 hours (range 6–24 hours, rarely longer) for the diarrhoeal syndrome. *B. cereus* is not considered communicable from person-to-person because of the high infectious dose required, which is about $10^5/g$. People at increased risk of severe infection include those with sickle cell disease, patients with intravascular catheters, intravenous drug users and those with immunosuppressive or debilitating medical conditions.

Prevention

• Store cooked foods at above 60°C or below 10°C before re-heating or consumption.
• Limit storage time and re-heat thoroughly.

Surveillance

• Infection by *B. cereus* should be reported to local public health departments and to national surveillance systems.

• Ensure laboratories test for *B. cereus* when an increase in cases of vomiting or diarrhoea with abdominal pain is noted.

Response to a case

• Collect data on food consumption in 24 hours before onset of symptoms. Ask particularly about meals out of the house.
• Although secondary spread of *B. cereus* does not occur, it is prudent to exclude risk groups with diarrhoea or vomiting. Microbiological clearance is not necessary before return.
• No need to screen contacts unless as part of an outbreak investigation.

Response to a cluster

• Discuss further investigation (e.g. serotyping and toxin production) with microbiologist.
• Undertake hypothesis-generating study covering food histories particularly restaurants, social functions and other mass catering arrangements.

Control of an outbreak

Identify and rectify faults with temperature control in food preparation processes.

Suggested case-definition for an outbreak

Clinical
Either:
1 Vomiting occurring 1–6 hours; *or*
2 Diarrhoea occurring 6–24 hours
after exposure to potential source.
Confirmed
As above, plus *B. cereus* of correct serotype cultured from stool or vomit.

Box 3.3.1 Other *Bacillus* species

The *Bacillus subtilis–licheniformis* group are recently recognised food-borne pathogens transmitted via inadequate post-cooking temperature control of foods such as meat or vegetable pastry products, cooked meat or poultry products, bakery products, sandwiches and ethnic meat/seafood dishes.

   B. subtilis causes a predominantly emetic illness with an incubation of 10 minutes to 4 hours (median = 2.5 hours) and *B. licheniformis* a predominantly diarrhoeal illness with incubation 2–14 hours (median 8 hours). *Bacillus thuringiensis* causes occasional food-borne outbreaks. *Bacillus mycoides, Bacillus amyloliquifacians* and *Bacillus pumilis* are rarely reported.

   Investigation and control measures are similar to *B. cereus*.

3.4 Botulism

Botulism is caused by a neurotoxin produced by *Clostridium botulinum*. In Europe it is a rare cause of food-borne infection with a potentially high mortality. One suspected case warrants immediate investigation. It is also a potential bioterrorism agent and a cause of severe illness in intravenous drug users.

Suggested on-call action

A suspected case of botulism should be viewed as an emergency for investigation:
• Ensure that the case is admitted to hospital.
• Obtain food history as a matter of urgency.
• Obtain suspect foods.
• Identify others at risk.
• Inform appropriate local and national authorities.
For more details see 'Response to a case' section.

   If deliberate release is suspected see 'Response to deliberate release' section at end of this chapter.

Epidemiology

A total of 100–200 cases of botulism are reported in the EU each year, giving a reported incidence of 0.03 cases per 100,000 population. The highest incidence in EU countries over the last 10 years has been from Romania, Poland and Lithuania, and multiple outbreaks have been reported from France, Germany, Italy and Spain since 1988.

The age, sex and ethnic distribution of cases will usually reflect the consumption patterns of the implicated foods (or drugs).

In recent years, cases of wound botulism have been reported in intravenous drug users in Europe. This is now the most common type of botulism in some European countries, such as the UK and Ireland.

Infant botulism is very rare in Europe. It affects children under 2 years of age, with most being under 6 months old.

Clinical features

Botulism is characterised by symmetrical, descending flaccid paralysis of motor and autonomic nerves. This initially affects cranial nerves and patients may present with a dry mouth, difficulty in swallowing, double vision, slurred speech and blurred vision. Weakness in the neck and arms follows, after which the respiratory muscles and muscles of the lower body are affected. Respiratory dysfunction may be severe enough to require ventilation. Autonomic symptoms may include dry mouth and gastrointestinal, cardiovascular and urinary dysfunction. There is usually no fever or sensory loss. Mortality of up to 10% is reported. Other syndromes have been confused with botulism (Table 3.4.1): deep

Table 3.4.1 Differential diagnosis of botulism

Disease	Distinguishing features
Guillain–Barré and Miller–Fisher syndromes	Anteceding febrile illness, paraesthesia, paralysis may be ascending, early loss of reflexes, increased CSF protein, EMG findings
Myasthenia gravis	Recurrent paralysis, sustained response to anticholinesterases, EMG findings
Stroke	Usually asymmetric paralysis, abnormal CNS image
Intoxication (carbon monoxide, organophosphates, mushrooms)	Drug detected in body fluid
Tick paralysis	Paraesthesias, ascending paralysis, tick bite (or tick *in situ*)
Poliomyelitis	Anteceding febrile illness, asymmetric paralysis, CSF changes
Viral syndrome	No bulbar palsies or flaccid paralysis
Psychiatric illness	EMG findings
Paralytic shellfish poisoning	Food history (onset <1 hour), paraesthesia

CSF, cerebrospinal fluid; CNS, central nervous system; EMG, electromyography.

tendon reflexes (may be present initially but diminish or disappear in ensuing days in botulism), brain scan, cerebrospinal fluid (CSF) examination, nerve conduction tests and Tensilon test for myasthenia gravis may help eliminate these other diseases.

Patients with food-borne botulism may present with gastrointestinal symptoms, such as nausea, vomiting, constipation, diarrhoea and abdominal cramps, or neurological symptoms.

Wound botulism cases may present with local inflammation at an injection site, followed by hypotension and circulatory collapse, as seen during the outbreak in the UK and Ireland in 2000. There was usually a very high white blood cell count, cases usually had a temperature of less than 40°C and they often looked and felt quite well before deteriorating dramatically over a period of a few hours.

Infants with botulism may present with constipation, lethargy, feeding difficulties, hypotonia, increased drooling and a weak cry.

Laboratory confirmation

Urgent confirmation of the diagnosis is important. Laboratory confirmation is usually by detection of toxin in faeces, serum, stomach contents or wound swab, or by detection of the organism in faeces, stomach contents or wound swab (rapid PCR testing is available). Sensitivity of tests decrease with time since onset (particularly for toxin). Suspect food samples may also be tested (10 g usually required). The aid of the relevant reference laboratory should be enlisted and suspect foods (or drugs) and clinical specimens sent immediately by courier. As *C. botulinum* is present in the environment, any isolate in food should be shown to be of the same 'cultural group' or produce the same toxin type as the cases (there are seven toxin types, designated by letters A–G). Toxin types A, B, E and F are associated with human disease, with type B being the most common in Europe. It may take up to 5 days for negative results to be available, although this does not exclude the diagnosis.

For wound botulism, pus (or wound swab) and tissue biopsy (from surgical débridement) should also be sent for anaerobic culture.

Transmission

Clostridium botulinum spores are ubiquitous in the environment and can be found in dust, soil, untreated water and the digestive tracts of animals and fish. Toxin type E is particularly associated with fish products. There are three naturally occurring forms of botulism: food-borne botulism, wound botulism and infant botulism.

Food-borne illness results from the ingestion of preformed toxin. Although boiling inactivates the toxin, spores may resist 100°C for many hours. These may multiply (producing toxin) when conditions are favorable, i.e. anaerobic, above pH 4.6 and at room temperature (usually 10–50°C, but in some cases as low as 3°C). Underprocessed foods or foods contaminated after processing that are then held at room temperature in anaerobic, non-acidic conditions are at particular risk. The contaminated food may be consumed directly or used as an ingredient for another product.

Food vehicles reported in outbreaks include meat products such as sausage and cured ham; canned, vacuum-packed, smoked or fermented fish products; vegetable products preserved by canning or storing in oil; and baked potatoes, honey and cheese. Many outbreaks are associated with home-preserved foods.

Intestinal or infant botulism usually results from the ingestion of *C. botulinum* spores, which then germinate in the gut, producing toxin. The source of the organism may be food-borne (e.g. from contaminated honey). Wound botulism usually results from the inoculation of *C. botulinum* spores, which then germinate in the anaerobic conditions of the wound, producing toxin that can cause systemic symptoms. Inhalation of toxin may also cause disease, but this is extremely rare under natural conditions.

Acquisition

The incubation period ranges from a few hours to at least 8 days and there are reports of potentially longer incubations. Most cases occur between 12 hours and 3 days after exposure. Gastrointestinal symptoms may precede neurological signs by a few hours and shorter incubations may be associated with higher doses and more severe disease. The incubation for wound botulism may be longer (4–21 days following trauma) and for inhala-tional botulism may be shorter (a few hours up to 4 days).

Although *Clostridium botulinum* may be found in the faeces of cases, botulism is not communicable from person to person. The dose of toxin needed to cause symptoms is very low with illness resulting from nanogram quantities of ingested toxin. Type F toxin is about 60 times more toxic than type B (order: F > C > A > D > B). Estimated lethal doses of type A toxin are 0.1 µg given intravenously or intramuscularly, 0.8 µg inhaled and 70 µg ingested. Therapeutic botulinum toxin preparations contain only about 2% of the lethal intravenous dose. There appears to be no acquisition of immunity to botulinum toxin, even after severe disease. Repeated illness is well recognised.

Prevention

• Care with commercial or home canning processes and with home preservation of fish, to ensure spores destroyed before storage.
• Avoid consumption from food containers that appear to bulge (possible gas from anaerobic organisms) or containers that are damaged. Avoid tasting potentially spoilt food.
• Refrigeration of incompletely processed foods. Boiling for 10 minutes before consumption would inactivate toxin in home-canned foods.
• High index of clinical suspicion and urgent investigation and response to cases.
• Prevention work with intravenous drug users.

Surveillance

• Botulism is statutorily notifiable in almost all EU countries.
• Clinicians should report suspect cases to local public health authorities for urgent investigation.
• Laboratories should report positive toxin or culture results from patients to the relevant local and national centres as a matter of urgency.

Response to a case

• Clinicians or laboratories should report suspected cases immediately to the relevant public health officer for urgent investigation.
• Take urgent food history from the patient or, if not possible, other reliable informant (e.g. spouse). Take details of all goods consumed in 5 days before illness. Ask specifically about any canned or preserved foods.
• Inform others who ate the suspect foods with the patient to seek medical help if symptoms develop.
• Obtain any leftovers of any foods eaten in last 5 days, including remains from uncollected domestic waste and unopened containers from the same batch. This prevents further consumption and allows storage under refrigeration by the laboratory in case later testing appropriate.
• Organise testing of foods at highest suspicion (e.g. canned food eaten 12–72 hours before onset) with reference laboratory.
• Inform appropriate national public health authority and, if a commercial food product is suspected, the national food safety agency.
• Case-finding: any other suspected cases in local hospitals or laboratories or known to national centre? If so, compare food histories.
• Ensure the patient is admitted to hospital for investigation and treatment.
• Antibiotics are not effective against preformed toxin, such as occurs in food-borne disease. Botulinum antitoxin is available and reduces duration of illness and fatality rate. Antitoxin can have serious side-effects, although these may be less severe with modern preparations and doses. It can be given without waiting for microbiological confirmation if a strong clinical diagnosis has been made, as toxin binding to motor nerves is irreversible. Appropriate antibiotics (e.g. penicillin and metronidazole) and surgical débridement is also indicated for wound botulism.
• Person-to-person spread is unlikely, but taking universal precautions is sensible for carers, laboratory staff and at post-mortems.
• No exclusions required for cases or contacts if well enough to work.

• If no obvious food source, consider intravenous drug use via contaminated illegal drugs; intestinal botulism, especially if child under 2 years of age; mis-injection of pharmaceutical preparation; or a deliberate bioterrorism incident.

Investigation of a cluster

• Treat individual cases as indicative of a significant public health risk and investigate as above.
• Instigate case-finding with local clinicians and laboratories, and national centre.
• Compare food histories: specifically ask *each* case about *each* food reported by all other cases.
• Organise laboratory testing of *any* food reported by more than one case.
• Check preparation details of any food reported by more than one case to see if anaerobic conditions could have been created for any component and/or it was stored at room temperature after cooking.
• Remember, as well as canned, bottled or preserved produce, unexpected food vehicles have been reported from recent incidents, including sautéed onions (kept under butter), hazelnut yogurt (canned purée used in preparation), baked potatoes (kept in foil) and honey.
• Consider the possibility that cases may be intravenous drug users exposed to contaminated illegal drugs (cases may not just be young males or homeless people).
• Consider the possibility of bioterrorism: this could be via air-borne release or contamination of foodstuffs. Consider if cases have similar geographical exposure but no common food exposure; multiple simultaneous outbreaks with no obvious common source; unusual toxin type (C, D, F or G, or E without exposure to aquatic food); or similar cases in animals (liaise with veterinary agencies).

Control of an outbreak

• Identify and remove any implicated food.

• If commercially produced food, organise recall of product.

• If food vehicle identified, organise medical assessment of others that have consumed it.

• If linked to intravenous drug use, liaise with local community drug workers to get public health messages on safer drug use out to users and to promote early diagnosis and treatment of cases.

Response to deliberate release

• Activate local and national plans and procedures.

• Decontamination of exposed people, clothing and fomites if air-borne release.

• Identify and monitor exposed individuals, including those who may have left the scene.

• No prophylaxis is indicated for those exposed if they remain asymptomatic.

• Ensure access to antitoxin and supportive therapy for those who develop symptoms.

• Full biological protective equipment for those entering 'exposed zone'.

• Contaminated area to be made out-of-bounds for a few days after release (toxin loses activity during this period).

Suggested case-definition for an outbreak

Confirmed: clinically compatible case with demonstration of botulinum toxin in blood, faeces, vomit or gastric aspirate.

Clinical: acute bilateral cranial neuropathy with symmetrical descending weakness, no sensory loss and afebrile.

Provisional: any three from dysphagia, dry mouth, diplopia, dysarthria, limb weakness, blurred vision or dyspnoea in an alert, non-febrile patient with no sensory deficit. Review when clinical investigations are complete.

If exposure known (e.g. food vehicle), then this can be added to the case-definition.

• Household bleach solution or 0.5% solution of hypochlorite (5000 ppm) are adequate decontamination.

• More general information is given in Chapter 4.15 and more specific information is available on the Health Protection Agency (HPA) website.

3.5 Brucellosis

Brucellosis is a transmissible zoonosis caused by a Gram-negative coccobaccillus of the genus *Brucella*. A wide variety of mammals are susceptible to *Brucella* species. *Brucella abortus* (cattle, camels), *Brucella melitensis* (goats, sheep, camels) and *Brucella suis* (pigs) are the usual causes of brucellosis (undulant fever, Malta fever, Mediterranean fever) in humans. Other *Brucella* species such as *Brucella canis* (dogs) and those associated with marine mammals are rare causes of human disease.

Epidemiology

Human brucellosis has a worldwide distribution with the Middle East and Central Asia having the highest reported incidence. In 2007, 836 cases were reported in Europe. The highest rates were reported from Greece (0.9 per 100,000 population) Italy, Portugal and Spain. Males aged 25–44 years have the highest rates suggesting an occupational risk factor. In much of northern Europe brucellosis in domestic animals has been eradicated and most cases are now acquired abroad. In countries where *Brucella* is still endemic, farmers, veterinarians, abattoir workers and consumers of unpasteurised milk products are at risk. In 2009, outbreaks of human infection were reported from Mexico (unpasteurised cheese), Russia and Kyrgyzstan (infected livestock).

Clinical features

In acute brucellosis there is a systemic febrile illness with hepatosplenomegaly which may be complicated by bone and joint manifestations, orchitis, epididymitis, neurological involvement and endocarditis. Most cases will recover but some develop chronic or relapsing disease characterised by malaise, depression and localised infection.

Laboratory confirmation

Serological methods are used, including specific IgG/IgM enzyme immunoassays. Interpretation of results is often difficult and should be informed by clinical and local prevalence data. Definitive diagnosis is by culture of *Brucella* from blood, bone marrow or pus but yield is often poor. Extended culture may be necessary although rapid culture technologies may be helpful.

Transmission

Transmission is by contact with infected animals or tissues (blood, urine, aborted fetus, placenta) as a result of inoculation, mucous membrane exposure, aerosol inhalation or consumption of unpasteurised dairy products. Infection can follow accidental self-inoculation by veterinarians with animal vaccine strains.

Brucella is a potential bioterrorism agent because it survives well in the environment and is highly infectious in aerosol form or as a contaminant of food, milk and water or by direct inoculation.

Acquisition

The incubation period is 5–60 days and depends on the species, route of transmission and infective dose which may be as low 10–100 organisms. Person-to-person transmission is rare. The duration of acquired immunity is uncertain.

Prevention

• The prevention of human disease depends on the control of brucellosis in food animals by vaccination, testing and slaughter of infected animals and pasteurisation of dairy products. Pastures and animal accommodation on farms may remain contaminated for prolonged periods.
• *Brucella* infection is a significant biohazard for laboratory workers and guidelines should be followed.
• Others at occupational risk (veterinarians, abattoir workers and farmers) should take suitable precautions. This includes people who handle marine mammals.
• Visitors to endemic countries should avoid unpasteurised dairy products.

Surveillance

• Brucellosis is a notifiable disease in many countries. In the UK it is statutorily notifiable if occupationally acquired.
• Cases should be reported to public health authorities.

Response to a case

• Cases should be investigated to determine the source of infection, including travel and food history.
• If the case has not been abroad, possible animal exposure should be sought in collaboration with veterinary authorities. Suspect animals may be tested.
• Contacts who may have been exposed to the source of infection should be offered investigation.
• Following laboratory exposure all workers at risk should be monitored for symptoms and offered repeated serological testing over a 6-month period. Post-exposure prophylaxis may be offered with an appropriate antibiotic.
• Following the accidental inoculation of animal vaccine, antibiotic chemoprophylaxis is recommended.

Investigation of a cluster

• As most cases in northern Europe are imported, a cluster usually results from a common exposure at a single point.
• A search should be made for the source of infection, usually milk or cheese from an infected herd.
• Implicated products should be recalled, production should cease and pasteurisation should be enforced.

Control of an outbreak

Control requires the identification and eradication of infected livestock, pasteurisation of dairy products, and control of domestic animals and animal products moving between countries.

Suggested case-definition for an outbreak

Clinical: an acute illness characterised by fever, night sweats, undue fatigue, anorexia, weight loss, headache and arthralgia.

Confirmed: clinical case with isolation of Brucella spp. from a clinical specimen, or demonstration by immunofluorescence of *Brucella* spp. in a clinical specimen, or fourfold or greater rise in *Brucella* agglutination titre between acute and convalescent serum specimens obtained at least 2 weeks apart.

3.6 *Burkholderia*

Burkholderia are Gram-negative, bipolar, aerobic, motile, rod-shaped bacteria. *Burkholderia mallei* is the cause of glanders and *Burkholderia pseudomallei* causes melioidosis. *Burkholderia cepacia* is important as a cause of pulmonary infections in those with cystic fibrosis. Both

B. mallei and *B. pseudomallei* are potential agents for biological terrorism.

Suggested on-call action

If you or reporting clinician/ microbiologist know of associated cases, report to the public health authorities.

Epidemiology

Glanders is endemic in parts of Africa, Asia, the Middle East and Central and South America and primarily affects horses. Natural cases in humans are rare, but occasional cases occur from laboratory exposures. Melioidosis is most common in South-East Asia and northern Australia with occasional cases in the South Pacific, Africa, India and the Middle East. Cases are rare in Europe and are imported. In the UK in the past 10 years fewer than 25 imported cases of *B. pseudomallei* have been confirmed.

Clinical features

Burkholderia mallei and *B. pseudomallei* cause pulmonary infections (pneumonia, abscess) and septicaemia. A localized, pus-forming, cutaneous infection with lymphadenopathy is also seen. The mortality of melioidosis is 20–50% even with treatment. Antibiotic resistance is common. The incubation period is 1–21 days.

Laboratory confirmation

Glanders: isolation of *B. mallei* from blood, sputum, urine or skin lesions. Melioidosis: isolation of *B. pseudomallei*. Molecular methods (PCR), latex agglutination assay and rapid immunofluorescence are available.

Transmission

Glanders: contact with tissues or body fluids of infected animals; contaminated aerosols or dust. Sporadic cases have been documented in veterinarians, horse caretakers and those who work in laboratories.

Melioidosis: *B. pseudomellei* is found in the soil, rice paddies and stagnant water. Acquisition is through inhalation or contact with contaminated soil. Rare person-to-person transmission associated with close contact is seen in melioidosis.

Prevention

Identification and elimination of the infection in the animal population.

Surveillance

Cases should be reported to the public health authorities.

Response to a case

Consider the possibility of deliberate release.

Response to a cluster and an outbreak

Consider the possibility of deliberate release.

3.7 *Campylobacter*

Campylobacter species cause diarrhoeal and systemic illnesses in humans and animals, and are the most common bacterial cause of infectious intestinal disease in developed countries. Although food-borne outbreaks are rarely identified, occasional outbreaks due to contaminated milk or water may occur.

> **Suggested on-call action**
>
> • Exclude symptomatic cases in high-risk groups (Box 2.2.1).
> • If you or the reporting clinician/microbiologist are aware of potentially linked cases, consult the Outbreak Control Plan.

Epidemiology

About 45 cases of *Campylobacter* infection per 100,000 population are reported annually in Europe although the true community incidence is much higher at an estimated 870 per 100,000. Deaths are rare. Infections occur at all ages, but are highest in children under 5 years and there is a secondary peak in young adults. Reported cases are higher in men and in some ethnic groups (e.g. south Asians in the UK).

Campylobacter infections occur all year round, but with highest incidence from June to September; this peak is slightly earlier than that seen for *Salmonella* (Figure 2.2.1). In Scandinavian countries, the peak is later, probably related to travel abroad. Outbreaks are rarely identified.

Certain groups are at increased risk of *Campylobacter* infection due to increased exposure, including those with occupational contact with farm animals or meat, travellers abroad, men who have sex with men (including infection with other *Campylobacter* species) and family contacts of cases. *Campylobacter* infection is the most commonly identified cause of traveller's diarrhoea in Scandinavia and the second most common (after enteropathogenic *Escherichia coli*) in the UK. *Campylobacter* infection is hyperendemic in developing countries.

Clinical features

Campylobacter infection may vary from asymptomatic (estimated 25–50% of cases) to a severe disease mimicking ulcerative colitis or acute appendicitis. Most diagnosed cases present with acute enteritis with symptoms of diarrhoea, abdominal pain and fever. There may be a prodromal period of fever, headache, myalgia and malaise for approximately 12–24 hours before onset of intestinal symptoms. Diarrhoea varies from loose stools to a massive volume of watery stools. About one-quarter have blood in the stool (usually appearing on the second or third day) and a similar number have vomiting. Abdominal pain may be prominent, is often described as constant or cramping rather than colicky and may be relieved by defaecation.

Most cases settle after 2–3 days of diarrhoea and 80–90% within 1 week. However, some cases may be prolonged or severe. Complications include reactive arthritis (1–5% of cases), Guillain–Barré syndrome (0.1% of cases) and haemolytic uraemic syndrome.

Although difficult to distinguish from other causes of intestinal infection in individual cases, *Campylobacter* might be suspected as the cause of an outbreak due to the combination of abdominal pain and fever, and/or the presence of bloody diarrhoea or faecal leukocytes. However, *E. coli* O157 may cause a similar picture.

Campylobacter jejuni is responsible for most campylobacteriosis and *Campylobacter coli*, which may be less severe, for most of the rest. Other species such as *Campylobacter fetus* and *Campylobacter lari* are uncommon causes of diarrhoea in immunocompetent individuals, but can cause severe systemic illness in debilitated or immunosuppressed patients.

Laboratory confirmation

The mainstay of diagnosis is culture of the organism from faecal samples. Sensitivity is increased if samples are delivered to the laboratory on the day of collection: if this is not possible, samples should be either refrigerated or stored in a suitable transport medium. Culture of *Campylobacter* requires different conditions than for other enteric pathogens. Provisional results may be available after overnight incubation. Confirmation that the colonies are *Campylobacter* requires simple microscopy, but identification of the species depends upon latex agglutination (quick but costly) or biochemical tests (takes 1–2 days).

Strain identification (by serotype, phagetype and/or genotype) of *C. jejuni* or *C. coli* may be available from reference laboratories if required for epidemiological purposes; however, more than one subtype can occur in outbreaks. Serological tests are in development.

Microscopic examination of fresh diarrhoeal stool specimens may permit a rapid presumptive diagnosis, although sensitivity is only 60% compared to culture. *Campylobacter* is sometimes isolated from blood cultures in acute illness. Resistance to antibiotics, especially fluoroquinolones, is high in southern Europe as well as from many holiday destinations outside Europe. *Campylobacter* may be isolated from food or environmental specimens after enrichment culture.

Transmission

Campylobacteriosis is a zoonosis. It is found worldwide in the gastrointestinal tract of many animals, including poultry, cattle, pigs, birds, wild mammals and domestic pets. Humans are not an important reservoir. Transmission from animals to humans occurs predominantly via ingestion of faecally contaminated food or water. *Campylobacters* are sensitive to drying, acid, high salt concentrations, chlorine and temperatures over 48°C.

The main routes of infection are as follows.

Water-borne

Campylobacter excretion by wild birds causes contamination of open waters, and the organisms can survive for several months in water below 15°C. Large outbreaks have occurred from the use of untreated surface water in community water supplies. There may also be failures in 'treated' water supplies. Smaller outbreaks have occurred from the storage of water in open-topped tanks. Deliberate or accidental ingestion of raw water can cause infection in those undertaking outdoor activities (e.g. trekkers and canoeists).

Milk-borne

Campylobacters are commonly found in bulked raw milk samples. Infected animals may contaminate milk with faeces or excrete the organism via infected udders. Campylobacters can survive in refrigerated milk for 3 weeks and, when ingested, milk protects the organisms from the effect of gastric acid. Properly conducted pasteurisation destroys the organism. Consumption of raw or inadequately pasteurised milk has caused large outbreaks of campylobacteriosis, and contributes to endemic infection.

Contamination of milk after pasteurisation may also occur. In the UK, home delivery of milk in foil-topped bottles left on the doorstep may be contaminated by pecking by wild birds.

Poultry and other foods

In the majority of sporadic cases in developed countries, *Campylobacter* probably entered the kitchen on contaminated meat. Chicken carcasses are the most commonly contaminated, but pork, lamb and beef (including meat products such as sausages) may also be affected. Contamination of these meats is usually with *C. jejuni*, with the exception of pork for which almost all are *C. coli*. The contamination can lead to illness in one of three ways: contamination of hands leading to accidental ingestion; inadequate cooking, especially of chicken and a particular risk for barbecues; and cross-contamination of foods, which will not be cooked, either via hands or via utensils such as knives and chopping boards. Fortunately, *Campylobacter* does not multiply on food, which reduces the risk of large food-borne outbreaks. Normal cooking kills *Campylobacter*, and viable organisms are reduced 10-fold by freezing, although freezing cannot be assumed to have made contaminated poultry safe.

Other food vehicles that have been reported include shellfish contaminated by sewage and mushrooms contaminated by soil.

Consumption of contaminated food and water is the likely cause of most cases of travel associated campylobacteriosis.

Direct transmission from animals

Approximately 5% of cases in the UK and the USA are thought to occur through contact with infected pets. The most likely source is a puppy with diarrhoea or, less often, a sick kitten and the most likely victim a young child. Transmission from asymptomatic pets has also been reported. Children may also be exposed to excreting animals on farm visits. Occupational exposure to excreting animals or contaminated carcasses is also well recognised.

Person-to-person spread

Although the transmissibility of *Campylobacter* is low, person-to-person spread does occur. The index case is usually a child who is not toilet trained. The victim may be the person responsible for dealing with soiled nappies. Vertical transmission has also been documented as has spread by blood transfusion.

Secondary spread has not been documented from asymptomatic food handlers or hospital staff.

Acquisition

The incubation period is inversely related to the dose ingested. Most cases occur within 2–5 days of exposure with an average of 3 days, but a range of 1–10 days incubation is reported.

The infectious period lasts throughout the period of infection, although once the acute symptoms have passed the risk of transmission is very low if adequate hygiene is practised. The average duration of excretion is 2–3 weeks, with some cases excreting for 2 months and occasional cases for 3 months. Antibiotic treatment (e.g. with erythromycin) usually terminates excretion but it is rarely necessary to attempt to do this. The infective dose is usually 10^4 organisms or above, but food vehicles that protect the organism against gastric acid (e.g. fatty foods, milk, water) can result in an infectious dose of as little as 500 organisms. Immunity develops in response to infection, with antibodies that protect against symptomatic infection against the similar strains. Patients with immune deficiencies or chronic illnesses may develop severe disease and those with HIV infection may suffer repeated illness with the same strain.

Prevention

• Chlorination of drinking water supplies and prevention of contamination.
• Pasteurisation of milk for retail sale.
• Reducing infection in poultry and animal farms.
• If unable to prevent contaminated meat leaving the slaughterhouse, gamma-irradiation of carcasses is effective, although not popular with the public.
• Adequate hygiene in commercial and domestic kitchens, particularly the avoidance of cross-contamination.
• Adequate cooking of meat, especially poultry.
• Protecting doorstep milk against birds.
• Handwashing after contact with faeces, nappies, meat or animals, including on farm visits.
• Conventional disinfectants are active against *Campylobacter*.
• Advice to travellers abroad and to HIV positive patients to reduce exposure.

Surveillance

• *Campylobacter* infection is statutorily notifiable in almost all European countries. In England, clinicians should notify as suspected 'Food Poisoning'.
• Laboratory isolates of *Campylobacter* species should be reported to local public health departments and the national surveillance system.
• Surveillance schemes may also incorporate typing data.

Response to a case

• Enteric precautions for case (see Chapter 1.2).
• Report to public health authorities (by clinician and laboratory).
• Exclude from work/nursery if in risk group (Box 2.2.1) until 48 hours after first normal stool. No microbiological clearance necessary.
• Antibiotic treatment unnecessary unless severe or prolonged illness.
• Obtain history of food consumption (particularly chicken, unpasteurised milk or untreated water), travel and contact with animals.
• Investigate illness in family or other contacts.

Investigation of a cluster

• Discuss further microbiological investigations of epidemiological relevance with the reference laboratory (e.g. typing of strains to see if similar). Ensure that local laboratories retain isolates for further investigation.
• Obtain details from cases on:
  (a) source of water supply (failure of treatment?);
  (b) source of milk supply (failure of pasteurisation?);
  (c) functions attended (food-borne outbreak?);
  (d) foods consumed, particularly consumption of undercooked chicken or, if *C. coli*, pork;
  (e) bird-pecked milk;
  (f) farm visits (age-distribution of cases may support this);
  (g) occupation/school/nursery; and
  (h) travel.

Control of an outbreak

• Exclude symptomatic cases if in risk groups and ensure enteric precautions are followed.
• Re-enforce food hygiene and handwashing.
• Transmission is usually thought to be food-borne or, occasionally, water-borne, so check for ways in which food or water could have become contaminated.
• Prevent use of unpasteurised milk, un-treated water or undercooked poultry.

Suggested case-definition for an outbreak

Clinical: diarrhoea or any two symptoms from abdominal pain, fever, nausea/vomiting, with onset 2–5 days after exposure in person with link to confirmed case.

Microbiological: isolate of outbreak strain from faeces or blood. As carriage of any type of *C. jejuni* in asymptomatic controls in the UK is only about 1% but 25–50% of cases of *Campylobacter* infection are asymptomatic, clinical component of case-definition could be waived if appropriate typing results are available.

3.8 Chickenpox and shingles (varicella-zoster infections)

Chickenpox is a systemic viral infection with a characteristic rash caused by varicella-zoster virus (VZV), a herpes virus. Its public health importance lies in the risk of complications in immunosuppressed and pregnant patients, and the potential for prevention by vaccination. Herpes zoster (shingles) is caused by re-activation of latent VZV whose genomes persist in sensory root ganglia of the brainstem and spinal cord.

Suggested on-call action

Assess clinical status of close contacts and arrange for exclusion/VZIG if appropriate (see 'Response to a case' section below).

Epidemiology

Chickenpox occurs mainly in children. There are epidemics every 1–2 years, usually in winter/spring. More than 90% of adults have natural immunity. Herpes zoster occurs mainly in middle or older age. Mortality is low (in Europe around 0.1 per million), although it increases with age.

Clinical features

There is sometimes a prodromal illness of fever, headache and myalgia. The diagnostic feature is the vesicular rash, which usually appears first on the trunk. The rash starts as small papules, which develop into clear vesicles, become pustules and then dry to crusts. There are successive crops of vesicles over several days. The hands and feet are relatively spared.

A more fulminant illness including pneumonia, hepatitis or disseminated intravascular coagulation may affect the immunocompromised, neonates and occasionally healthy adults, particularly smokers and pregnant women. Congenital varicella syndrome occurs following infections in the first 5 months of pregnancy. Although most fetal risk appears to be in weeks 13–20, pregnant women are at most risk between weeks 27 and 33.

Herpes zoster begins with pain in the dermatome supplied by the affected sensory root ganglion. The trunk is a common site. The rash appears in the affected area and is vesicular and rapidly coalesces. It is very painful and persists for several days and even weeks in elderly people.

Laboratory confirmation

This is rarely required as the clinical features are so specific. If necessary, VZV is readily demonstrable from vesicular fluid in both chickenpox and shingles; serology is also available and can be used to demonstrate immunity.

Transmission

Man is the only reservoir. Carriage does not occur. Chickenpox is highly infectious; up to 96% of susceptible people exposed develop the disease. Herpes zoster is much less infectious. Transmission is by direct person-to-person contact, by air-borne spread of vesicular fluid or respiratory secretions and by contact with articles recently contaminated by discharges from vesicles and mucous membranes.

Acquisition

The usual incubation period for chickenpox is 14–16 days (range 7–24 days). Cases are infectious for up to 5 days before the onset of the rash (usually 1–2 days) until 5 days after the first crop of vesicles. Infectivity may be longer in immunosuppressed patients. Most transmission occurs early in the disease.

Patients with herpes zoster are usually only infectious if the lesions are exposed or disseminated. Infectivity is increased in immunosuppressed patients.

Prevention

• Live attenuated vaccines are available either as monovalent vaccines or in combination with measles/mumps/rubella (MMR).
• In most European countries a selective vaccination policy has been adopted; however, in some countries (e.g. Germany, parts of Italy) universal vaccination of children is recommended. Vaccination schedules can

be found at the EUVAC website (www. euvac.net/graphics/vaccination/var.html).
• The aim of selective vaccination is to prevent varicella among those in close contact with individuals who are most at risk from complications of the disease (e.g. non-immune healthcare workers and household contacts of the immunosuppressed). In addition, those who are likely to be exposed to cases of varicella (laboratory and clinical infectious disease staff) may be considered for vaccination if not immune.
• The schedule is one dose in children (although the need for a second dose is under consideration) and two doses in adults.
• A live attenuated vaccine is available for the prevention of shingles and post-herpetic neuralgia in adults over 50 years.

Surveillance

• Chickenpox is notifiable in many EU countries (in the UK, only notifiable in Scotland and Northen Ireland).
• Laboratory diagnosis is rare, so local surveillance depends on informal sources such as schools. The public health practitioner may also be contacted with a request for specific immunoglobulin in an immunosuppressed or pregnant contact. Trend data can be obtained from sentinel general practices.

Response to a case

• Exclude children with chickenpox from school/nursery until 5 days from the onset of rash. Healthcare workers with chickenpox should stay off work for the same period.
• Non-immune healthcare workers with significant exposure to VZV should be excluded from contact with high-risk patients for 8–21 days after exposure, or report to the occupational health department if they feel unwell or develop a fever or rash.
• No exclusion criteria need be applied to individuals with herpes zoster in the community. Healthcare workers with shingles should inform their Infection Control Team; they

may continue working if the lesions are localised and covered with a bandage or clothing. If they are in contact with high-risk patients an individual risk assessment should be carried out.

• In most circumstances, no further action is required. However, there are some situations in which post-exposure prophylaxis with human varicella-zoster immunoglobulin (VZIG) is indicated. VZIG is indicated for non-immune individuals with a clinical condition that increases the risk of severe varicella (e.g. immunocompromised individuals, neonates, very premature or low birth weight infants, pregnant women especially before 20 weeks and in the 3 weeks before delivery) and who have significant exposure to chickenpox or herpes zoster (but only if disseminated or in an exposed area or if the case is immunosuppressed). Significant exposure is defined as at least 15 minutes in the same room, face to face or on the same ward, from 48 hours before onset of rash to crusting (chickenpox) or from day of rash to crusting (shingles). A positive history of varicella is usually reliable; a negative history requires confirmation by serology. Detailed advice on the use of VZIG is available in a number of European countries; supplies are often limited.

Investigation of a cluster

Look for links to institutions with high levels of susceptible individuals.

Response to an outbreak

• In most outbreaks there will be no specific action in addition to the exclusion criteria and issue of VZIG described above.
• Hospital outbreaks pose special problems because of the risk of transmission to immunosuppressed and pregnant patients. All staff in contact with these high-risk groups should be screened for VZV antibody. Non-immune staff could then either be vaccinated or be excluded from contact with high-risk

patients for 8–21 days after exposure (see above).

Suggested case-definition for an outbreak
Physician diagnosis of chickenpox or herpes zoster.

3.9 Chikungunya

Chikungunya is a mosquito-borne viral disease caused by an alphavirus of the family Togaviridae and first described during an outbreak in southern Tanzania in 1952.

Suggested on-call action
None usually required.

Epidemiology

Chikungunya is endemic in Africa and Asia. Occasional cases are reported. Large outbreaks have been described in the Democratic Republic of the Congo (1999–2000), on islands of the Indian Ocean (2005–2007), India (2006–2007) and in Gabon (2007). In 2007 transmission was reported for the first time in Europe during an outbreak in northern Italy.

Clinical features

A variety of clinical manifestations may occur. Symptoms are often mild; the infection may go unrecognised, or be misdiagnosed in areas where dengue fever is endemic. Classically, there is abrupt onset of fever with joint pain, which can be very debilitating; often combined with muscle pain, headache, nausea, fatigue and rash. It usually lasts for days or weeks. Most patients recover fully. In some cases joint pain may persist for months or years. Cases of eye, neurological, heart complications and gastrointestinal complaints have been reported. Serious complications are uncommon. Nevertheless, in elderly patients it has been described as contributing to the cause of death.

Laboratory confirmation

During the first few days of infection it is possible to isolate the virus from blood. Serological tests, such as enzyme-linked immunosorbent assay (ELISA), may confirm the presence of IgM and IgG anti-chikungunya antibodies. IgM antibody levels are highest 3–5 weeks after the onset of illness and persist for approximately 2 months.

Transmission

The virus is transmitted by the bite of female mosquitoes, most commonly *Aedes aegypti* and *Aedes albopictus* which bite throughout daylight hours with peaks of activity in the early morning and late afternoon. Person-to-person transmission has not been reported.

Acquisition

The incubation period varies between 2 and 12 days. Person-to-person transmission is unlikely.

Prevention

Reduce the proximity of mosquito vector breeding sites to human habitation. For protection during outbreaks, clothing that minimises skin exposure to the vectors is advised. Repellents can be applied to exposed skin or to clothing.

Surveillance

• As a newly emerging disease in Europe it is notifiable in only some European countries (e.g. Italy).
• Cases should be reported to the Public Health Authorities so that assessments of risk can be made.

Response to a case

• Treatment is directed primarily at relieving the symptoms, including joint pain. There is no vaccine commercially available.
• No public health action is usually necessary.

Investigation of a cluster and control of an outbreak

If clusters arise from areas where chikungunya has not previously been recognised, the national authorities should be informed.

Suggested case-definition
Compatible clinical illness with laboratory confirmation of chikungunya.

3.10 *Chlamydophila pneumoniae*

Chlamydophila (previously classified as *Chlamydia*) *pneumoniae*, also known as Taiwan acute respiratory agent (TWAR), is a recently recognised pathogen and is a relatively common cause of atypical pneumonia and other respiratory infections.

Suggested on-call action
None required unless an outbreak is suspected.

Epidemiology

Infection probably occurs worldwide and has been demonstrated in many European countries. Data from the USA shows annual incidence rates of 6–9% in 5–14-year-olds falling to 1.5% for adults, leading to an overall seroprevalence of 50% by about 30 years of age. Incidence is low in under 5 year olds, but infection/re-infection may occur at any age. No seasonal pattern has been demonstrated but there is evidence of 2–3 year cycles of high and low endemicity.

Clinical features

The most commonly identified manifestations of *C. pneumoniae* infection are pneumonia and bronchitis, which are usually mild but often slow to resolve. Approximately 7–10% of community-acquired pneumonia is caused by this organism. Pharyngitis and sinusitis may occur in isolation or together with chest infection and these together with a usually insidious onset, prolonged cough and a high incidence of laryngitis may help to distinguish an outbreak from other causes of atypical pneumonia. Acute asymptomatic infection occurs, but carriers are rare.

Laboratory confirmation

Diagnosis is usually confirmed by serology or direct antigen detection. Serology is based on demonstration of a fourfold rise to genus-specific IgG on complement fixation testing which therefore cross-reacts with *C. psittaci* and *C. trachomatis*. Microimmunofluorescence detection of *C. pneumoniae* specific antibody, including an IgM test for diagnosis of acute infection is required for confirmation. IgM rises can be detected after about 3 weeks and IgG 6–8 weeks after onset. Re-infection provides an IgG response in 1–2 weeks without an IgM response. Direct antigen and PCR tests have been developed. *C. pneumoniae* is difficult to culture, but throat swabs may be positive on special cultures. There is limited genotypic or phenotypic variation, so typing is not possible. Co-infection with other respiratory pathogens is relatively common.

Transmission

No zoonotic or environmental reservoir has been discovered. Spread is likely to be person-to-person, presumably via respiratory tract secretions. Transmission appears to be slow but outbreaks, particularly in institutions such as nursing homes, schools and the military, do occur.

Acquisition

The incubation period is unclear: estimates range from 10 to 30 days. The infectious period is also unclear but appears to be prolonged. It is possible that asymptomatic cases may also play a part in transmission. Although strong antibody responses occur, re-infection is common (sometimes even within the same outbreak). Most severe cases or deaths occur in those with underlying disease.

Prevention

General measures for respiratory infection including the following:
- Stay away from work or school when ill;
- Cover mouth when coughing or sneezing;
- Sanitary disposal of respiratory secretions;
- Handwashing; and
- Avoid overcrowding.

Surveillance

Sporadic infection with *C. pneumoniae* is not statutorily notifiable in most countries. However, possible outbreaks or clusters should be reported to local Public Health departments. Laboratories should report all clinically significant infections to national surveillance systems.

Response to a case

• Hygiene advice to cases and advice to stay at home whilst coughing/sneezing.
• Check for links to other cases.

Investigation of a cluster

• Seek microbiological advice to confirm as *C. pneumoniae* infection.
• Look for direct contact between cases or attendance at same functions or institutions.

Control of an outbreak

Control is likely to be difficult because of asymptomatic infectious cases, re-infection, prolonged infectivity and long incubation period. It could include hygiene measures, case-finding and treatment, but effectiveness is not known.

> **Suggested case-definition for an outbreak**
>
> Demonstration of *C. pneumoniae* specific IgM or fourfold rise in specific IgG.

3.11 *Chlamydophila psittaci*

Psittacosis (or ornithosis) is a potentially fatal systemic disease caused by *Chlamydophila* (previously classified as *Chlamydia*) *psittaci*. It is a zoonotic infection particularly associated with birds.

> **Suggested on-call action**
>
> • If linked cases are suspected, institute outbreak plan.
> • If not, ensure the case is investigated promptly on the next working day.

Epidemiology

Much of the reported epidemiology of psittacosis is based on a combination of respiratory symptoms and demonstration of Chlamydiaceae group antigen on serology: it therefore requires re-examination in the light of the discovery of the more common *Chlamydophila pneumoniae* (see Chapter 3.10) which also causes disease fitting such a case-definition.

Around 60 cases of psittacosis are reported a year in Britain, about 40 in the Netherlands and about 25 in Germany, but all are likely to be considerable underestimates. Cases occur worldwide and are more common in those exposed to birds occupationally or as pet owners. Cases occur mostly in adults and more often in males. There is no distinct seasonal pattern.

Clinical features

Onset may be insidious or non-specific with fever and malaise, followed by an atypical pneumonia with unproductive cough, fever and headache, with 20% mortality if untreated. Other syndromes resemble infectious mononucleosis and typhoid. Asymptomatic infection may occur. Most cases report fever and most (eventually) develop a cough. Headache, myalgia and chills are each reported in about half of cases. Relapses may occur. *Chlamydophila abortus* (also previously classified as *Chlamydia psittaci*) may cause serious infection in pregnant women, resulting in late abortion, neonatal death and disseminated intravascular coagulation in the mother.

Laboratory confirmation

Culture is rarely used because of the risk of laboratory-acquired illness and diagnosis is usually based on serology. As routine complement fixation tests (CFTs) cross-react with *C. pneumoniae*, further testing may be necessary to confirm which species is responsible. Acute and convalescent samples of serum are usually collected 2–3 weeks apart. Microimmunofluorescence (MIF) tests are now available and are specific for *C. psittaci*. Antigen or PCR tests may be possible in some laboratories. Typing may also be available to assist public health investigation.

Transmission

Chlamydophila psittaci is a zoonotic disease. Animal reservoirs include psittacine birds such as cockatiels, parakeets, parrots, macaws and lovebirds; other birds, particularly ducks, turkeys and pigeons; and less commonly mammals, especially sheep (*C. abortus*). Infection is transmitted to humans by inhalation of infected aerosols contaminated by droppings, nasal discharges or products of conception in which it may survive for months at ambient temperatures. Birds may be asymptomatic carriers of the organism. *C. psittaci* is destroyed by routine disinfectants such as bleach (1:100), quaternary ammonium (1:1000) and 70% isopropyl alcohol.

Groups at increased risk of disease include those in the pet trade, bird fanciers, poultry workers, abattoir workers, veterinarians and laboratory workers. Owners of pet birds are also at risk: psittacosis in the UK and Sweden has been linked to importation of exotic birds for pets.

If human-to-human spread of *C. psittaci* occurs at all (earlier reports may actually have been *C. pneumoniae*) then it is rare.

Acquisition

The incubation period has been reported as anything from 4 days to 4 weeks. Most cases probably occur 5–15 days after exposure. Infection may result from only brief, passing exposure to infectious birds. The infectious period in birds may last for months. Human cases are not considered infectious for practical purposes. Protective immunity to re-infection is short lived. Those at risk of severe infection include pregnant women (especially to *C. abortus*) and the elderly.

Prevention

• Quarantine and other controls on imported birds.
• Masks, good ventilation and measures to avoid contamination in poultry plants and other areas where workers might be exposed.
• Pregnant women to avoid exposure to sheep, especially during lambing (*C. abortus*).

Surveillance

• Psittacosis should be reported promptly to local public health authorities. It is formally notifiable in many European countries, including Germany, the Netherlands, Belgium, Sweden, Denmark and Norway.
• Laboratories should report all clinically significant infections to national surveillance systems.

Response to a case

• All cases should be reported promptly by the clinician or microbiologist for investigation by local public health officers.
• Look for exposure to psittacines, poultry, other birds and mammals. Trace the source back to pet shop, aviary, farm, etc. Involve veterinary and microbiological colleagues to test animals for infection. Infected birds should be treated or destroyed and the environment thoroughly cleaned and disinfected.
• Ensure other potential cases are tested.
• No need for isolation. Cough into a paper towel for safe disposal.

Investigation of a cluster

• Discuss further investigation with a microbiologist to confirm *C. psittaci* as the cause, and to see if typing is possible. Different serovars are associated with different animal sources (e.g. A and F with psittacines, B with pigeons and doves, C with ducks and geese and D with turkeys).
• Conduct hypothesis-generating study to include pet birds (possibly illegal); pet mammals; hobbies (e.g. pigeon racing); visits to pet shops, farms, bird centres, etc; and occupational exposure to animals. Document less defined exposures, for example walking through fields (potentially contaminated pasture?), roofing (exposure to pigeons?), etc. Check if any institution or home visited had a pet bird.

Control of an outbreak

Work with veterinary colleagues:
• Look for infected birds or mammals.
• Treat or destroy infected birds.
• Thoroughly clean and disinfect environment.
• Case-finding to ensure those infected receive prompt treatment.
• Action to prevent recurrence.

Suggested case-definition for an outbreak

Confirmed
Compatible clinical illness plus:
• Culture of *C. psittaci*; *or*
• Fourfold increase in specific IgG by MIF; *or*
• Demonstration of specific IgM by MIF (titre $\geq$16); *or*
• PCR positive.
Suspected
Compatible clinical illness plus:
• Epidemiological link to confirmed case; *or*

• Fourfold increase by CFT antibody testing; *or*
• Single high IgG title by MIF.
In an epidemiological investigation, may wish to include asymptomatic individuals with clear microbiological evidence of recent infection (see criteria for confirmed cases) to help identity exposure.

3.12 *Chlamydia trachomatis* (genital)

Bacteria in the family Chlamydiaceae are obligate intracellular organisms that can infect mammals and birds. Of the two genera (*Chlamydia* and *Chlamydophila*) four species can affect humans: *Chlamydia trachomatis, Chlamydophila pneumoniae, Chlamydophila psittaci* and *Chlamydophila abortus*. One group of biovars of *C. trachomatis* cause genital infection, neonatal ophthalmia, pneumonia and adult ocular infection; different biovars cause lymphogranuloma venereum (LGV; L1, L2 and L3) and endemic trachoma. Genital *Chlamydia* infection is the most commonly diagnosed sexually transmitted infection (STI) in Europe.

Suggested on-call action

Not usually applicable.

Epidemiology

In Europe, genital chlamydial infection is the most frequently diagnosed STI (see Table 3.28.1). The highest rates of infection are in males aged 20–24 years and females aged 16–24 years. In England, amongst females aged 16–19 years, annual incidence exceeds 1%. Surveys among sexually active women in the UK have found prevalences of 4–12%.

Similar results have been reported in European and North American studies. Risk factors for infection include age 25 years or less, recent change of sexual partner, use of oral contraceptives and low socio-economic status.

Lymphogranuloma venereum is endemic in Africa, Asia, South America and Caribbean America, but until recently has been rare in Western Europe. Since 2004, outbreaks have occurred amongst men who have sex with men (MSM) in major cities in Europe. At the end of 2009, the UK reported a doubling of the normal monthly incidence of LGV with most cases presenting as proctitis in HIV-positive white MSM, often with multiple sexual partners.

Clinical features

Many cases of infection in men and women are asymptomatic. In women there may be cervicitis and urethritis which may be complicated by pelvic inflammatory disease, tubal damage, infertility and ectopic pregnancy. In men there is urethritis which may be complicated by epididymitis.

Unlike other forms of *C. trachomatis*, LGV is invasive. It is a chronic disease that starts with a painless sore that develops into swollen lymph glands and haemorrhagic proctitis.

Laboratory confirmation

A range of tests are available for the laboratory diagnosis of *C. trachomatis* including culture and nucleic acid amplification tests (NAATs) on urine or swab samples. Less sensitive enzyme immunoassay tests should no longer be used.

A new variant of *C. trachomatis* (nvCT) was reported from Sweden in 2006. It is of public health importance because it is not detected by some NAATs and therefore gives false negative results. Currently, nvCT is rare outside Sweden. Laboratories should ensure

they are using a NAAT capable of detecting nvCT.

Transmission

Transmission is usually by direct sexual contact. Adult eye infection can be spread indirectly by fingers contaminated with infected genital discharges.

In the recent increase in LGV cases, knowledge of the reservoir of infection and mode of transmission is incomplete as asymptomatic cases and urethral infection are uncommon. However, high-risk sexual behaviour including use of sex toys and attendance at sex parties have been described.

Acquisition

The incubation period is 7–14 days and the case will remain infectious until treated. Only limited short-term immunity occurs and re-infection rates are high.

Prevention

• Programmes of opportunistic selective screening, case finding and partner notification are cost-effective. Universal population screening is not recommended.
• In the UK, selective screening is offered to men and women under 25 years who are sexually active, annually or after a change of sexual partner. Urine or self-taken lower vaginal swabs are tested with NAATs. The service is available in a variety of community settings.
• Use of condoms during sexual intercourse and avoiding shared use of sex toys will reduce individual risk.
• In the UK, diagnostic testing is recommended for men and women with symptoms and women undergoing gynaecological surgery.
• Testing for LGV should be offered during routine clinical care to HIV positive MSM who have symptoms of LGV infection and have a positive test for *C. trachomatis*.

Surveillance

• It is not necessary to report individual cases to local health protection teams, but anonymised or aggregated data should be reported to national surveillance systems.
• Cases who attend genitourinary medicine (GUM) clinics are reported through the GUM-CAD system (see Chapter 2.7) in England and Wales. However, many cases are treated in general practice.
• Laboratories should report positive results through laboratory reporting systems.

Response to a case

• Treatment is with a 7-day course of doxycycline or erythromycin or a single dose of azithromycin.
• Cases should avoid sexual intercourse for 7 days after the completion of treatment.
• Patients identified with *C. trachomatis* should have partner notification discussed at time of treatment by a trained healthcare professional.

Investigation of a cluster and control of an outbreak

This is not generally applicable but contact tracing, mapping sexual networks, treatment and education may be appropriate.

Suggested case-definition

Cases are defined by the results of appropriate laboratory tests.

3.13 Cholera

Cholera is a life-threatening secretory diarrhoea resulting from infection with toxin-producing *Vibrio cholerae* O1 or O139.

Suggested on-call action

• Cases should normally be admitted to an infectious diseases unit and enteric precautions instituted.
• Confirm diagnosis and the toxin production status of the isolate.
• Exclude cases in risk groups 1–4 (Box 2.2.1) for 48 hours after the first normal stool.
• Identify household contacts and those with common exposure, place under surveillance for 5 days from last contact and exclude from food handling.

Epidemiology

Cholera is rare in Europe. In 2007, 17 confirmed cases were reported by France (4), the UK (4), the Netherlands (3), Germany (2), Spain (2), Slovenia (1) and Norway (1). Worldwide, cholera has become more widespread as the virulent El Tor biotype has spread, encouraged by international migration and the breakdown of public health measures especially associated with war, famine and other disasters. European visitors are unlikely to visit areas where cholera is common. *V. cholerae* O139 has recently been identified as causing epidemic cholera.

Clinical features

Cholera is characterised by a sudden onset of copious watery diarrhoea and sometimes vomiting. Stool volumes of up to 30 L a day lead to rapid dehydration. There may be severe muscle pain as a result of hypokalaemia. This dramatic presentation is distinctive, but mild or subclinical infections are more common. The outcome depends on the amount of fluid and electrolyte loss and replacement; severe untreated cases have 50% case-fatality, but with correct treatment, less than 1% die.

Laboratory confirmation

Vibrios are small, comma-shaped, motile, Gram-negative bacilli, which may be seen on direct microscopy of stools or cultured from stool or a rectal swab. Various media have been described for culture; colonies can be recognised by fermentation reactions or by using antisera or fluorescent antibody tests. *V. cholerae* O1 is divided into two biotypes: classical and El Tor. Determination of toxin production is important, non-toxin-producing organisms are not of public health significance (most *V. cholerae* isolated in the UK are not toxin producers). More recently, polymerase chain reaction (PCR) and other nucleic acid-based rapid techniques have been described.

Transmission

Infection is faeco-oral, commonly through contaminated water. Undercooked seafood can also act as a vehicle. Cholera vibrios are sensitive to acidity. Most die in the stomach, but achlorhydria increases susceptibility to infection. Following colonisation of the small bowel, an enterotoxin that interferes with intestinal epithelial cell metabolism is produced, causing secretion of electrolytes and water into the intestinal lumen. Person-to-person spread should not occur where sanitary conditions are acceptable.

Acquisition

The incubation period is 6–48 hours. Cases are infectious during the period of diarrhoea and up to 7 days after.

Prevention

Control by sanitation is effective but may not be feasible in endemic areas.

• A parenteral vaccine of whole killed bacteria has been used widely, but is relatively ineffective and is not generally recommended.
• Antibiotic prophylaxis is feasible for small groups over short periods in high-risk situations.
• Breastfeeding in endemic areas protects infants from disease.

Surveillance

• Cholera is a notifiable disease, and the public health authorities should be informed of any case.
• WHO should be informed by the national agency.
• Illnesses caused by strains of *V. cholerae* other than toxigenic *V. cholerae* O1 or O139 should not be reported as cases of cholera.

Response to a case

• See on-call box above.
• Individual cases should be investigated to determine the source.
• Microbiological clearance: when indicated, two consecutive negative stools taken at intervals of at least 24 hours are required.
• Hygiene advice to the case and contacts.

Investigation of a cluster

• Clusters should be investigated in case there is secondary transmission within the household or community. This is rare in Europe.
• Obtain history of foreign travel.

Control of an outbreak

Outbreaks are rare in developed countries and are controlled through the provision of safe drinking water supplies.

<table>
</table>

Suggested case-definition for an outbreak
Clinical: an illness characterised by diarrhoea and/or vomiting in a contact of a case. *Confirmed*: clinical case with isolation of toxigenic *Vibrio cholerae* O1 or O139 from stool or vomitus.

3.14 Creutzfeldt–Jakob disease and other human transmissible spongiform encephalopathies

Human transmissible spongiform encephalopathies (TSEs) are a group of conditions characterised by progressive fatal encephalopathy with typical spongiform pathological appearances in the brain. They include classic Creutzfeldt–Jakob disease (CJD), variant Creutzfeldt–Jakob disease (vCJD), kuru and fatal familial insomnia. These conditions are believed to be caused by prion proteins, known as PrP in the case of vCJD.

Suggested on-call action
• Undertake risk assessment. • May need to prepare for media interest.

Epidemiology

CJD in its classic form is the most common of the human TSEs but is still rare, with an annual incidence worldwide of 0.5–1.0 cases per million population.

The first case of vCJD was identified in 1996. Cases have occurred in several Euro-

Table 3.14.1 Variant Creutzfeldt–Jakob disease (vCJD) cases worldwide (October 2010)

Country	Total
UK	174
France	25
Spain	5
Ireland	4
Netherlands	3
USA	3
Italy	2
Portugal	2
Canada	1
Japan	1
Saudi Arabia	1

Source: EuroCJD.

pean countries, but particularly in the UK where 174 cases had been reported by October 2010 (Table 3.14.1). The number of cases peaked in 2000, and has been declining since then; in 2010 only three from EuroCJD cases of vCJD were reported in the EU. The age distribution of vCJD is younger than in classic CJD and cases have a different symptom profile and a different appearance of brain tissue on post-mortem. There may be genetic differences in susceptibility: all cases of vCJD (except one) tested to date are homologous for methionine at codon 129 of the prion protein gene, this is similar to cattle, where codon 129 codes for methionine – about 38% of the UK population are of this genotype. Regarding the one confirmed case in a heterozygote, by analogy with scrapie, it is believed that heterozygosity will increase the incubation period. No relationship with occupation is apparent.

Kuru is a disease that occurs exclusively in Papua New Guinea; it has now almost disappeared.

Clinical features

The onset of vCJD is with variable psychiatric symptoms. This is typically followed by abnormal sensation at 2 months, ataxia at 5 months, myoclonus at 8 months, akinetic mutism at 11 months, with death at 12–24 months.

Laboratory confirmation

The diagnosis of vCJD is made on the basis of typical clinical features (see case-definition) and post-mortem findings of spongiform change and extensive PrP deposition with florid plaques throughout the cerebrum and cerebellum.

Transmission

Most cases of classic CJD are sporadic, about 15% are inherited and around 1% are ia-trogenic, transmitted from human pituitary-derived growth hormone injections, corneal transplants and brain surgery involving con-taminated instruments. Classic CJD is not thought to be transmissible via blood trans-fusion.

The most likely source of vCJD in hu-mans is cattle infected with bovine spongi-form encephalopathy (BSE). The PrP causing vCJD and BSE are indistinguishable from each other, but are different from those causing classic CJD or scrapie. The route of spread is unknown although consumption of infected bovine neural tissue is thought to be the most likely. Such exposure is likely to have been at its greatest before the introduction of effec-tive control measures in 1990. In addition to the CNS tissues (including eye and pituitary) that are infectious in all types of TSE, vCJD also involves the lymphoreticular system and so tissues such as tonsils, appendix, thymus, lymph nodes, spleen, Peyer's patches and pos-sibly bone marrow could all be infectious. Cases possibly associated with blood trans-fusion have been reported; iatrogenic trans-mission from contaminated surgical instru-ments is also theoretically possible, with CNS and back of eye operations likely to pose the highest risk. Although scrapie, the main TSE of sheep, is not thought to be transmissible to humans, it is possible that sheep infected with BSE could have entered the food chain.

Kuru is transmitted by cannibalistic con-sumption of infected human brain tissue; there is some suggestion that transmission may have occurred by spreading infected brain material over superficial cuts.

Acquisition

The incubation period for vCJD is unknown, but is probably several years; for iatro-genic CJD and kuru the mean incubation is 12 years. The infective dose is unknown, but is likely to be affected by route of exposure. Cattle under 30 months of age are thought to be significantly less likely to be infectious.

Prevention

• Prevent BSE in cattle and transmission of infected tissues to humans. This includes banning consumption of potentially infected feed to cattle, avoiding human consumption of nervous and lymphoreticular tissues, safe preparation of carcasses and slaughter of af-fected herds.
• Effective decontamination of surgical in-struments according to best practice. Single use disposable instruments should be used where possible.
• Incinerate surgical instruments used on def-inite or probable CJD cases and high-risk groups.
• Quarantine of surgical instruments used on possible cases.
• Effective tracking system for surgical instru-ments.
• Use of leukodepleted blood for transfusions.
• Use of non-UK-sourced plasma and blood products.
• Avoid transplant and tissue donations and blood transfusions from certain high-risk groups.
• Infection control guidance for CJD pa-tients undergoing surgery have been drawn up by the Advisory Committee on Dangerous Pathogens (ACDP) (available via Health Pro-tection Agency website).
• Pentosan polysulphate is under evaluation as a potential post-exposure prophylactic.

Surveillance

In Europe, surveillance of CJD (including vCJD) is undertaken by the European Creutzfeld–Jakob Disease Surveillance Network (EuroCJD, www.eurocjd.ed.ac.uk). The network undertakes surveillance which includes identification of risk factors, routes of transmission and identification of novel forms of human prion disease. It also provides advice on diagnosis including review of clinical data and examination of tissue samples.

Response to a case

• Neurologists should report to the local public health department who will report to EuroCJD.
• Investigate patient's medical history, especially recent surgery or organ or tissue donation and blood donations. Advise on infection control measures.
• A look back exercise should be considered in any case of vCJD who has undergone an invasive procedure, particularly if involving nervous or lymphoid tissue. This should be based upon a risk assessment considering the type of exposure and how long previously the exposure occurred. Advice is available from EuroCJD. Those at highest risk are probably those exposed to instruments on the first few occasions of use after the potential contamination.

Investigation of a cluster

• Seek advice from national public health institute and EuroCJD.
• The uncertain and prolonged incubation period make the identification and investigation of clusters difficult. For vCJD, look for common exposures over a wide period of time, particularly common sources of beef and bovine products since 1980, and consider the possibility of iatrogenic transmission.

Suggested case-definition

Definite: progressive neuropsychiatric disorder and neuropathological confirmation of vCJD on post-mortem.
Probable: progressive neuropsychiatric disorder, lasting more than 6 months, with routine investigations not suggesting an alternative diagnosis and no history of iatrogenic exposure *and* either (a) or (b):
(a) Four from following list:
Early psychiatric symptoms; persistent painful sensory symptoms; ataxia, myoclonus *or* chorea *or* dystonia; dementia; *and* EEG does not show changes typical of sporadic CJD;
and bilateral pulvinar high signal on magnetic resonance imaging (MRI) scan.
(b) Positive tonsil biopsy.

3.15 *Clostridium difficile*

Clostridium difficile is an anaerobic spore-forming bacterium widely distributed in soil and the intestinal tracts of humans and animals which was identified as the cause of pseudomembranous colitis (PMC) in the 1970s. *C. difficile* infection (CDI) is an important healthcare-associated infection (HCAI) which in 1996, in the UK, was estimated to cost £4000 per case due to prolonged hospital stay and additional treatment costs.

Suggested on-call action

• Hospital outbreaks will be managed by the infection control doctor. Local health protection team should be prepared to participate in meetings of the outbreak control group.
• Local health protection team may be called upon to investigate and manage incidents involving CDI in community nursing homes.

Epidemiology

Elderly, hospitalised patients are at greatest risk. There is a background rate of CDI in most hospitals and outbreaks may occur. From the late 1990s, CDI rates and severity increased in Europe and North America. A number of reasons have been proposed for this increase including greater awareness on the part of health professionals leading to increased testing and reporting, an older population, an increase in community-acquired CDI and the emergence of the more virulent ribotype O27 strain. In England, in 2007–2008, 55% of isolates were O27 but this had fallen to 36% by 2008–2009. CDI rates in the UK are now declining. There were 25,604 cases of CDI in patients aged 2 years and over in 2009–2010, a reduction of 29% compared with the 36,095 cases in 2008–2009 and a 54% reduction compared with the 55,498 cases reported in 2007–2008.

Clinical features

CDI is a spectrum of disease, often triggered by antibiotic exposure, comprising colonisation, toxin production, diarrhoea and severe colitis. *C. difficile* causes 25% of cases of antibiotic-associated diarrhoea and a greater proportion of more severe disease. In a typical case of CDI, diarrhoea starts within a few days of commencing antibiotics, although antibiotics taken 1–2 months previously may still predispose to infection. There may be abdominal pain (occasionally without diarrhoea) and fever. Complications include dehydration, PMC, toxic megacolon and perforation.

Laboratory confirmation

Laboratories test specimens for *C. difficile* toxin using either an immunoassay detecting both toxin A and toxin B, or a neutralised cell cytotoxicity assay. Culture (which in the absence of toxin is insufficient for diagnosis) is required if typing is to be performed to establish which strains are present in a ward or hospital and for antibiotic sensitivity testing.

Transmission

C. difficile is present in the faeces of 3% of healthy adults, 7% of asymptomatic care-home residents and 20% of elderly patients on long-stay wards. *C. difficile* is transmitted from patients with symptomatic CDI either directly, via the hands of healthcare workers, through the accumulation of spores in the environment or on contaminated fomites such as commodes. Spread does not occur from an asymptomatic carrier in the absence of diarrhoea. Transmission to medical and nursing staff has been reported, although this is unusual and the disease is usually mild and short-lived. Community-acquired CDI does occur and is probably under-diagnosed.

Acquisition

CDI occurs when a pathogenic strain of *C. difficile* colonises the gastrointestinal tract of a susceptible patient. Once established, CDI is a toxin-mediated condition. Risk factors that predispose to CDI are age, antibiotic treatment, cytotoxic agents, intensive care, nasogastric intubation, concurrent illness and alteration in gut motility.

Prevention

• Control of antibiotic usage: in hospitals there should be an antimicrobial management team (AMT) including an antimicrobial pharmacist and restrictive antibiotic guidelines that promote the use of narrow-spectrum agents.
• Standard infection control procedures, including staff training and a high level of environmental cleanliness.

Surveillance

• Clinicians and other healthcare practitioners should have a high index of suspicion and should submit faecal specimens for laboratory testing when diarrhoea may be due to CDI.
• Laboratories should test diarrhoeal specimens for toxins A and B from patients aged 2 years and over.
• Include CDI in the mandatory surveillance of HCAI.

Response to a case

• Involve the hospital infection control team.
• Side room isolation with enteric precautions, use of gloves and aprons and attention to handwashing by all staff. There should be adequate accommodation for single-room isolation or cohort nursing on normal wards.
• Bowel function should be monitored daily using the Bristol Stool Chart (http://www .sthk.nhs.uk/library/documents/stoolchart .pdf) and patients care should be overseen by a multidisciplinary clinical review team.
• Thorough environmental cleaning: the use of environmental disinfectants is unnecessary.

Investigation of a cluster

• All patients with diarrhoea should be identified, risk factors should be documented and faecal samples submitted for toxin tests, culture and ribotyping. In a hospital outbreak, typing may help to determine whether all patients are infected with the same strain, whether relapses are due to the original outbreak strain and whether patients are infected with more than one strain at a time.
• Routine environmental sampling is not recommended but may form part of an investigation, especially if isolates can be typed.

Control of an outbreak

• Strict adherence to antibiotic policies.
• Case finding through enhanced surveillance.

• Side room isolation.
• Enteric precautions and handwashing.
• Restrict movements and transfers of patients.
• Environmental cleaning.
• Disinfection and sterilisation of equipment.
• Correct handling of infected linen.
• Screening for and treatment of asymptomatic patients who are *C. difficile* carriers is unnecessary.
• There is no need to screen asymptomatic staff for carriage of *C. difficile*: staff who are asymptomatic carriers do not present a risk to patients and they can continue in their normal duties.
• Staff who are on antibiotics can remain at work even if CDI is affecting patients.

Suggested case-definitions

C. difficile infection: one episode of diarrhoea (stool loose enough to assume shape of sample container or Bristol Stool Chart types 5–7), not attributable to any other cause or medication, with positive toxin assay (with or without a positive *C. difficile* culture) and/or endoscopic evidence of PMC.
Period of increased incidence of CDI: two or more new cases (occurring >48 hours post-admission, not relapses) in a 28-day period on a ward.
Outbreak of CDI: two or more cases caused by the same strain related in time and place over a defined period that is based on the date of onset of the first case.

3.16 *Clostridium perfringens*

Clostridium perfringens (formerly *Clostridium welchii*) is primarily a food-borne pathogen, which causes a mild gastrointestinal illness due to an enterotoxin. It is a cause of outbreaks, usually associated with mass catering.

Epidemiology

The incidence of *C. perfringens* food poisoning presenting to general practice in England is about 1.3 per 1000 person years. *C. perfringens* is identified as the cause of 1.4% of all gastroenteritis outbreaks reported in the UK, but this rises to 8% of those thought to be foodborne. There is little known variation by age, sex, ethnicity, occupation and geography. Reported cases are higher in autumn and winter months (especially December) than in summer, perhaps because of seasonal consumption of the types of foods often associated with infection. The association of infection with institutions or large gatherings likewise probably reflects patterns of food preparation. Outbreaks often have a high attack rate.

A much more serious disease (enteritis necrotans) is caused by different strains and is rare in Europe. *C. perfringens* is also the major cause of gas gangrene.

Clinical features

Almost all cases of *C. perfringens* food poisoning have diarrhoea (watery, often violent), usually with colicky, often severe, abdominal pain. Nausea may occur and a small proportion may have fever or vomiting. Blood in the stool is rare. Most cases recover within 24 hours, although elderly or debilitated patients may be more severely affected and occasional deaths are reported.

Laboratory confirmation

Clostridium perfringens can be isolated from anaerobic culture of stool samples. They are divided into five types (A–E) on the basis of toxin production. Those most frequently associated with food poisoning are the A2 strains, which form markedly heat-resistant spores. A1 strains, whose spores are relatively heat sensitive, may also cause illness.

As asymptomatic carriage of *C. perfringens* is extremely common in healthy humans and carriage of heat-resistant organisms not uncommon, isolation of the organism from sporadic cases is of little value. However, serotyping, which allows cases to be linked to each other and to strains from potential food vehicles, is useful in outbreak investigation. Other factors that may help separate cases from carriers are a quantitative culture of organisms (over 10^6/g faeces usually significant) or the demonstration of enterotoxin in faeces. More than one serotype can be present in the same specimen.

Transmission

C. perfringens is ubiquitous in soil and in the gastrointestinal tracts of mammals and birds. Many opportunities exist for spores to contaminate food, particularly meat and meat products, but provided contamination remains low, illness does not result. *C. perfringens* can grow at temperatures between 15°C and 50°C with optimal growth at 43–45°C, when a generation time of 10 minutes can be achieved. Spores, particularly those of the A2 strains, can survive normal cooking, including boiling for longer than 1 hour. These 'heat-activated' spores will then germinate in the protein-rich environment as the food cools: the longer the food remains at the organism's preferred temperature, the larger the number of resulting organisms. If the food is not then reheated to at least 70°C for 2 minutes throughout its bulk to kill the vegetative cells before eating, then a potentially infectious dose is ingested. The ingested organisms sporulate in the gut and (probably as a result of the initial heat shock) produce the enterotoxin, which causes disease. Bulk cooking of meat/poultry stews, roasts, pies and gravies appear to be particularly vulnerable to this chain of events.

Acquisition

The incubation period is usually 8–18 hours, although a range of 5–24 hours has been reported (possibly occasionally shorter). *C. perfringens* gastroenteritis is not spread from person to person, and asymptomatic food handlers are not thought to be infectious to others. The infectious dose in food is usually greater than 10^5 organisms. There is no evidence of effective immunity post-infection.

Prevention

• Prevention is dependent upon adequate temperature control of food after (initial) cooking. Meat dishes should be served whilst still hot from initial cooking *or*, if not served immediately:
   (a) refrigerate to below 10°C within 2 hours of end of cooking; and
   (b) reheat to achieve 70°C for at least 2 minutes throughout the bulk of the food; and
   (c) cook and reheat as small a quantity of food as is practicable.
• Take particular care in large functions, or if consumers likely to include elderly or debilitated people.

Surveillance

Report cases of food poisoning to local public health authorities and positive samples from cases to national surveillance systems.

Response to a case

• As with all cases of diarrhoea, hygiene advice should be given and it is best if the case does not attend work or school until he/she has normal stools.
• Occupational details should be sought: cases in risk groups 1–4 (Box 2.2.1) should be excluded until 48 hours after the first normal stool. No microbiological clearance is necessary.
• No action is necessary with asymptomatic contacts of cases.

Investigation of a cluster

A laboratory identified cluster is currently a rare event. Should one occur in a group of individuals with a compatible clinical illness, then analysis of person/place/time variables should be followed by a semistructured questionnaire aimed at identifying common foods, especially cooked meat/poultry products and meals eaten outside the home.

Control of an outbreak

• As secondary spread from cases is unlikely, the aim of the outbreak investigation is to discover how it happened so that lessons can be learnt. In practice this means trying to identify how an infectious dose resulted in a food presented for consumption.
• The vehicle of infection is identified by microbiological analysis of remaining food to find the same serotype as the cases (make sure you know how the food was stored after serving but before sampling) or by an analytical epidemiological study to show that cases were statistically significantly more likely to have eaten the food than controls.
• The environmental investigation will concentrate on how the food was cooked, stored and reheated. It is worth remembering that type A1 spores should not survive adequate initial cooking.

Suggested case-definition for analytical study of *C. perfringens* outbreak

Clinical: diarrhoea or abdominal pain with onset between 8 and 18 hours of exposure.
Confirmed: clinical case with one of: isolate of outbreak serotype; demonstration of enterotoxin in faeces; spore count $>10^5$/g.

3.17 Coxsackievirus infections

Human coxsackieviruses are a diverse group of enteroviruses. Historically, groups A and B were described, each comprising several serotypes. Modern taxonomy groups coxsackieviruses with other enteroviruses and echoviruses in three species of human enterovirus: A, B or C. Coxsackieviruses cause a range of clinical syndromes, including hand, foot and mouth disease (HFMD).

Suggested public health on-call action

None generally needed.

Epidemiology

Infection may be sporadic or epidemic. In recent years, in England and Wales, laboratory reports of confirmed coxsackievirus isolates have declined due to the use of newer molecular diagnostic tests. In 2007, non-polio enterovirus was confirmed in 295 cases presenting with neurological symptoms. Detection rates are highest in children. The clinical conditions associated with virus detection are typically meningitis and other more serious infections as milder clinical syndromes do not normally merit laboratory diagnosis. Most cases occur between July and December, and viral activity peaks at intervals of 2–5 years. There is evidence of spread of epidemic serotypes across Europe in certain years. Outbreaks of A9 were reported in the UK in 1976 and 1985, and A16 was epidemic in 1981. An outbreak of viral meningitis due to B5 was reported in Cyprus in 1996. According to general practice data from England and Wales, the mean weekly incidence of HFMD in 2009 was 1.15 per 100,000 per week but this overall rate disguises age and seasonal variations, for example the rate in 1- to 4-year-olds in October was 51.1.

Clinical features

Infection may be clinical (Table 3.17.1) or subclinical. HFMD is usually due to coxsackievirus A16 and is a mild illness with fever and a vesicular rash in the mouth and on the palms, soles and buttocks. HFMD due to a closely related virus, enterovirus 71, has been reported from several Asian countries and was associated with occasionally fatal neurological involvement in Taiwan in 1998. There is interest in a possible link between Type 1 diabetes and B1 infection.

Laboratory confirmation

Coxsackieviruses may be isolated in tissue culture from faeces or other clinical specimens and serological tests are available. Molecular methods are now widely used.

Transmission

Human clinical and subclinical cases are the reservoir of infection. Spread is by direct contact with faeces, blisters and respiratory droplets. Enteroviruses may also spread indirectly via environmental water and sewage.

Acquisition

The incubation period is 3–5 days and a person will be infectious during the acute illness and while the virus persists in the faeces.

Infection generally leads to immunity although infection with different serotypes may occur.

Prevention

• Standard and enteric precautions, particularly handwashing and hygienic disposal of faeces, will reduce exposure.

Table 3.17.1 Clinical syndromes caused by coxsackievirus infection

Acute haemorrhagic conjunctivitis	Subconjunctival haemorrhages and lid oedema. Often due to serotype A24.
Epidemic myalgia (Bornholm disease)	Chest or abdominal pain, aggravated by movement and associated with fever and headache. Outbreaks have been reported.
Hand, foot and mouth disease	A mild infection with ulcers in the mouth and a maculopapular or vesicular rash on the hands, feet and buttocks. Often due to serotype A16. Systemic features and lymphadenopathy are absent and recovery is uneventful.
Herpangina	Fever, painful dysphagia, abdominal pain and vomiting with vesicles and shallow ulcers on tonsils and soft palate.
Meningitis	Fever with signs and symptoms of meningeal involvement. Encephalitic signs may be present.
Myocarditis Pericarditis	B1–B6 are most often associated with heart disease. Heart muscle necrosis varies in extent and severity. Heart failure may follow. Most patients with viral myocarditis recover fully. Treatment is largely supportive.
Skin	Rashes are common including a fine pink rubella-like rash or petechial, purpuric, vesicular, bullous or urticarial rashes. Onychomadesis (complete nail shedding) has been described.

• Pregnant women may wish to avoid exposure, as a possible risk of abortion has been suggested.

Surveillance

Sporadic cases will not normally be reported to public health authorities, but clusters of cases and outbreaks should be reported.

Response to a case

Children with HFMD may attend school or nursery when well enough.

Investigation of a cluster and control of an outbreak

The local public health team may wish to alert local schools and general practitioners if an outbreak of HFMD occurs.

Suggested case-definition

Characteristic clinical appearance with or without laboratory confirmation.

3.18 Cryptosporidiosis

Cryptosporidia are protozoan parasites, which usually cause an acute self-limiting diarrhoeal illness. Their main public health importance lies in the severe illness caused in immunocompromised individuals, the lack of specific treatment and the potential to cause outbreaks, including large water-borne outbreaks.

Suggested on-call action

• If case in risk group for onward transmission (Box 2.2.1), exclude from work or nursery.
• If you or reporting laboratory/clinician are aware of other potentially linked cases, consult local outbreak plan.

Epidemiology

Cryptosporidium is the fourth most commonly identified cause of gastrointestinal infection in the UK, with around 5000 isolates reported a year. There is significant under-reporting in many European countries, but evidence of past infection is common with seroprevalence rates of 20–35% reported. Diagnosed infection rates are highest in children aged 1–5 years and low in those over 45 years (Table 3.18.1). Males and females are affected equally. The most common source for outbreaks are drinking water and swimming pools.

Cryptosporidiosis has a marked seasonal pattern in Europe with a peak in autumn and, in some countries (e.g. UK and Ireland), an earlier peak in spring (mainly *Cryptosporidium parvum*) (Figure 2.2.2). Groups at particular risk of infection include animal handlers (*C. parvum*), travellers abroad (particularly to developing counties), contacts of cases, men who have sex with men and those who are immunosuppressed. Rates may also be higher in rural areas. The reported incidence of cryptosporidiosis in some AIDS centres is as high as 20%, although this is not universal. The age profile of cases in immuno-suppressed patients is higher than that shown in Table 3.18.1.

Clinical features

The main presenting symptom is diarrhoea, which in immunocompetent individuals may last from 2 days to 4 weeks, with an average of 2 weeks. The diarrhoea may contain mucus but rarely blood, may be profuse and may wax and wane. The diarrhoea may be preceded by anorexia and nausea, and is usually accompanied by cramping abdominal pain. Vomiting, fever, fatigue, headache, anorexia or myalgia may also be reported.

Immunosuppressed patients have difficulty in clearing the infection, particularly HIV infected individuals with CD4 T-lymphocyte counts below 200 cells/mm^3. Many such individuals have a prolonged and fulminant illness which may contribute to death.

Laboratory confirmation

The mainstay of diagnosis is microscopy of stool samples to detect cryptosporidia oocysts. It is important that such microscopy be undertaken by experienced personnel, both to maximise ascertainment and because a wide variety of microscopic structures can be confused with *Cryptosporidium* oocysts. Repeat sampling may improve ascertainment. Individual cases are sometimes diagnosed by intestinal biopsy. Serological methods have been used in epidemiological studies and outbreaks. Antigen detection or polymerase chain reaction (PCR) tests may be available from specialist laboratories.

Genotyping is available and splits infections into *Cryptosporidium hominis* ('genotype 1'), which is found only in humans and accounts for approximately 40% of cases; *C. parvum* ('genotype 2'), found in animals and humans (about 50%); and other cryptosporidia (3%, although higher in the immunosuppressed).

Transmission

Cryptosporidium parvum has been demonstrated in a wide variety of animals including cattle, sheep, goats, horses, pigs, cats, dogs, rodents and humans. Clinical disease and most oocyst excretion are thought to occur mainly in young animals. Transmission to humans is by faeco-oral spread from animals or other

Table 3.18.1 Age-distribution of sporadic cryptosporidiosis (UK)

Age-group (years)	Percentage of total cases
Under 1	6
1–4	39
5–14	17
15–24	13
25–34	13
35–44	7
45–54	3
55–64	1
65 plus	2

Source: PHLS Study Group, 1990.

humans. The main routes of spread are as follows.

Person to person

Cryptosporidiosis can be transmitted by cases to family members, nursery contacts, carers and sexual partners. Spread can be direct faeco-oral or via contaminated items such as nappies. *C. hominis* cases have higher excretion levels than *C. parvum*, although both are transmissible. Aerosol or droplet spread from liquid faeces may also occur. Secondary spread in households is common and may occur after resolution of clinical symptoms in the index case. Many outbreaks have been reported in nurseries.

Animal to person

Human infection with *C. parvum* can occur from contact with farm or laboratory animals and, occasionally, household pets. In addition to agricultural and veterinary workers, those at risk include children visiting farms on educational or recreational visits where they may handle lambs or calves. A number of outbreaks associated with such visits have been reported.

Drinking water

Contamination of drinking water may occur from agricultural sources or human sewage contamination. Oocysts passed in faeces can survive in the environment for months. They are resistant to chlorination and their removal relies on physical methods of water treatment such as filtration, coagulation and sedimentation. Over 50 drinking water related outbreaks have been reported in the UK, but the largest such outbreak occurred in Milwaukee, USA, in 1993 when an estimated 400,000 people became ill. A review of the UK outbreaks found a common thread of an inadequacy in the treatment provided or of the operation of the treatment process.

Other

Infection has been reported via food and milk. Many swimming pool outbreaks have been reported, usually as a result of faecal contamination of water and inadequate pool maintenance. Transmission has been reported from healthcare workers to patients (both immunosuppressed and immunocompetent) and between patients. The source of much cryptosporidiosis in the UK remains unclear. *C. hominis* may be associated with travel abroad.

Acquisition

The incubation period is unclear: 4–7 days would seem to be average, but a range spanning 1–28 days has been reported. The infectious period commences at onset of symptoms and may continue for several weeks after resolution. Asymptomatic infection has also been reported.

The infective dose can be as low as 10 oocysts in some cases (thus enabling autoinfection) with a median infective dose (ID_{50}) of around 100 oocysts. The UK Expert Group found it was not possible to recommend a health-related standard for *Cryptosporidium* in drinking water. In immunocompetent individuals the immune response successfully limits the infection. Patients with AIDS are at increased risk of acquisition and increased severity. Relative immunosuppression due to chickenpox and malnutrition has also been associated with infection, but renal patients do not appear to be at increased risk. Oocyst excretion may be very high in the immunosuppressed.

Prevention

- Handwashing after contact with faeces, nappies and animals (take particular care in contact with these if immunosuppressed).
- Safe disposal of sewage, taking particular care to avoid water sources.
- Risk assessment for water supplies, protection against agricultural contamination,

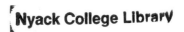

adequate water treatment (e.g. coagulation aided filtration) and monitoring of water quality, particularly turbidity.
- Enteric precautions for cases (Chapter 1.2) and exclusion of those in at-risk groups (Box 2.2.1).
- Immunosuppressed patients to boil water (both tap and bottle) before consumption and avoid contact with farm animals and infected humans.
- Guidelines for farm visits by children have been developed and can be adapted for local use (Health and Safety Executive, UK). Guidelines have also been developed for swimming pools (Pool Water Advisory Group, UK).
- *Cryptosporidium* is resistant to many common disinfectants. Ammonia, sodium hypochlorite, formalin, glutaraldehye and hydrogen peroxide may be effective. Heating to 72°C for 1 minute inactivates the parasite.

Surveillance

- All gastrointestinal infections thought to have been acquired from food, water or public areas should be reported to local public health authorities and confirmed *Cryptosporidium* cases to national surveillance systems.
- The most important function of surveillance of cryptosporidiosis is the detection of outbreaks, particularly water-borne outbreaks. All diarrhoeal samples should be examined for oocysts (unless a bacterial or viral cause has already been identified) and all positives reported. Home postcode should be collected on all cases to be plotted on water supply zone maps, which can provided by water providers and need regular updating. Trigger levels can be calculated for districts and regions. A seasonal baseline can be set, based on historical data with confidence intervals. High figures for 1 week only may be the result of reporting delay (look at dates of onset). The age distribution of cases should also be monitored.
- Water providers should also undertake appropriate monitoring of water quality and inform the local public health authorities of po-

tentially significant failures (e.g. levels of one oocyst per 10 L of water; see Box 3.18.1).

Response to case

- Enteric precautions for case (see Chapter 1.2).
- Exclude from work/school if in risk group (Box 2.2.1) until 48 hours after first normal stool. No microbiological clearance necessary.
- Cases should not use swimming pools until 2 weeks after first normal stool.
- Investigate illness in family or other contacts.
- Obtain history of raw water consumption (including postcodes of premises on which consumed and any consumption from private water supplies), contact with other cases, contact with animals, nurseries, swimming pools, travel and milk consumption in previous 14 days.

Investigation of cluster

- Check to see if neighbouring areas, particularly those sharing a water supply, have an increase.
- Check age range of affected cases: an increase in cases in adults could suggest water-borne infection, or link with immunosuppressed patients. If most cases in school age children, consider visits to farms or swimming pools or, if under 5 years, links to nurseries.
- Epidemic curve may suggest point source, continuing source or person-to-person spread.
- Check with water provider whether any recent evidence of increased contamination or failure of treatment.
- Plot cases by water supply zones. Check with water provider how cases relate to water sources (e.g. reservoirs, treatment centres) during relevant period. Supply zones are not fixed and some areas may also receive water from mixed sources.
- Collect and review risk factor details from individual cases for hypothesis generation

---

Box 3.18.1 Response to detection of oocysts in water supply

The relationship between oocyst counts and the health risk to those who drink the water is unclear. However, the water companies in the UK will inform public health authorities of breaches in water quality standards. An appropriate response would be (based on Hunter, 2000):

Collect information for risk assessment:
- When and where sample taken.
- Number of oocysts detected and results of any viability testing.
- Results of repeat testing (should be carried out urgently).
- Source and treatment of affected water supply.
- Any recent changes in source or treatment.
- Distribution of water supply.
- Any treatment failure or high turbidity identified.
- How long water takes to go through distribution system.
- History of *Cryptosporidium* sampling and results for this supply.
- Any previous outbreaks associated with this supply.

For a low oocyst count in a supply in which oocysts are frequently detected and not associated with previous outbreaks, further action may not be necessary.

Call the incident management team if significant exposure is likely, e.g.:
- unusually high oocyst count or demonstration of viability;
- evidence of treatment failure or increased turbidity;
- groundwater source; or
- association with previous outbreaks.

Possible actions:
- None.
- Advice to particular groups.
- Enhanced surveillance for human cases.
- Provision of alternative water supply.
- Boil water notice to affected area.

Boil water notices are issued if risk is thought to be ongoing, e.g.:
- repeat samples positive;
- treatment or turbidity problems continue; or
- contaminated water not yet cleared from distribution system.

---

and further investigation as appropriate (see Chapter 4.2). Case finding may also be necessary.
- Organise confirmatory testing and genotyping by reference laboratory. If *C. hominis*, look for potential humans sources; if *C. parvum*, consider animal and human sources.

Control of an outbreak

- If a water-borne outbreak is likely then:
  (a) Issue 'boil water' notice if contamination is likely to be ongoing. A communications plan should already exist for public information. Water needs only to be brought to the boil: prolonged boiling is not necessary.

(b) Organise Outbreak Control Team to include relevant water company specialists/managers and Local Authority. If potentially serious, add appropriate experts. The addition to the team of an individual who has dealt with such an outbreak before should be considered.

(c) Consult Bouchier report (Box 3.18.2) for more detailed advice.

Box 3.18.2 Selected recommendations of Bouchier report

1.2.6	Water providers to develop local liaison arrangements with Health Authority (HA) and Local Authorities for rapid appraisal of potential health risk.
1.2.8	Water utilities to provide Consultant in Communicable Disease Control (CCDC) with water supply zone maps. HA to make early contact with water provider if outbreak of cryptosporidiosis suspected.
1.2.9	Human cryptosporidiosis to be laboratory reportable disease.
1.2.10	HA to make postcode of cases available to water providers for mapping.
1.2.40	Criteria should be in place for identifying outbreaks and activating control teams.
1.2.55	All parties to simulate incident/outbreak events to rehearse emergency procedures.
1.2.61	Outbreak Control Team to use guidance on Epidemiological Investigation of Outbreaks of Infection (Appendix A4 of report).
1.2.63	All water to be used by immunocompromised persons should be boiled first.

Further reading: Bouchier I.T. (Chairman). *Cryptosporidium in water supplies. Third report of the group of experts to: Department of Environment, Transport and the Regions and the Department of Health.* London: Department of Environment, Transport and the Regions, 1998.

- Exclude symptomatic cases in risk groups (Box 2.2.1).
- Advise public on how to prevent secondary spread.
- Institute good practice guidelines at any implicated nursery, farm, swimming pool or hospital.

Suggested case-definition for analytical study of an outbreak

Cohort study (e.g. nursery, school class):
- Clinical: diarrhoea within 1–14 days of exposure.
- Confirmed: diarrhoea and oocysts seen in faecal specimen.

Case–control study (e.g. general population): diarrhoea plus oocysts (of correct genotype, if known) in faeces, with no other pathogen isolated, no previous cases of diarrhoea in family in last 14 days and date of onset since commencement of increase in cases.

3.19 Cyclosporiasis

Cyclospora cayetanensis is a protozoan that causes human gastroenteritis.

Epidemiology

Infection occurs worldwide. In the UK about 60 cases are reported annually, the major risk factor being travel abroad: risk areas include Central America, South America, the Indian subcontinent and South-East Asia. A probable food-borne outbreak has occurred in Germany and cases have been acquired in Turkey, but the large outbreaks seen in North America have not been reported in Europe.

Clinical features

Cyclosporiasis presents with watery diarrhoea, often associated with weight loss, nausea, abdominal cramps, gas, anorexia and fatigue. Diarrhoea may be prolonged but is self-limiting. Diagnosis is confirmed by detection of oocysts in faeces. If *Cyclospora* is suspected, inform the laboratory so that stool concentration can be carried out. Laboratories with little experience of *Cyclospora* should refer putative positives to more experienced laboratories for confirmation, as pseudo-outbreaks have occurred.

Transmission and acquisition

Humans are so far the only host species identified for *C. cayetanensis*. Oocysts are excreted in a non-infective unsporulated form; sporulation takes about 7–15 days in the environment (preferably at 22–32°C) and infection results from ingestion of mature sporulated oocysts. Spread is therefore indirect via vehicles such as drinking water, swimming pools and food; person-to-person spread is unlikely. Outbreaks in developed countries have been associated with berries, salads and herbs, usually imported from endemic countries. The incubation period is 1–14 days (median 7 days).

Prevention

Prevention and control in developed countries relies on sanitary disposal of faeces and advice to travellers. Should a cluster of cases occur within Europe, ask each case about travel abroad: if no history of travel, than take a food history asking specifically about raw fruit, salad, vegetables, herbs and imported food.

3.20 Cytomegalovirus

Cytomegalovirus (CMV, human herpesvirus 5 (HHV-5)), a herpes virus, causes a variety of infections. Its major impact is on the newborn and the immunocompromised.

> **Suggested on-call action**
>
> No person-to-person spread under normal conditions, therefore no need for urgent action.

Epidemiology

The prevalence of CMV rises with age; 60–90% of adults have antibodies.

Clinical features

Most infection is asymptomatic. Occasionally, a glandular fever-like illness occurs. Congenital infection may cause stillbirth, perinatal death, cytomegaloviruria in an otherwise normal infant, or fever, hepatitis, pneumonitis and severe brain damage. CMV is a major cause of morbidity in immunocompromised patients. Disease may result from reactivation of latent infection. There may be pulmonary, gastrointestinal or CNS involvement, CMV causes retinitis and ulcerative disease of the gastrointestinal tract in the terminal phase of AIDS.

A post-transfusion syndrome, resembling infectious mononucleosis, can develop following transfusion with infected blood.

Laboratory confirmation

CMV may be isolated from urine, other body fluids or tissues. CMV may be excreted by individuals without active disease; a positive culture must be interpreted with caution. The demonstration of active disease may require biopsy. New techniques for rapid diagnosis demonstrating CMV antigens or DNA are being developed.

Transmission

CMV is transmitted through body fluids, blood or transplanted organs. In the newborn, infection may have been acquired transplacentally or during birth.

Pathogenesis

The incubation period for transfusion of CMV mononucleosis is 2–4 weeks. Infectivity of body fluids may persist for many months.

Prevention

• Screening of transplant donors for active disease.
• Risk assessment for those receiving transplantation and consideration of prophylaxis.

Surveillance

No need to report individual cases, other than through routine laboratory surveillance.

Response to a case

No public health response is usually necessary.

Investigation of a cluster and control of an outbreak

Investigate to ensure that it is not caused by exposure to contaminated blood or blood products.

Suggested case-definition for an outbreak

Neonatal: clinically compatible disease with isolate or PCR positive.
Adult: clinically compatible disease with isolate or CMV DNA detection or antigen detection or specific IgM-positive or fourfold rise in antibody titre.

3.21 Dengue fever

Dengue is a febrile disease caused by a flavivirus with four distinct serogroups and is transmitted by the bite of *Aedes* mosquitoes.

Suggested on-call action

None usually necessary.

Epidemiology

Endemic throughout the tropics and subtropics. The WHO estimates that every year between 50 and 100 million people develop dengue fever, 500,000 with severe clinical symptoms, and that approximately 22,000 individuals die, most of whom are children.

Almost half the dengue imported into Europe comes from Asia. Dengue haemorrhagic fever (DHF) is most common in children younger than 10 years from endemic areas.

Some recent studies suggest that some illness labelled as dengue may have been caused by flaviviruses such as Zika virus or alphaviruses.

Clinical diagnosis

Dengue presents with an abrupt onset of fever, chills, headache, backache and severe prostration. Aching in the legs and joints occurs during the first hours of illness. Fever and symptoms persist for 48–96 hours, followed by rapid defervescence, after about 24 hours a second rapid temperature rise follows (saddleback temperature). Typical dengue is not fatal.

In DHF bleeding tendencies occur with shock 2–6 days after onset. Mortality for DHF ranges 6–30%; most deaths occur in infants less than 1 year old.

Laboratory confirmation

Serological diagnosis may be made by haemagglutination inhibiting and complement fixation tests using paired sera.

Transmission

Spread by mosquito bites (e.g. *Aedes aegypti*). No person-to-person spread.

Acquisition

The incubation period is 3–15 days. Human-to-human spread of dengue has not been recorded, but people are infectious to mosquitoes during the febrile period.

Prevention

• Avoidance of mosquito bites (e.g. with bed nets and insect repellent).
• Control or eradication of the mosquito vector.
• To prevent transmission to mosquitoes, patients in endemic areas should be kept under mosquito netting until the second bout of fever has abated.

Surveillance

Public health officials should be informed of individual cases.

Response to a case

• Isolation is not required.
• Specimens should be taken using universal precautions and the laboratory informed.

Investigation of a cluster and control of an outbreak

Not relevant to European countries.

Suggested case-definition
A clinically compatible case confirmed by: • growth from or demonstration of virus in serum and/or tissue samples by immunohistochemistry or by viral nucleic acid detection; *or* • demonstration of a fourfold or greater rise in IgG or IgM antibody titres to one or more dengue virus antigens in paired serum samples.

3.22 Diphtheria

Diphtheria is an infection of the upper respiratory tract, and sometimes the skin. It is caused by toxin-producing (toxigenic) strains of *Corynebacterium diphtheriae*, and occasionally by toxigenic *Corynebacterium ulcerans*. It is a rare infection, but potentially fatal if untreated.

Suggested on-call action
• Obtain full clinical details, travel and vaccination history. • Liaise with both local and reference laboratories to ensure rapid diagnosis and toxigenicity testing. • Prepare a list of close contacts. • If diagnosis is strongly suspected, arrange for immediate swabbing, chemoprophylaxis and vaccination of close contacts. • Ensure the case is admitted to a specialist unit.

Epidemiology

Diphtheria is rare in countries with well-established immunisation programmes. In the EU, 47 cases were reported in 2008, of which 62% were from Latvia. Many cases were mild, in vaccinated individuals. The case fatality rate is 5–10%. Indigenous cases are very rare, although several countries in Europe (France, Germany, Italy, the Netherlands, Romania, Sweden and the UK) have reported sporadic cases due to toxigenic *C. ulcerans* in recent years.

There has been a rise in infections due to non-toxigenic strains of *C. diphtheriae* in recent years; these cases have presented with a mild sore throat only.

A large epidemic of diphtheria occurred in countries of the former USSR during the 1990s; there were more than 150,000 cases and 5000 deaths. A number of cases are still reported every year in the Baltic states.

Clinical features

Diphtheria is rarely recognised on clinical grounds, as many cases are in vaccinated individuals. In classic respiratory diphtheria there is sore throat, fever, enlarged cervical lymph nodes and swelling of the soft tissues of the neck – the 'bull neck' appearance. The pharyngeal membrane, which is not always present, is typically grey, thick and difficult to remove. There may be hoarseness and stridor. Nasal diphtheria usually presents with a blood-stained nasal discharge. Cutaneous diphtheria causes small ulcers, often on the legs. The disease is caused by a toxin that particularly affects the heart and nervous system. The effects of this toxin are irreversible and so early treatment (with antitoxin) is essential.

Laboratory confirmation

It is usually the identification of a *Corynebacterium sp.* from a nose or throat swab or skin ulcer that alerts the public health physician to the possibility of diphtheria. Any isolate of a potentially toxigenic *Corynebacterium* should be referred promptly to the national reference laboratory for confirmation and toxigenicity testing. Where the diagnosis seems likely, an acute serum specimen should be obtained before giving antitoxin, and any skin lesions should be swabbed.

Transmission

Humans are the only reservoir for *C. diphtheriae* and carriers are rare in vaccinated populations, so an infectious case is the usual source. Transmission is usually by air-borne droplets or direct contact with infected respiratory discharges or skin ulcers; rarely from contact with articles contaminated by discharges from infected lesions. Diphtheria is not highly infectious, although exposed cutaneous lesions are more infectious than nasopharyngeal cases.

The normal reservoir for *C. ulcerans* is cattle; human infections are usually acquired through animal contact or by eating or drinking unpasteurised dairy products.

Acquisition

The incubation period is 2–5 days, occasionally longer. Cases are no longer infectious after 3 days of antibiotic treatment. Untreated cases are infectious for up to 4 weeks. The infectious dose is not known. Natural immunity usually (although not always) develops after infection. A substantial proportion of adults are non-immune (50% in the UK in 2000) and the proportion increases with age.

Prevention

• Vaccinate with diphtheria toxoid (usually combined with tetanus, pertussis and Hib). A full primary course is three doses in the first year of life. Booster doses are recommended at varying intervals; the aim is to have five doses eventually. The current European schedules can be found at http://www.euvac.net/graphics/euvac/index.html.
• Boosters are recommended for travellers to countries where diphtheria is endemic or epidemic, and for laboratory and clinical infectious staff.

Surveillance

• The disease is notifiable throughout the EU, and since March 2010 co-ordination of European surveillance activities is undertaken by the European Centre for Disease Prevention and Control (ECDC).
• Report immediately to the public health authorities on suspicion.
• Laboratory reporting should specify whether the organism is a toxin producer.

Response to a case

• Secure confirmation from reference laboratory. The priority is to determine whether the strain is toxigenic; this can be done within a few hours by PCR.
• All cases must be assessed by a suitably experienced physician. Unless there is strong clinical suspicion, other control measures can await confirmation of toxigenicity.
• No control measures required for infections due to non-toxigenic strains.
• For confirmed or strongly suspected toxigenic infections, action is outlined below for case and contacts.

Measures for the case

• Arrange strict barrier nursing until microbiological clearance has been demonstrated (minimum two negative nose and throat swabs, at least 24 hours apart, the first at least 24 hours after stopping antibiotics).
• Secure microbiological clearance with a 7-day course of erythromycin (or other macrolide antibiotic) or parenteral penicillin. Give a booster or primary vaccination course (depending on vaccination status). The effects of diphtheria toxin are irreversible, so early diagnosis and treatment with antitoxin is vital. It is important to know how to access supplies of diphtheria antitoxin, including out of hours.

Measures for close contacts

• Close contacts include household and kissing contacts; this may be extended further (e.g. to school contacts) if many of these less close contacts are unvaccinated.
• Obtain swabs from nose and throat, and any skin lesions, for culture.
• Monitor for 7 days from last contact with case (daily measurement of temperature and examination of throat).
• Exclude food handlers and those with close contact with unvaccinated children from work until all swabs shown to be negative.
• Give a 7-day course of erythromycin (or other macrolide antibiotic).
• Obtain further nose and throat swabs after course of antibiotics, and repeat course if still positive.
• Give a booster or primary vaccination course (depending on vaccination status). Current WHO guidance for Europe recommends a booster for contacts if more than 12 months have elapsed since the last dose.
• Infections due to toxigenic *C. ulcerans* should be treated the same as *C. diphtheriae*, as there is some evidence that person-to-person transmission may occur.
• No public health action is required for infections due to non-toxigenic *C. diphtheriae*, although the patient should be treated with penicillin or erythromycin if symptomatic.

Investigation of a cluster

Obtain travel history or links to travellers.

Response to an outbreak

As for an individual case, but in addition consider the need for a community-wide vaccination programme.

Suggested case-definition for an outbreak
Laboratory evidence of infection due to toxigenic *C. diphtheriae* or *C. ulcerans*, in a patient with compatible symptoms. Sore throat only in a vaccinated individual is a compatible symptom.

3.23 Encephalitis, acute

Suggested on-call action

The causes of acute encephalitis are unlikely to cause outbreaks and do not require public health action unless rabies is suspected.

Acute encephalitis is inflammation of the brain, caused by a variety of viruses. The most common cause in Europe is herpes simplex type 1, which is a severe infection mainly affecting adults; the case fatality rate may be as high as 70%. The incidence of acute encephalitis in Western countries is estimated to be 10.5 per 100,000 in children and 2.2 per 100,000 in adults.

Herpes simplex encephalitis is intrinsically acquired, so no public health action is required.

Tick-borne encephalitis (see Chapter 3.77) occurs in many European countries, and there are several mosquito-borne encephalitides in the USA. Other causes of acute encephalitis are Japanese B encephalitis (see Chapter 3.41), West Nile Virus (see Chapter 3.87) and rabies (Chapter 3.62). Encephalitis also occurs as an acute complication of measles and chickenpox.

3.24 Enterococci, including glycopeptide-resistant enterococci

Enterococci, including the species *Enterococcus faecalis* and *Enterococcus faecium*, are normally present in the gastrointestinal tract. They are of low virulence but can cause a range of infections in immunocompromised hospital patients, including wound infection, urinary tract infection, septicaemia and endocarditis. Enterococci may also colonise open wounds and skin ulcers. Enterococci readily become resistant to antibiotics. By the mid-1980s resistance to commonly used antibiotics was widespread, leaving only glycopeptides (vancomycin and teicoplanin) available for treatment. In 1987, vancomycin-resistant enterococci (VRE) were reported and have since spread to many hospitals. Vancomycin resistance may be coded by transferable plasmids and there is concern that it may transfer to other more pathogenic bacteria. Transfer to methicillin-resistant *Staphylococcus aureus* (MRSA) has been reported.

Suggested on-call action

The local health protection team should be prepared to assist the infection control doctor to investigate and control nosocomial outbreaks of glycopeptide-resistant enterococci (GRE).

Epidemiology

In EU countries, hospitals take part in the Hospitals in Europe Link for Infection Control through Surveillance (HELICS) network's surveillance of nosocomial infections in intensive care units (ICUs). The proportion of ICU bacteraemias that are caused by *Enterococcus* spp. varies from 20% in Romania, 16% in Germany, 5.6% in Italy to 0% in Slovakia. In England, Wales and Northern Ireland, bloodstream infections caused by *Enterococcus* spp. fell from a peak of 7628 in 2006 to 6155 in 2008. In England, there has been mandatory reporting of bacteraemias caused by GRE since 2003. Numbers peaked at 911 in 2007 but declined to 559 in 2009. There are different strains of GRE and hospital outbreaks have been reported from dialysis, transplant, haematology and ICUs.

Clinical features

Enterococcal infection should be suspected in any case of sepsis in critically ill hospitalised patients, particularly those with severe underlying disease. GRE bacteraemias may be associated with a poorer clinical prognosis than non-GRE bacteraemia.

Laboratory confirmation

Appropriate microbiological investigation is essential to identify accurately enterococci and detect glycopeptide resistance. Enterococci are often detected in mixed culture where the clinical significance is unclear. Typing of strains is available.

Transmission

• The lower gastrointestinal tract is the main reservoir: most infection is endogenous.
• Spread can occur from infected or colonised patients, either directly or indirectly via the hands of medical and nursing staff, contaminated equipment or environmental surfaces.
• Animal strains of GRE may colonise the gastrointestinal tract of humans via contaminated food.

Acquisition

• Most infection is endogenous.
• Stool carriage may persist for months or years.
• Risk factors include prior antibiotic therapy (glycopeptides or cephalosporins), prolonged hospital stay, admission to ICU or other specialist units.

Prevention

• Prudent use of antibiotics in medical and veterinary practice.
• Prompt diagnosis of GRE by the microbiology laboratory (routine screening for vancomycin resistance among clinical isolates). Heightened awareness in those who have received medical care overseas.

• Implementation of appropriate control of infection measures (standard precautions and source isolation).
• Selective screening for VRE in ICUs, etc.
• Periodic antibiotic sensitivity surveys.

Surveillance

Cases should be reported to national surveillance schemes and isolates may be submitted to the appropriate Antibiotic Reference Unit.

Response to a case

• Treatment is with a combination of antibiotics guided by sensitivity testing (colonisation is more frequent than infection).
• Removal of catheters and drainage of abscesses may be necessary.
• Attempted clearance of carriage by oral therapy is usually unsuccessful and is not recommended.
• Screening staff for stool carriage is of no value.
• Emphasise hand hygiene and ward cleaning.
• Implement infection control measures based on clinical risk assessment.
• Patients with GRE (especially where there is diarrhoea or incontinence) should be isolated in single rooms or cohort nursed in bays on the open ward.
• When a patient with GRE is transferred to another institution, inform clinical and infection control staff.

Investigation of a cluster

Isolates from both infected and colonised patients should be typed: hospital outbreaks can involve a single strain whereas community strains are usually of multiple types.

Control of an outbreak

• Reinforce measures for a single case.

• Screening to identify colonised patients (faecal sample most useful screening specimen).

Suggested case-definition

Cases are defined microbiologically, based on the results of culture and antibiotic sensitivity.

3.25 Epstein–Barr virus

Epstein–Barr virus (EBV), also known as human herpesvirus 4 (HHV-4), a member of the herpesvirus family, is the cause of infectious mononucleosis (glandular fever). EBV is also associated with Burkitt's lymphoma in African patients, and other neoplasias.

Suggested on-call action

Not generally applicable.

Epidemiology

In countries where there is overcrowding and poor hygiene, 90% of children have serological evidence of EBV infection by the age of 2 years. In developed countries, infection is delayed until adolescence and early adult life.

Clinical features

The clinical features of infectious mononucleosis are fever, tonsillitis, lymphadenopathy, splenomegaly and hepatitis. Treatment with ampicillin leads to a temporary erythematous maculopapular skin rash. Young children generally have a mild non-specific illness.

Laboratory confirmation

Diagnosis is confirmed by the finding of atypical mononuclear cells in the peripheral blood. Heterophile antibody tests such as the Paul–Bunnell or Monospot tests are often used as first line tests. Tests for IgM and IgG to EBV viral capsid antigen and tests for EBV nuclear antigen are also available.

Transmission

Most cases are spread from asymptomatic carriers by oro-pharyngeal route as a result of contact with saliva, either directly during kissing or indirectly on hands or fomites. Attack rates may be as high as 50%. EBV can also be spread in blood transfusions.

Acquisition

The incubation period is 4–6 weeks. After recovery a person may remain infectious for several months because EBV persists in the lymphoid tissue of the oropharynx and is excreted in saliva. Lifelong immunity follows infection, although latent infection can reactivate.

Prevention

Health education and hygienic measures where practical may reduce exposure to saliva, especially from infected persons.

Surveillance

Reporting of cases is not generally required.

Response to a case

Exclusion of cases is not necessary. Splenic enlargement is common in infectious mononucleosis and spontaneous splenic rupture is a rare, potentially fatal complication occurring in 0.1–0.5% of patients. Although evidence is lacking, it is prudent to recommend that strenuous physical exercise is avoided for 3–4 weeks after the onset of illness and that contact sports are avoided until there is no evidence of splenomegaly.

3.26 *Escherichia coli* O157 (and other *E. coli* gastroenteritis)

Many different strains of *Escherichia coli* are associated with gastrointestinal illness, which can be classified into seven main syndromes. The most serious illness is that caused by verocytotoxic *E. coli* (VTEC), also known as enterohaemorrhagic *E. coli* (EHEC) or Shiga toxin producing *E. coli* (SHEC), although the terms are not strictly synonymous), which has the potential to cause haemolytic uraemic syndrome (HUS) (the most common cause of acute renal failure in children) and death. The other syndromes are summarised in Table 3.26.1.

The most common VTEC strain in most European countries is *E. coli* O157:H7 (others are given in Box 3.26.1). It may be food-borne and can cause large outbreaks with the potential for secondary spread.

Suggested on-call action

If *E. coli* O157 or other VTEC:
• Exclude if in high-risk group (Table 2.2.1).
• If other cases known to you or reporting clinician or laboratory, implement outbreak plan.
• If no other cases are known, ensure risk factor details are collected on the next working day at the latest.
If other *E. coli* gastroenteritis: exclude if in high-risk group (Table 2.2.1).

Epidemiology

The reported incidence of VTEC infection in Europe is 0.7 per 100,000 population per year, although many additional cases are likely to not be identified by surveillance systems. Much higher rates are recorded in Ireland, Sweden, Denmark and the UK. The highest reported incidence is seen in children under 5 years, with little gender difference. VTEC infections tend to increase in the summer, with a peak in September (Figure 2.2.2). Incidence may be higher in rural areas.

Most cases are sporadic. Outbreaks may affect communities (often via food vehicles), nurseries/daycare centres, schools, restaurants, nursing homes, hospitals, open farms, campsites and swimming pools/lakes. In 2011 a large outbreak took place in Northern Germany with more than 4000 reported cases. In some countries, a significant proportion is associated with foreign travel.

HUS has an incidence of about 8 per 100,000 children under 5 years, of which 90% are 'typical' (diarrhoea-associated; Box 3.26.1).

Clinical features

Infection with *E. coli* O157 may cause no symptoms; a diarrhoeal illness, often accompanied by abdominal cramps; haemorrhagic colitis with bloody diarrhoea and severe abdominal pain, often without fever; HUS with renal failure, haemolytic anaemia and thrombocytopaenia, particularly in children; and thrombocytopaenic purpura, particularly in adults, which may add neurological complications to the features of HUS. About one-third of diagnosed cases are admitted to hospital.

HUS may occur 2–14 days after the onset of diarrhoea (usually 5–10 days). It affects 2–8% of all reported cases, although it may be higher in young children. VTEC, especially *E. coli* O157:H7 is the most common cause of HUS and causes the more common glomerular ('typical') form of the disease (Box 3.26.1). The case fatality rate of severe

Table 3.26.1 *E. coli* causing diarrhoea (other than VTEC)

Designation	Epidemiology	Illness	Incubation	Sources	Main 'O' serogroups
Enteropathogenic (EPEC)	Sporadic cases and outbreaks in children, usually aged less than 2 years, especially in developing countries Outbreaks reported in schools, neonatal units, food premises, hotels	Watery diarrhoea, abdominal pain, nausea, vomiting and fever Fatigue, myalgia or headache may occur. Duration 6 hours to 4 days (but diarrhoea may be prolonged)	2–73 hours (median 8–18 hours)	Faeco-oral, e.g. via fomites and hands in nurseries and hospitals Cases excrete for up to 2 weeks, but infectious dose fairly high Contaminated infant foods in developing countries	18, 25, 26, 44, 55, 86, 111, 114, 119, 125, 126, 127, 128ab, 142, 158, 608
Enterotoxigenic (ETEC)	Major cause of traveller's diarrhoea Dehydrating diarrhoea in children in developing countries Outbreaks associated with restaurants/caterers	Watery diarrhoea and abdominal pain. Headache, fatigue, nausea, anorexia, vomiting or fever may occur Average duration 6 days	1–166 hours (median 10–50 hours)	Food and water contaminated by humans. Nosocomial outbreaks reported Cases excrete for up to 7 days, but infectious dose high	6, 8, 11, 15, 20, 25, 27, 63, 78, 80, 85, 114, 115, 128ac, 148, 149, 153, 159, 167, 173
Enteroinvasive (EIEC)	Occasional cause of traveller's diarrhoea or outbreaks in developed countries. Serious infection common in children in developing world	Watery diarrhoea, often with blood and mucus Abdominal pain, fever Lasts up to 2 weeks	1–156 hours (mean 35 hours)	Contaminated food Probable human reservoir Infectious dose probably high	28ac, 29, 52, 112ac, 115, 124, 136, 143, 144, 145, 147, 152, 159, 164, 167

Enteroaggregative (EAggEC)	Common in developing countries (inc. Indian subcontinent) and a risk for travellers. Children more commonly affected. Outbreaks reported in Europe (schools, neonatal units, restaurants, hotels)	Diarrhoea, usually watery, often prolonged. May be blood or mucus, abdominal pain, low grade fever, nausea or vomiting. Often chronic in children or AIDS	8–18 hours (possibly longer)	Contaminated food and possibly water. Infectious dose probably high	3, 15, 19, 44, 62, 73, 77, 86, 98, 111, 113, 127, 134
Diffuse-adherence (DAEC) or Diarrhoea-associated haemolytic (DHEC)	Preschool children in developing countries	Diarrhoea (mucoid and watery). Fever, vomiting. Lasts about 8 days	Unclear	Probably food. Infectious dose may be lower	–
Cytolethal distending toxin-producing (CDT-producing)	Importance as yet unclear	Diarrhoea	Unclear	Unclear	–

Control:
- Enteric precautions for cases, personal hygiene.
- Exclude risk groups until 48 hours after first normal stool.
- Advice to travellers abroad.
- Good food hygiene and safe water.
- Handwashing and environmental cleaning in nurseries.

Box 3.26.1 Causes of haemolytic uraemic syndrome

Typical ('post-diarrhoeal', 'epidemic', 'D+'):
- *E. coli* O157:H7 and O157:H
- Other *E. coli* (e.g. O26, O55, O91, O103, O104, O111, O113, O116, O119, O128, O130, O145, O157)
- Viruses (e.g. coxsackie)
- *Shigella* dysentery
- *Campylobacter*
- *Streptococcus pneumoniae*
- Influenza

Atypical ('sporadic', 'D–'):
- Inherited disorders
- Systemic lupus erythematosus
- Cancer
- Drugs (e.g. mitomycin C, ciclosporin, quinine, crack cocaine)
- Pregnancy
- Oral contraceptives
- Idiopathic

---

infection (HUS or thrombotic thrombocytopaenic purpura (TTP)) is reported as 3–17%. Mortality may be particularly high in outbreaks affecting elderly care patients.

Laboratory confirmation

Diagnosis is usually based on stool culture and is more likely to be successful if specimens are obtained within 4 days of onset of symptoms. Most *E. coli* O157 differ from other *E. coli* in not fermenting sorbitol, although VTEC infection due to sorbitol fermenting strains of O157 have been reported and non-O157 VTEC strains commonly ferment sorbitol.

VTEC strains produce one or both of two verocytotoxins (VT1 and VT2): tests for these toxins are available at reference laboratories and can help identify non-O157 VTEC strains. Phage typing and genotyping may be available from reference laboratories to aid epidemiological investigations. Serology can be used for retrospective diagnosis, and salivary testing is also possible.

Methods exist for examining food, water, environmental and animal samples for *E. coli* O157.

Transmission

The natural reservoir of *E. coli* O157 is the gastrointestinal tract of animals, particularly cattle, but also sheep, goats, deer, horses, dogs, birds and flies. Humans are infected via the following routes:
- Contaminated foods: the most commonly reported food vehicle is beef, particularly ground beef dishes such as beefburgers, followed by salad/fruit produce, such as lettuce, spinach, melon and apple juice. Dairy products and other foods have also been reported as vehicles of infection. Infection may result from inadequate cooking of already contaminated food (e.g. beefburgers), or from cross-contamination of food that will be eaten raw, such as cold cooked meats or salad. The organism is relatively resistant to acid, fermentation and drying.
- Direct contact with animals (e.g. at farm visitor centres). Excreting animals are usually asymptomatic. Soil and water contaminated by animal faeces has led to outbreaks in campers and is also linked to sporadic infection.
- Secondary faeco-oral spread from infected cases is common, particularly in families and institutions with children under 5 years

old, with attack rates of 20–38% reported in nursery outbreaks. Asymptomatic excretion is common in family contacts of cases.

• Drinking and bathing in contaminated waters have been linked with incidents of infection.

• Nursing and laboratory staff have acquired infection through occupational exposure.

Acquisition

The incubation period ranges from 6 hours to 10 days, although 2–4 days is most common. The incubation period may depend on the number of organisms ingested.

Patients can excrete the organism in the faeces for 2–62 days, with reported median excretion periods ranging 5–29 days. Excretion may be intermittent or prolonged and excreters commonly have at least 10^6 viable organisms per gram of stool. The infectious dose is low (possibly less than 100 organisms), so patients are presumed to be potentially infectious as long as the organism can be detected in the faeces. Microbiological clearance is usually viewed as two consecutive negative faecal samples, taken at least 24 hours apart.

Immunity is thought to develop following exposure to *E. coli* O157.

Prevention

• Minimise contamination of carcasses at slaughter.

• Adopt the hazard analysis critical control point (HACCP) approach in both food processing and food service industries to prevent survival of or contamination by *E. coli* O157.

• Good kitchen practices including separation of raw and cooked foods to avoid cross-contamination, washing of fruit and vegetables and storage of foods below 10°C.

• Cook beef, lamb and other meat products so that any contaminating organisms are subjected to minimum of 70°C for 2 minutes. Cook beefburgers until juices run clear and no pink bits remain inside.

• Pasteurisation of milk and dairy products.

• Handwashing is effective at reducing the risk of gastroenteritis from many organisms and has been shown to be effective for *E. coli* O157. Antibacterial soap may increase the effectiveness of handwashing.

• Adequate hygiene and toilet facilities in nurseries, schools and healthcare premises. Routine disinfectants are effective against *E. coli* O157. Supervised handwashing in nurseries and infant schools.

• Precautions during farm visits by children, including:

(a) handwashing after touching animals;

(b) avoid eating and drinking whilst visiting animals;

(c) keep face away from animals;

(d) do not put hand to mouth;

(e) do not touch animal droppings; and

(f) clean shoes after visit.

• Keep animals off fields for 3 weeks before allowing their use for recreation.

• Protection and treatment of drinking water supplies.

• Good hygiene practices at public swimming pools.

Surveillance

• All cases of infectious bloody diarrhoea or HUS should be reported to the local public health authority as a matter of urgency.

• All isolates of VTEC should be reported to local public health authorities and national surveillance systems: statutorily notifiable in most EU countries.

• Laboratories should test all samples from cases of diarrhoea or bloody stools for *E. coli* O157 and should report provisional isolates (and send for confirmation and typing).

Response to a case

The severity of disease, particularly in children and the elderly, the small infectious dose and the ability to spread person to person and via contaminated food means that even single cases require prompt investigation and control.

• Enteric precautions during diarrhoeal phase.

• Adequate fluid and electrolyte replacement and monitoring for the development of HUS. Antimotility agents are usually not recommended. Referral to hospital if complications such as bloody diarrhoea occur.

• The use of antibiotics in the treatment of *E. coli* O157 is not usually recommended. There is no evidence that antibiotics reduce the duration of infection, diarrhoea or bloody diarrhoea. There is some evidence that quinolones and fosfomycin may prevent the development of HUS or TTP, but there are also studies that suggest that antibiotics, particularly (but not exclusively) co-trimoxazole, may increase the risk of HUS/TTP and even increase mortality. At the time of writing more studies are required before antibiotics can be routinely recommended.

• Report to public health authorities: compulsorily notifiable in most European countries.

• Hygiene advice should be given to cases and contacts, particularly on handwashing. Suggest remaining off work/school until normal stools for 48 hours for those in non-high-risk groups.

• If case is in a high-risk group for further transmission (Box 2.2.1) exclude from work or nursery until asymptomatic and two consecutive negative faecal specimens taken at least 24 hours apart.

• Cases in infant school children may be considered as risk group 4 (Box 2.2.1) and may also be excluded until microbiological clearance.

• Household contacts in high-risk groups to be screened. Exclude those in all high-risk groups (Box 2.2.1) until two negative faecal specimens obtained from the contact and, for risk groups 3 and 4 only, until the index case becomes asymptomatic.

• Detailed history from all cases for all 10 days before onset, covering food, water, animal contact, farms, swimming, nursery/school, other institutions and travel. Compare with previous cases. Potential sources of infection should receive follow up appropriate to the risk.

Investigation of a cluster

• Organise phage typing, toxin typing and genotyping with reference laboratory.

• Undertake hypothesis-generating study to cover all food and water consumed in 10 days before the onset of illness, and all social, school and work activities and visits undertaken. Include exposure to farm animals, pets and cases of gastroenteritis. Ask specifically about minced beef or lamb products, cooked meats and milk. Trace common foods back to source.

• Investigation of social networks may reveal potential for person-to-person spread via common (possibly asymptomatic) contacts.

Control of an outbreak

An outbreak of VTEC is a public health emergency and requires a prompt and thorough response. Particular actions include the following:

• Hygiene advice to all cases and contacts.

• Exclude cases as detailed above.

• Enhanced cleaning in all institutional outbreaks.

• Supervised handwashing for children in affected nurseries and infant schools.

• Exclude all cases of diarrhoea from affected (non-residential) institutions, until normal stools and two consecutive negative samples taken at least 24 hours apart received.

• In daycare establishments for children under 5 years (high risk of HUS and poor hygiene) screen all attenders. Exclude all positives until microbiological clearance is achieved. Adopt a similar approach for confused or faecally incontinent elderly attending daycare facilities.

• In residential accommodation for children under 5 years or the elderly, screen all residents. Maintain enteric precautions for all positives until microbiological clearance is achieved. Preferably nurse in a private room with own washbasin and exclusive use of one toilet whilst diarrhoea continues.

• Institute *urgent* withdrawal of any implicated food. If a local supplier is involved,

ensure personally that this is done. If national or regionally distributed food, contact the relevant government department (e.g. Food Standards Agency in the UK).
• Issue 'boil water notice' for contaminated drinking water.
• Ensure adequate precautions are taken at any implicated farm open to the public, including restricting access to animals whilst appropriate control measures are implemented (HSE guidance available in UK).
• Monitor cases at increased risk of HUS or TTP to ensure prompt referral.
• Antibiotic prophylaxis is not generally recommended.

Suggested case-definition for an outbreak

Confirmed: diarrhoea with demonstration of *E. coli* O157 of outbreak strain in stools.
Presumptive: HUS occurring after diarrhoea with no other cause identified.
Clinical: diarrhoea in person epidemiologically linked to outbreak (e.g. onset within 9 days of consuming vehicle) with further investigations awaited.

3.27 Giardiasis

Giardia lamblia, also known as *Giardia intestinalis* or *Giardia duodenalis*, is a protozoan parasite that causes intestinal infection throughout the world. In developed countries the illness is particularly associated with waterborne outbreaks, nurseries and other institutions, and travel abroad.

Suggested on-call action

• Exclude symptomatic cases in risk groups.
• If linked cases, consult outbreak control plan.

Epidemiology

Prevalence rates (including asymptomatic excretion) of 2–7% have been demonstrated in developed countries. A study in England and Wales found only about one-fifth of cases were reported to national surveillance. The annual rate for reported cases in most of Europe is about 5 per 100,000, with much higher rates in Romania. Children under 5 years have the highest incidence. Cases occur throughout the year, with small peaks in spring and autumn. Refugees, residents of institutions, travellers abroad and men who have sex with men are reported to be at higher risk.

Clinical features

About one-quarter of acute infections are asymptomatic excretors. Symptomatic diarrhoea may be accompanied by malaise, flatulence, foul-smelling greasy stools, abdominal cramps, bloating, nausea, anorexia and weight loss. Prolonged diarrhoea, malabsorption and weight loss may be particularly suggestive of giardiasis. The duration of illness is variable, with a range of 1–90 days reported (average 2–3 weeks).

Laboratory confirmation

Giardia infection is usually confirmed by microbiological examination of fresh stool samples for cysts. A single stool sample will identify only about 60% of those infected but three samples (preferably taken on non-consecutive days) will identify over 90%. Cysts may not yet be present at the onset of disease. Antigen assays are reported to be highly sensitive and specific, although they are not yet universally available. They may have a role in cohort screening during outbreaks.

Transmission

Giardiasis results from faeco-oral transmission of *Giardia* cysts. This can occur directly or via food or water. Humans appear to be the main source for *G. lamblia* infection in other humans, although zoonotic transmission does occur. *Giardia* cysts are environmentally resistant and survive well in cold water. Water-borne transmission appears to be the most common route through faecal contamination of recreational or drinking water. Direct person-to-person spread is the other main route, particularly in children, both in families and nurseries. Outbreaks are also reported from nursing homes and daycare centres. Food-borne outbreaks, often linked to infected food handlers, occur, but are not common.

Acquisition

The incubation period is usually 5–16 days (median 7–10 days), but extremes of 1–28 days have been reported. Although average duration of excretion is about 2 weeks, it may persist for up to 6 months and may be intermittent. The exact risk from asymptomatic excretors is unclear, but as few as 10 cysts may cause infection (although 100–10,000 cysts are usually needed). Breastfeeding has a protective effect; there is increased susceptibility in those with reduced immunity or gastric acidity.

Prevention

Prevention of giardiasis is dependent on:
• Adequate treatment of water supplies: standard chlorination is not sufficient to destroy cysts and should be supplemented by filtration, flocculation or sedimentation.
• Adequate control of infection and food hygiene practices in institutions, especially those dealing with children.
• Handwashing after toilet use and before preparing food.
• Advice to travellers abroad on safe food and water.

Surveillance

Diagnosed cases should be reported to public health authorities. Notification is compulsory in many EU countries.

Response to a case

• Hygiene advice should be given. Ideally, the case should not attend work or school until he/she has normal stools.
• Cases in risk groups 1–4 (Table 2.2.1) should be excluded until 48 hours after the first normal stool. Microbiological clearance is not necessary before return. Schoolchildren should ideally not attend school until they have had no diarrhoea for 24 hours.
• Treatment of symptomatic cases. Metronidazole for 5 days or single dose tinidazole are both effective.
• Enteric precautions for cases in hospitals and care homes.
• Screening of symptomatic household contacts may identify individuals needing treatment.

Investigation of a cluster

Enquiries should include water consumption (compare to water supply zones), food sources, swimming pools or other recreational water, contact with day centres (especially for children) or other institutions, travel and (if cases mainly adult men) sexual contact.

Control of an outbreak

• Water-borne outbreaks are usually due to use of untreated surface water, inadequate water treatment (e.g. ineffective filtration) or sewage contamination. Geographic mapping of cases can help the local water company identify areas for further investigation.
• Outbreaks in nurseries and other institutions are controlled by enhanced infection

control, especially supervised handwashing for all children, and exclusion and treatment of all symptomatic children. Some would also recommend treatment of asymptomatic carriers: while this will help control the outbreak and prevent spread to community and family contacts, the benefit to the asymptomatic individual is unclear.

Suggested case-definition for an outbreak

Demonstration of cysts plus:
• Diarrhoea; *or*
• Three from bloating/flatulence, abdominal cramps, weight loss, nausea, smelly stools and fatigue; *or*
• Common exposure with acute cases (outside of family).

3.28 Gonorrhoea, syphilis and other acute STIs

Sexually transmitted infections (STIs) are defined by their route of transmission: they are transmitted by direct sexual contact. For HIV infection, see Chapter 3.39 and for genital *Chlamydia* infection, see Chapter 3.12.

Suggested on-call action

On-call action is rarely required; however, the public health team may be alerted to clusters of cases of STI (e.g. syphilis or gonorrhoea) and should be prepared to initiate or assist with an investigation.

Epidemiology

In recent years in the UK, annual total diagnoses of STIs have increased. Similar increases

have been seen in other Western European countries and there have been large increases in Eastern Europe and countries of the former Soviet Union. There is evidence of a substantial burden of STI morbidity, particularly among men who have sex with men, young men and women, those of black ethnic origin and those living in urban areas. More detail is given in Table 3.28.1.

Diagnosis

See Table 2.7.1.

Transmission

STIs are spread by direct, usually sexual, contact with infectious discharges or lesions. Syphilis may also be spread *in utero* and via blood transfusions.

Acquisition

Incubation periods vary (see Chapter 2.7).

Prevention

The prevention of STIs depends on the following:
• Health and sex education to discourage multiple sexual partners and casual sexual activity and to promote correct and consistent use of condoms.
• Early detection of cases and prompt effective treatment.
• Identification, examination and treatment of the sexual partners of cases.
• Opportunistic or routine screening and treatment of certain subgroups of the population who may be at increased risk of STIs or their complications. An example is the routine use of syphilis serological tests in pregnancy, to prevent congenital syphilis. Increasingly in the UK screening for gonorrhoea and *Chlamydia* is being promoted at genitourinary medicine (GUM) clinics and

Table 3.28.1 Epidemiology of acute STIs in England and Wales

Chlamydia infection	*Chlamydia* is the most frequently notified STI in Europe. The overall rate of 122.6 (per 100,000 population) conceals wide variations. For example, the rate in the UK is 201 while that in Belgium is 23. Notification rates are more likely to reflect screening practices and testing volume rather than true incidence. Sweden reported a rate of 517 and a 45% increase in the number of cases from 2006. This increase is due to new testing methods that are able to detect a new variant of *C. trachomatis.* An EU-wide survey revealed that the spread of this variant was restricted to Sweden or to Swedes' sexual partners in other countries.
	In the UK, genital chlamydial infection is the most frequently diagnosed STI. In 2009, there were 217,000 reports from GUM clinics and other community-based settings that screen for *Chlamydia,* a 7% rise compared with 2008 but double the number seen 10 years ago. The increase in *Chlamydia* diagnoses in recent years has been due in part to increased testing with more sensitive tests. In the UK, in 2009–2010, 22.1% of the 15- to 24-year-old population were tested for *Chlamydia* with 1,524,339 tests performed outside of GUM clinics by the NCSP.
Gonorrhoea	The gonorrhoea notification rate varies widely among European countries, ranging from less than one case (per 100,000) in Italy, Poland and Portugal to approximately 30 cases in Latvia and the UK. Variations in surveillance systems prevent meaningful comparisons.
	In the UK, gonorrhoea incidence peaked in 2002 but since then has fallen although in 2008–2009 new cases increased by 6% from 16,451 to 17,385. There is a disproportionately high incidence of gonorrhoea in young men and women, homosexual and bisexual men, those of Afro-Caribbean ethnic origin and those living in urban areas.
	In the UK, amongst gonococci there is widespread resistance to antimicrobial agents including ciprofloxacin, penicillin, tetracycline and azithromycin, particularly in isolates from MSM and persons who have acquired infections abroad. Cefixime or ceftriaxone are the treatment of choice for gonorrhoea. In 2009, in the UK 1.2% of gonococcal isolates demonstrated decreased susceptibility to cefixime and 0.3% to ceftriaxone. This highlights the need for prevention rather than treatment. In 2008–2009 resistance to ciprofloxacin increased from 28% to 35%. In 2009, no isolates were resistant to spectinomycin.
Infectious syphilis	Over the past 10 years, Western European countries experienced a rise in the rate of syphilis cases, first among MSM and then amongst sex workers, migrants and among heterosexual adults. In Central and Eastern Europe high rates of syphilis were seen in the early 1990s as a consequence of the socio-economic changes occurring at that time. Currently, in Europe there are wide variation in syphilis notification rates due to differences in national surveillance systems.
	Although relatively rare in the UK, there was a marked increase in syphilis in 1999–2005 but since then numbers have been stable and in 2008—2009 there was a fall of 1% from 3309 to 3273. The past increases and the recent falls have affected both MSM and heterosexual men and women. Syphilis (and gonorrhoea) may cluster geographically and may disproportionately affect certain population groups, notably black ethnic minorities and MSM.
Genital herpes simplex virus infection	In the UK, cases of genital herpes have been rising gradually for many years. However, recent rises have been particularly marked and are due to the much greater use of sensitive molecular tests. In 2007–2008 diagnoses of first episode genital herpes at GUM clinics increased by 5% from 26,270 to 28,957. As infection is more commonly symptomatic in women, they consistently have a higher incidence than males.
Genital warts	Cases of genital warts cases reported from GUM clinics in UK have risen gradually in recent years. In 2008–2009 the number of new cases was unchanged at 91,000. The incidence is consistently higher in males than females.

GUM, genitourinary medicine; MSM, men who have sex with men; NCSP, National Chlamydia Screening Programme.

in other community settings exploiting non-invasive specimen collection and new molecular tests.

Surveillance

See Chapter 2.7.

Response to a case

• Individual cases of STIs are not generally reported to the local health protection team.
• The case should receive prompt effective treatment and should refrain from sexual intercourse until treated.
• Sexual contacts should be identified, examined and treated as appropriate.

Investigation of a cluster and control of an outbreak

An STI outbreak has been defined as:
• observed number of cases greater than expected over a defined time period in a particular setting;
• linked cases of STIs;
• the need for additional resources to manage the cases; and
• any case of congenitally acquired infection.

The underlying principles of outbreak investigation can be applied to outbreaks of STIs but there are some differences. STIs are often associated with a degree of stigma, confidentiality issues may restrict the availability of patient data and although patients and sexual contacts may be identified and treated relatively easily, effective control may require sustained behavioural change to reduce

Table 3.28.2 Managing STI outbreaks at local level

Identification	Increase in number of cases in local area
	Recognise potential outbreak
	Review local surveillance data
	Compare with national disease trends
	Confirm local increase
	Identify cases and contacts
	Descriptive epidemiology
	Describe those affected and possible source
Response	Discuss with colleagues
	Establish Outbreak Control Group
	Case finding
	Analytic epidemiology
	Microbiological investigation
	Further research
Secondary prevention	Partner notification
	Investigate networks
	Publicity campaigns to encourage those at risk to come forward for screening
	Alert local practitioners (GUM and general practice)
	Additional clinic sessions
Primary prevention	General health promotion campaigns
	Targeted health promotion campaigns
	Outreach work
Evaluate control measures	Monitor surveillance data
	Outbreak report
	Key lessons

GUM, genitourinary medicine.

spread in sexual networks. Compared with other outbreaks, STI outbreaks will usually take longer to investigate and control.

The management of STI outbreaks requires a multiagency approach involving the GUM physician, sexual health advisers, health protection team, microbiologist and director of public health and sexual health lead at the local primary care trust. Ideally, these participants should meet at least annually and should draw up an STI outbreak contingency plan.

Guidelines on investigating STI outbreaks have been published at http://www.hpa.org.uk/web/HPAwebFile/HPAweb_C/121455300 2033 (accessed March 2010) (Table 3.28.2).

3.29 Hantavirus

Hantavirus infection is an acute zoonotic viral disease.

Suggested on-call action
None is usually required.

Epidemiology

Hantavirus infections are found where there is close contact between people and infected rodents. Regions especially affected include China, the Korean peninsula, Russia and Northern and Western Europe. In Europe, foci are recognised in the Balkans, the Ardennes and the Nordic countries. Sweden reported approximately 200 cases, Finland 1000, Germany more than 1500, Russia more than 10,000 cases annually and more than 1000 cases have been documented in the former Yugoslavia.

Clinical features

The clinical picture depends upon the subtype causing the infection and is characterised by haemorrhagic fever with renal syndrome (HFRS) or acute pulmonary oedema (hantavirus pulmonary symdrome (HPS)). HFRS manifests as fever, thrombocytopenia and acute renal failure, and HPS as fever with respiratory difficulty. A number of different subtypes exist, each of which is associated with a particular rodent species. Of the two European subtypes, Puumala tends to cause milder disease (nephropathia epidemica), but Dobrava HFRS is often severe (Table 3.29.1).

Laboratory confirmation

Specific antibodies (IgM or IgG) can be identified by enzyme-linked immunosorbent assay (ELISA) or indirect immunofluorescent antibody test (IFA). IgM is often present on hospitalisation. Polymerase chain reaction (PCR) for specific RNA may be available.

Transmission

Aerosol transmission from rodent excreta is common. Human-to-human transmission has been reported in South American (Andes virus) HPS.

Table 3.29.1 Main hantavirus serotypes

Syndrome	Serotype	Geography
HFRS	Dobrava	Balkans
	Puumala	Northern Europe
	Hantaan	Asia
	Seoul	Worldwide
HPS	Sin Nombre	North America
	Various other serotypes	North and South America

HFRS, haemorrhagic fever with renal syndrome; HPS, hantavirus pulmonary syndrome.

Acquisition

The incubation period is 1–6 weeks. The infectious period for HPS is unclear.

Prevention

In areas that are known to be endemic, rodents should be excluded from living quarters.

Response to a case

• HFRS is not transmitted person to person and there is no need for urgent public health action.
• In view of the possibility of person-to-person spread in HPS, suspected cases should be nursed in isolation.

Suggested case-definition
HFRS or HPS is confirmed by IgM or PCR.

3.30 Head lice

Head lice (*Pediculus humanus capitis*) are wingless insects that live close to the scalp where they feed on blood. The female head louse lives for approximately 1 month and lays 50–150 eggs during her lifetime. The eggs are tear-shaped, 1 mm in length and are securely glued to the hair shaft close to the scalp. The eggs hatch after 7–12 days and the emerging nymphs moult three times before reaching maturity in 9–12 days when mating occurs. The full-grown louse is 2–3 mm long. Empty egg sacks (nits) are white and shiny, and may be found some distance from the scalp as the

hair grows out. Although there may be a large number of lice on an affected head, the average number is about 10.

Suggested on-call action
Not generally applicable.

Epidemiology

Data from surveys amongst children in the UK suggest a point prevalence of 4–8%. According to UK GPs, the mean weekly incidence of head lice has declined steadily from 4.9 per 100,000 population in 2000 to 1.46 in 2009. Anyone with head hair can get head lice but children aged 3–12 years are particularly affected.

Clinical features

Head lice infestation is associated with little morbidity but causes high levels of anxiety amongst parents. Many early infestations are asymptomatic. Itching and scratching of the scalp may occur after 4–6 weeks due to sensitisation to head lice excretions and secondary bacterial infection may occur.

Laboratory confirmation

Diagnosis depends on finding live lice on the head. Empty eggshells (nits) are not proof of active infestation. Lice move rapidly away from any disturbance, and examination of dry hair is unreliable. Lice can only be reliably detected by combing wet lubricated hair with a 'detector' comb. If lice are present they fall out or are stuck to the comb. If necessary, lice and nymphs can be examined with a magnifying glass or low-power microscope to confirm their presence.

Transmission and acquisition

Transmission is by direct contact with the head of an affected person. Lice cannot jump or fly but move readily through dry hair and cross from person to person when heads touch. Transmission occurs in schools, at home and in the wider community. Indirect spread when personal items are shared is possible, but head lice do not survive for more than 48 hours away from the scalp. A person will remain infectious for as long as there are adult lice on the head and re-infestation may occur. Humans are the only source of head lice, which are host-specific and do not spread from or to animals.

Prevention

• It is probably impossible to completely prevent head lice infestation.
• A number of preventative measures have been promoted including repellents such as piperonal, regular brushing and electronic combs, but evidence for their effectiveness is lacking.
• Reducing head lice infestation depends on case finding by regular diagnostic wet combing followed by prompt treatment of cases if active infestation is found.
• Contacts of cases must also be examined and treated if appropriate.

Surveillance

• Pharmaceutical data may provide some insight into pediculocide prescribing patterns.
• If head lice are causing particular problems in community settings, such as schools, the local public health team should be informed.

Response to a case

• There are three main methods of treatment (Box 3.30.1).
• The role of other agents such as 'natural' products and flammable or toxic substances is unclear.
• No treatment method is 100% effective. In one study the overall cure rate for wet combing was 38% compared with 78% for malathion lotion.
• Treatment may fail because of misdiagnosis, non-compliance, re-infestation, pediculocide resistance or use of an ineffective preparation.
• Contacts of a case should be examined for head lice by wet combing and treated if necessary.
• It is not necessary to exclude children with head lice from school or nursery (Table 3.30.1).

Investigation of a cluster

• Clusters of cases of head lice may be reported from schools or other institutional settings.

Box 3.30.1 Treatment of head lice

• *Chemical pediculocides.* A number of chemical pediculocides are available including carbaryl, malathion and the pyrethroids (permethrin and phenothrin). Lotions and liquids are preferred and contact time should be 12 hours. A single application may not kill unhatched eggs and a second application is advised after 7 days. After treatment, wet combing should be carried out to check for lice. Pediculocides should only be used if live lice are confirmed and should never be used prophylactically.
• *Occlusive agents.* These agents suffocate lice by obstructing their respiratory spiracles. In some trials 4% dimethicone lotion has proved effective.
• *Mechanical removal.* Lice and larvae as they hatch can be mechanically removed by wet combing well lubricated hair with a detector comb every 4 days for 2 weeks. This process, which must be carried out meticulously, breaks the life cycle of the head louse.

Table 3.30.1 Head lice: suggested responsibilities

Parent	Brush or comb their children's hair each day
	Use detector comb to detect infestation
	Ensure recommended treatment has been carried out
Health visitor and school health nurse	Education of parents about head lice
	In case of outbreaks in schools and nurseries ensure policy is being correctly followed
	Advise families with recurrent problems and consider further measures
Head teacher	Agree a written policy on the management of head lice with the school nurse and public health team
	Publicise this policy to parents, pupils, staff and others
	Children who are found to have head lice should be managed confidentially by the school health nurse
	There is no need to exclude children from school because of head lice
	Letters to parent alerting them to head lice in school may be used
Specialist health protection staff and Community Infection Control Nurse	Receive reports of particular head lice problems in community settings and advise on management
	Involve other carers, such as community nurses, GPs and teachers as appropriate
	Make available information on head lice for the public and professionals
GP and practice staff	Explain the use of a detection comb and wet combing to confirm active infestation
	Discuss treatment options
	Make available patient information leaflet
	Prescribe pediculocides when appropriate; only those with confirmed infestations should be treated
Pharmacist	Explain the use of a detection comb and wet combing to confirm active infestation
	Discuss treatment options
	Offer for sale wet combing materials including detector combs or pediculocides as appropriate
	Pediculocide formulated as shampoos should not be offered for sale
	Patient information leaflet should be provided with all prescriptions and sales of head lice treatment

• The school health nurse is usually the most appropriate person to investigate and advise on control measures.

Control of an outbreak

• Parents may be alerted and asked to carry out case finding by wet combing.
• They should be advised to treat their child promptly if live lice are discovered, using one of the two treatment options.
• Accurate information, explanation and sympathetic reassurance will be required.

3.31 *Helicobacter pylori*

Helicobacter pylori causes a chronic infection associated with chronic upper gastrointestinal disease.

Epidemiology

Infection occurs worldwide. Prevalence in developed countries is 20–50% (up to 75% in socially deprived areas) and, in general, increases with age, with acquisition rates higher in children. However, there is also a cohort effect of decreasing incidence with time.

Despite high rates of infection in certain areas of the world, the overall frequency of infection is declining.

Diagnosis

Most infection is asymptomatic, but it may cause gastritis and both gastric and duodenal ulceration. Infection is also associated with gastric adenocarcinoma. The annual incidence of peptic ulcer disease is 0.2% and over 90% of these patients will have *H. pylori* infection. Diagnosis is by serology, breath testing with urea, culture from gastric biopsy/aspirate, or antigen testing of faeces. Treatment is with a mix of antibiotics and antisecretory drugs.

Transmission and acquisition

Transmission is unclear but probably by ingestion of organisms, most likely faeco-oral, but perhaps by oral–oral or gastro-oral routes. Spread via contaminated gastric tubes and endoscopes is recorded and endoscopists have increased risk. Infectivity is assumed to be lifelong and higher in those with achlorhydria.

Control

Other than routine hygiene and disinfection, there is insufficient evidence at present to recommend further preventative interventions. Eradication of infection is associated with remission of gastritis and peptic ulceration.

3.32 Hepatitis A

Hepatitis A virus (HAV) is an acute infection of the liver, which is primarily spread faeco-orally.

Suggested on-call action

- If a case is in a risk group for further transmission (Box 2.2.1), exclude from work or nursery.
- Exclude any contacts in risk groups who are known to be unwell.
- Refer household contacts for vaccination.
- If you or the referring clinician/ microbiologist are aware of potentially linked cases, refer to local outbreak plan.

Epidemiology

The incidence of hepatitis A has been decreasing in developed countries over the last 50 years. About 17,000 cases are reported each year in Europe (3.3 per 100,000). The incidence of HAV is lowest in Scandinavia, higher in Mediterranean countries and highest in Eastern Europe (Table 3.32.1). The decreased incidence in Europe has led to increased susceptibility in younger people. Cases are more common in those aged under 45 years and in men. High prevalence areas include most of Asia, Africa and Latin America, and many cases in Europe result from travel to these countries. Other groups at increased risk include those in contact with a case of HAV (e.g. household or nursery), men who have sex with men, intravenous drug users, ethnic minorities with links to high prevalence countries, haemophiliacs, and residents and workers in institutions for the mentally handicapped.

Clinical features

The clinical picture may range from no symptoms to fulminant hepatitis and is greatly influenced by age. Less than 10% of those aged under 6 years develop jaundice, but 40% have fever and dark urine and 60% have symptoms such as nausea/vomiting, malaise and diarrhoea. Around half of older children and

Table 3.32.1 General patterns of HAV infection in European countries

Endemicity	Countries	Age of cases (years)	Most common transmission
Very low	Scandinavia	Over 20	Travel abroad
Low	Germany	5–40	Common source outbreaks,
	Netherlands		person to person,
	UK		travel abroad
	Southwestern Europe		
Intermediate	Greece	5–24	Person to person,
	Balkan countries		common source outbreaks,
	Eastern Europe		contaminated food/water,
	Baltic states		travel abroad
	Turkey		

three-quarters of adults develop jaundice after a 2–3 day prodrome of malaise, anorexia, nausea, fever and dark urine. Overall case fatality is around 0.5% but is increased in those aged over 65 years. Chronic infection does not occur, but some cases may be prolonged and relapsing for up to a year.

Laboratory confirmation

Confirmation of acute HAV is dependent upon demonstration of specific IgM antibodies, which are usually present at onset of symptoms and persist for around 3 months. IgG antibody persists for life and so in the absence of IgM, a fourfold rise in titres in paired samples is required for diagnosis. Persistent IgG is taken as evidence of immunity due to past infection (or vaccination). Blood samples are usually used, but salivary IgM (and IgG) testing is available at specialist laboratories and may be useful in outbreak investigations. HAV-RNA can be detected in blood and stool early in the infection. Subtyping may also be available.

Transmission

HAV infection is spread primarily by the faeco-oral route from other humans. Up to 10^8 infectious units per millilitre are excreted in faeces during the late incubation period and the first week of symptoms. Viraemia also occurs during the prodromal phase of the illness but at much lower levels than in stool. Saliva and urine are of low infectivity.

Faeco-oral spread is likely to be responsible for secondary transmission to household (average secondary attack rate about 15%) and nursery contacts, perhaps aided by transmission via fomites. HAV can spread rapidly but silently among mobile, faecally incontinent children in nurseries and then cause illness in their contacts. Infection in illicit drug users has been reported in several European countries and is likely to be due to poor hygiene, although contamination of drugs and needle sharing may contribute. Travellers to endemic countries risk exposure via food or water. HAV can survive for 3–10 months in water, suggesting that even in Europe, shellfish harvested from sewage-contaminated waters are a potential source; shellfish concentrate viruses by filtering large quantities of water and are often eaten raw or after gentle steaming which is inadequate to inactivate HAV. Infected food handlers with poor personal hygiene may also contaminate food. Imported fruit and salad vegetables have also caused outbreaks.

Many cases of HAV do not have a recognised risk factor: it is likely that many of these contracted their infection from an undiagnosed or asymptomatic child case in their household. Such cases may be a factor in community outbreaks that evolve slowly over several months.

Acquisition

The incubation period is reported as 15–50 days (mean 28 days) and appears to be dose dependent. The infectious period is from 2 weeks before onset of symptoms until 1 week after, although some, particularly children, may excrete a week longer. Infectivity is maximal during the prodromal period.

Immunity to previous infection is lifelong, but because of the decreasing incidence over the last half-century, the majority of those under 50 years of age are susceptible. Those at increased risk of severe disease include those with chronic liver disease or chronic hepatitis B or C infection and older people.

Prevention

• Personal hygiene, including handwashing; ensuring toilet hygiene in nurseries and schools; care with food and water during travel to less developed countries; condom use and careful hygiene after anal sex.
• Sanitary disposal of sewage and treatment of water supplies.
• Vaccination of travellers (over 1 year of age) to countries outside of Northern or Western Europe, North America, Australasia or Japan, preferably at least 2 weeks before the date of departure (but can be given up to day of departure if necessary). This includes ethnic minority residents who are visiting relatives or friends in their family's country of origin. If time permits, those over 50 years of age or born in high endemicity areas or with a history of jaundice can be tested for immunity before vaccination. Immunoglobulin (HNIG) may be available for immunocompromised travellers.
• Vaccination of other risk groups, including patients with chronic liver disease or haemophilia, those with chronic hepatitis B or C, men who have sex with men, intravenous drug users, certain laboratory staff, staff and residents of certain institutions where good hygiene standards cannot be achieved, sewage workers and people who work with primates.

• Shellfish should be steamed for at least 90 seconds or heated at 85–90°C for 4 minutes before eating.
• Sodium hypochlorite, 2% glutaraldehyde and quaternary ammonia compound with 23% hydrogen chloride are effective on contaminated surfaces.

Surveillance

• Confirmed or suspected cases of acute infectious hepatitis should be reported to local public health authorities.
• All laboratory-confirmed acute cases (e.g. IgM positive) of hepatitis A should be reported to local public health authorities and national surveillance systems.

Response to a case

• Enteric precautions until 1 week after onset of jaundice (if no jaundice, precautions until 7 days after onset of first symptoms). Case should not prepare food for 14 days after onset.
• Exclude all cases in groups with increased risk of further transmission (Box 2.2.1) until 7 days after onset of jaundice. Preferable if all cases do not attend work or school for 7 days after onset.
• Exclude household and sexual contacts with symptoms as for cases.
• Personal hygiene advice to cases and contacts, particularly handwashing. Asymptomatic contacts who attend nursery or infant school should have handwashing supervised. Particular care with contacts who are food handlers until 40 days post-exposure.
• Vaccination should be offered to relevant household, sexual and other close contacts (see national policy). Vaccination of contacts aged 1–50 years is likely to be effective if given within 14 days of exposure. Contacts aged over 50 years or with pre-existing chronic liver disease, HBV, HCV or HIV infection or immunosuppression may benefit from receiving immunoglobulin in addition to vaccine. Some authorities (e.g. UK HPA) would

offer vaccine up to 8 weeks after exposure to prevent tertiary infection and offer immunoglobulin up to 4 weeks after exposure to those with chronic pre-existing liver disease or HBV/HCV infection to attempt to ameliorate severity of infection.

• If the case has attended pre-school childcare whilst potentially infectious, consider extending vaccination to close contacts. If the case is a food handler or attends primary school, a risk assessment will be required to assess risk of transmission.

• Collect risk factor data for 2–5 weeks before onset: contact with case, travel abroad, mental handicap or other institution, seafood, meals out of household, blood transfusion, occupation.

Investigation of a cluster

• Confirm that cases are acute (clinical jaundice and/or IgM positive).

• Describe by person, place and time. Does epidemic curve suggest point source, ongoing person-to-person transmission (or both) or continuing source? Are there cases in neighbouring areas?

• Collect risk factor data as for individual case and interview cases sensitively regarding sexuality, sexual activity, illicit drug use and imprisonment. Obtain full occupational and recreational history (e.g. exposure to faeces, nappies, sewage, untreated water). Obtain as full a food history as patient recall allows for 2–5 weeks before onset.

• Discuss with microbiologist use of salivary testing for case finding and availability of genotyping to confirm cases are linked.

Control of an outbreak

• Try to define if population at risk is suitable for immunisation (e.g. staff and pupils at a nursery).

• Hygiene advice to cases, contacts and any implicated institution. Ensure that toilet and hygiene facilities are adequate.

• For community outbreaks, re-inforce hygiene measures in nurseries and schools and vaccinate contacts of cases.

• For prolonged community outbreaks with disease rates of over 50 per 100,000 per annum, consult with relevant experts on appropriateness of vaccination of affected population.

Suggested case-definition for an outbreak

Confirmed: demonstration of specific IgM in serum or saliva.

Suspected: case of acute jaundice in at-risk population without other known cause (confirmation important in groups at risk of other hepatitis viruses, e.g. drug users).

3.33 Hepatitis B

Hepatitis B is an acute viral infection of the liver. Its public health importance lies in the severity of disease, its ability to cause long-term carriage leading eventually to cirrhosis and hepatocellular cancer, its transmissibility by the blood-borne route and the availability of vaccines and specific immunoglobulin.

Suggested on-call action (next working day)

• Arrange for laboratory confirmation.

• Identify likely source of infection for acute cases.

• Arrange for testing and vaccination of close household/sexual contacts.

Epidemiology

The incidence of acute hepatitis B varies considerably across Europe, and has been

---

Box 3.33.1 Risk groups for hepatitis B in Europe

- Injecting drug users
- Individuals who frequently change sex partners
- Close family and sexual contacts of cases and carriers
- Individuals who receive regular blood or blood products
- Patients with chronic renal failure and chronic liver disease
- Healthcare workers and laboratory staff
- Foster carers and people who adopt children from medium and high prevalence countries
- Staff and residents of institutions for those with learning difficulties
- Morticians and embalmers
- Prisoners and prison staff
- Long-term travellers to high prevalence countries
- Babies born to acutely infected or carrier mothers

---

declining in recent years. The overall notification rate in 2008 was 1.29 per 100,000. The highest rates are in Bulgaria (8.17 per 100,000) and Latvia (6.16 per 100); however, comparisons between countries should be made with caution because of a large variability in surveillance systems. The true incidence is higher, as about 70% of infections are subclinical and may not be detected. Most cases are in adults at high risk of infection (Box 3.33.1). Horizontal transmission within families also occurs in the higher incidence countries. The carriage rate is below 1% in most European countries, although there is considerable geographical variation within countries, with higher rates in inner cities amongst those of minority ethnic origin (especially South-East Asia and the Far East). Carriage rates are lowest in the UK and Scandinavia.

Clinical features

Hepatitis B is clinically indistinguishable from other causes of viral hepatitis. After a non-specific prodromal illness with fever and malaise, jaundice appears and the fever stops. The course of the disease is very variable and jaundice may persist for months. Liver failure is an important early complication.

Laboratory confirmation

The diagnosis and stage of infection can be determined from the antigen and antibody profile in the blood (Figure 3.33.1). Patients with detectable hepatitis B antigen at 6 months (surface antigen (HBsAg) and/or e antigen (HBeAg)) are considered to be carriers.

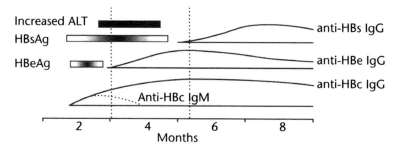

Fig. 3.33.1 Occurrence of hepatitis B virus markers and antibodies in the blood of infected patients. ALT, alanine aminotransferase; HBeAg, hepatitis B e antigen; HBsAg, hepatitis B surface antigen; IgG, immunoglobulin G.

Transmission

Humans are the only reservoir. Transmission is from person to person by a number of blood-borne routes, including sharing of drug-injecting equipment, transfusions of blood and blood products, needlestick injuries, skin piercing with inadequately sterilised equipment, mother-to-baby transmission during or soon after childbirth and sexual intercourse.

In low-prevalence countries, transmission occurs mainly through shared syringes, needlestick injuries, sexual contact, bites and scratches. In high prevalence countries, perinatal transmission is the most important route; ulcerating skin disease and biting insects also play a part in developing countries.

Acquisition

The incubation period ranges 40–160 days, with an average of 60–90 days. Carriers of HBsAg who are also e antigen positive and/or e antibody negative are much more infectious than those who are e antibody positive. Patients who do not become carriers and develop natural immunity are immune for life.

Approximately 10% of patients with acute HBV infection become chronic carriers. Long-term complications of being a carrier include cirrhosis and hepatocellular carcinoma.

Prevention

• Hepatitis B vaccination of infants and/or older children is recommended in most EU countries, except for the UK and a few other countries, where selective vaccination is recommended only for high-risk groups (Box 3.33.1). Vaccines are available as monovalent preparations, or in combination with hepatitis A and infant DTP-containing combinations. There are many different schedules; however, a primary course usually consists of three doses with or without a fourth dose. An accelerated schedule may be used when rapid protection is required (e.g. for travellers). The vaccine should not be given in the buttock as efficacy may be reduced. Higher dose formulations are available for patients with chronic renal failure.

• Protection is probably lifelong in a healthy adult who responds to the primary course. However, healthcare workers (HCW) and babies born to hepatitis B carrier mothers should have their antibody status checked 4–6 months after immunisation. Poor responders (anti-HBs 10–100 mIU/mL) should receive a booster dose, and in non-responders (anti-HBs <10 mIU/mL) a repeat course should be considered. Adults over 40 years of age and those with immunodeficiency are more likely to be non-responders.

• Ensure that all blood and blood products are screened and not derived from donors at risk of infection.

• Adopt universal procedures for the prevention of blood-borne virus transmission in hospitals and all other situations where needles and other skin-piercing equipment are used (e.g. acupuncture clinics, tattoo parlours, ear/body-piercing).

• Prevent infected HCWs from performing exposure-prone procedures.

• Promote condom use.

• The above general measures for the prevention of blood-borne virus infections are covered in more detail in Chapter 2.10.

• Screen all women in pregnancy. Babies born to mothers who are HBsAg positive and anti-HBe positive (i.e. low infectivity) should receive an accelerated course of vaccine. Babies whose mothers are e antigen positive, who have had acute hepatitis B in pregnancy, who have no e markers or whose e markers are not known should, in addition to a course of vaccine, receive 200 IU hepatitis B-specific immunoglobulin (HBIG) intramuscularly as soon as possible after birth.

• Offer post-exposure prophylaxis for significant exposures to a known or suspected HBsAg source (Table 3.33.1). A significant exposure is one in which HBV transmission may occur. This may be an injury involving a contaminated needle, blade or other sharp object, or blood contaminating non-intact skin or eyes. HBV does not cross intact skin. Exposure to vomit, faeces and sterile or

Table 3.33.1 Hepatitis B virus (HBV) prophylaxis for reported exposure incidents

HBV status of person exposed	Significant exposure			Non-significant exposure	
	HBsAg Positive source	Unknown source	HBsAg Negative source	Continued risk	No further risk
≤1 dose HB vaccine pre-exposure	Accelerated course of HB vaccine* HBIG × 1	Accelerated course of HB vaccine*	Initiate course of HB vaccine	Initiate course of HB vaccine	No HBV prophylaxis Reassure
≥2 doses HB vaccine pre-exposure (anti-HBs not known)	One dose of HB vaccine followed by second dose 1 month later	One dose of HB vaccine	Finish course of HB vaccine	Finish course of HB vaccine	No HBV prophylaxis Reassure
Known responder to HB vaccine (anti-HBs ≥10 mIU/mL)	Booster dose of HB vaccine	Consider booster dose of HB vaccine	Consider booster dose of HB vaccine	Consider booster dose of HB vaccine	No HBV prophylaxis Reassure
Known non-responder to HB vaccine (anti-HBs <10 mIU/mL 2–4 months post-vaccination)	HBIG × 1 Consider booster dose of HB vaccine	HBIG × 1 Consider booster dose of HB vaccine	No HBIG Consider booster dose of HB vaccine	No HBIG Consider booster dose of HB vaccine	No HBV prophylaxis Reassure

Source: From S. Handysides (1992) *Exposure to Hepatitis B Virus:Guidance on Post-Exposure Prophylaxis*. CDR Review. PHLS Communicable Disease Surveillance Centre, with permission.

HBIG, hepatitis B immunoglobulin; HBsAg, hepatitis B surface antigen.

* An accelerated course of vaccine consists of doses spaced at 0.1 and 2 months. A booster dose is given at 12 months to those at continuing risk of exposure to HBV.

uncontaminated sharp objects poses no risk. Transmission is not known to have occurred as a result of spitting or urine splashing.
• The dose of HBIG is 200 IU for children aged 0–4 years, 300 IU for children aged 5–9 years and 500 IU for adults and children aged 10 years or more.

Surveillance

• Acute hepatitis B is notifiable in most European countries.
• Surveillance should ideally be based on laboratory reports, as the disease is clinically indistinguishable from other causes of viral hepatitis. IgM and e antigen/antibody results should be included with notifications to facilitate public health action.

Response to a case

• Obtain laboratory confirmation, assess whether acute (IgM and/or clinical history) and how infectious (HBeAg, anti-HBe, HBsAg).
• If acute, determine possible source of infection.
• If infectious, give advice to case to limit infectivity to others and identify sexual and close household contacts. Arrange to have their hepatitis B markers checked to see if they have already been infected before vaccinating them. Contacts who are HBsAg, anti-HBs or anti-HBc positive do not need to be vaccinated, although for sexual partners the first dose of vaccine should be given while awaiting test results and the use of condoms advised until immunity is established.

Investigation of a cluster and response to an outbreak

• Look for a common source and take appropriate action.
• If an infected HCW is the source, a lookback investigation should be conducted to identify other cases associated with the HCW (see Chapter 4.6).

Suggested case-definition for an outbreak

Jaundice plus presence in serum of HBsAg, HBeAg or anti-HBc IgM.

3.34 Hepatitis C

Hepatitis C is a worldwide public health problem. Large numbers of people are chronically infected with hepatitis C virus (HCV) and a substantial proportion will develop chronic liver disease in the future.

Suggested on-call action

Only rarely will HCV cases, clusters or incidents be notified outside normal office hours.

Epidemiology

HCV was first identified in 1989 and an antibody test became available in 1990. Surveillance of HCV infection is influenced by the availability and extent of testing and reporting of results. Current tests do not differentiate between present and past infection and because most acute infections are asymptomatic it is not possible to distinguish incident from prevalent cases. The number of chronically HCV infected persons is substantial. For example, it is estimated that 185,000 persons in the UK (approximately 300 per 100,000 population) are chronically infected. Of the reports that included risk factor information, over 90% identified injecting drug use (IDU) as the main route of transmission.

In England, anti-HCV seroprevalence varies from 0.3% amongst pregnant women, 0.6% amongst those attending genitourinary medicine clinics to 22% in recent IDU. The annual overall notification rate for HCV infection in the EU is 9 cases per 100,000, with rates that vary widely from 35 per 100,000 population in Ireland to 27 in Sweden, 17 in UK, 7.5 in Germany and <0.1 in Austria (2008 figures). These variations probably reflect the extent to which case finding is encouraged rather than true differences in occurrence.

Clinical features

Acute hepatitis C is often asymptomatic. There may be elevated liver enzymes but jaundice is uncommon and serious liver disease is rare. Following infection, 20% will clear the virus in 2–6 months. Of those who are chronically infected, 75% will have some degree of active liver disease and of these 25% will progress to cirrhosis over the ensuing 20 years, of whom 1–4 % will develop liver cancer each year. After 25–30 years with HCV infection the risk of liver cancer is more than 40-fold compared to the general population.

Laboratory confirmation

HCV is a small enveloped single-stranded RNA virus. Anti-HCV IgG antibody tests are normally positive within 3 months of infection. To indicate whether the virus is still present quantitative and qualitative polymerase chain reaction (PCR) tests for HCV-RNA are used. Tests are available to distinguish between the six main HCV genotypes and many more subtypes. Genotypes and subtypes have differing geographical distributions and predict response to treatment. In the UK, genotype 1a and 3a are the most common genotypes while genotype 1b, and to a lesser extent genotype 2, are the common genotypes found elsewhere in Europe.

Transmission

HCV is spread by contact with blood or body fluids from an infected person. Those at greatest risk are current and past IDU, those who received blood products before heat treatment in 1986 and recipients of blood transfusions before testing was introduced in 1991. Other less efficient routes of transmission are vertical spread from mother to infant; unprotected sex with an infected partner; through medical and dental procedures abroad with contaminated equipment; during tattooing or skin piercing with blood-contaminated equipment; and horizontal spread in households as a result of sharing contaminated toothbrushes or razors. Incidents involving transmission of HCV from patient to healthcare worker (HCW) and from HCW to patient are being reported more frequently. In the UK, 1113 percutaneous exposures involving HCV positive source patients were reported in 2000–2007 and there were 14 seroconversions. There have been five cases reported in the world literature of transmission of HCV from HCWs resulting in infection in 13 patients and in the UK in 1994–2003 there were five incidents of HCV transmission from infected surgeons involving 15 patients.

Acquisition

The incubation period is 6–9 weeks. A person will remain infectious for as long as they are infected with the virus.

Prevention

Unlike hepatitis A and B, no vaccine is available for hepatitis C. Control of HCV infection depends on the following (Table 3.34.1):
• improved surveillance;
• raising public and professional awareness;
• case finding by more testing of defined risk groups;
• better treatment and care;

Table 3.34.1 Target groups for particular hepatitis C virus (HCV) prevention measures

Injecting drug users	Needle exchange schemes
	Supply of other injecting equipment such as spoons, filters, water and tourniquets
	Methadone and other maintenance programmes
	Health education targeted at younger IDUs and people injecting drugs for the first time
	Promote hygienic injecting practices
	Encourage other drug administration routes such as smoking and snorting
	Consider alcohol and hepatitis B (co-factors in development of liver disease)
	Established IDUs and ex-IDUs should have access to appropriate services
People with HCV infection, their sexual partners and household contacts	Access to information, counselling, testing and referral
	Adopt measures to reduce the risk of further transmission (see Chapter 1.2, universal precautions for blood-borne infections)
	Advise on alcohol to reduce risk of liver damage
	Develop clinical networks for diagnosis and treatment
Health and social care workers including staff of alcohol and drug agencies	Ensure good knowledge of HCV and other blood-borne viral infections
	Implement infection control measures, including universal precautions
	Guidelines on occupational aspects of HCV have been published
	Guidelines are available for staff in drugs services and renal dialysis centres
Prisoners, prison staff and probation service staff	Access to information and professional advice, including counselling, testing and referral
	Supply injecting equipment in prisons
General population, particularly young people	Ensure awareness of HCV and transmission
	Implement universal precautions to manage bleeding and blood spillages in the community
	Follow infection control guidelines for skin piercing, tattooing, etc.
Blood, organ and tissue donation	People with HCV and those who may have been exposed to HCV should not donate blood or carry a donor card
	Screening and heat treatment should be used where appropriate
HCV infection in mothers and infants	Universal antenatal screening for HCV is not recommended
	Pregnant women at risk of HCV infection should be offered hepatitis C testing
	Breastfeeding should be discouraged only if the mother is viraemic

IDU, injecting drug use/user.

• preventing transmission amongst IDUs, young people and in prisons by needle exchanges and targeted education; and
• promoting infection control measures in community and healthcare settings.

Surveillance

• Hepatitis C is a statutory notifiable disease in all EU countries except Spain and the UK. In the UK, viral hepatitis (unspecified) is notifiable.
• Cases of chronic HCV infection detected as a result of serological testing should be reported to national laboratory surveillance schemes.
• Rarely, acute cases are diagnosed and these should be reported to the local health authorities for investigation.
• In the UK, details of cases where the date of infection is known should be reported to the National Hepatitis C Register.

Response to a case

• The cases should receive information about the infection and advice on preventing further spread. Patient advice leaflets are available.

• For acute cases, enquire about the circumstances of exposure and the possibility of infection as a result of healthcare, acupuncture, other alternative therapy and blood transfusion.

• The case should be referred for further investigation and possible treatment if indicated, and longer term support and counselling.

• HCV is treated with pegylated interferon and ribavarin. Treatment guidelines are available in most countries. The regimens vary according to genotype. Sustained virological response (SVR), which is defined as HCV-RNA negative 24 weeks after cessation of treatment, may be achieved in 60–80% of cases.

Investigation of an incident or outbreak

• All those who have potentially been exposed should be identified and offered testing. Those with evidence of infection will need counselling and follow up by a liver specialist who can advise on treatment options.

• If a HCW who has performed exposure-prone procedures is found to have HCV infection, a look-back exercise may be required (see Chapter 4.6).

Suggested case-definition for an outbreak

An acute illness with:
• Discrete onset of symptoms (such as nausea, vomiting, abdominal pain and diarrhoea); *and*
• Jaundice or abnormal serum aminotransferase levels.
  Laboratory criteria for diagnosis:
• Elevated serum AST/ALT level and anti-HAV IgM negative; *and*
• Anti-HBc IgM negative or, if not done, HbsAg negative; *and*
• Anti-HCV screening test positive verified by an additional, more specific assay (e.g. RIBA for anti-HCV or HCV RNA).

3.35 Delta hepatitis

Delta hepatitis is caused by a satellite virus that only infects patients during the antigen-positive stages of acute hepatitis B or long-term HBsAg carriers. The epidemiology is thus similar to that of hepatitis B (see Chapter 3.33), although less common; worldwide about 5% of HBsAg carriers are infected with delta hepatitis. In Europe, prevalence rates are highest in Romania and the Mediterranean countries. Transmission is by the same routes as hepatitis B. The incubation period is 2–8 weeks. General control measures for blood-borne viruses will prevent spread of delta hepatitis. There is no specific vaccine or immunoglobulin.

3.36 Hepatitis E

Hepatitis E virus (HEV) is the main cause of enterically transmitted non-A non-B hepatitis worldwide.

Epidemiology

Although rare in Europe (an average of 30 cases per year are reported in the UK and 100 in Germany), HEV is responsible for around half of acute sporadic hepatitis in many developing countries and is most common in southern Asia, northern and western Africa and Central America. Most clinically reported cases occur in young or middle-aged adults.

Diagnosis

HEV causes an illness similar to hepatitis A (abdominal pain, anorexia, dark urine, fever, hepatomegaly, jaundice, malaise, nausea and vomiting) without chronic sequelae or carriage. The severity of hepatitis is dose-dependent. Case fatality is low, except in women infected in the third trimester of pregnancy, when it may reach 20%. Specific IgM testing is available in specialist laboratories, although a positive result should be treated with caution in those without risk factors. RNA tests may also be available.

Transmission and acquisition

HEV is transmitted faeco-orally, with most outbreaks linked to contaminated drinking water. Food-borne transmission also occurs. Person-to-person spread is inefficient (1–2% secondary attack rate), but nosocomial spread is described. Virus excretion in stools probably occurs before clinical onset and lasts up to 14 days afterwards. The incubation period is reported as 15–60 days (mean 30–40 days).

Control

Prevention relies primarily on provision of safe water supplies. European travellers to developing countries, particularly if pregnant, should take care with food and water. Confirmed or suspected cases in Europe should be notified to local public health authorities.

3.37 Herpes simplex

Infection with herpes simplex viruses (HSV) is characterised by a localised primary infection, latency and recurrence. HSV-1 is typically associated with gingivostomatitis and HSV-2 with genital infection (see Chapter 3.28). However, either may affect the genital tract and HSV-2 can cause primary infection of the mouth.

Suggested on-call action
Usually none required.

Epidemiology

The incidence of HSV-1 infection peaks first in preschool-aged children. There is a second lower peak in young adults. It is rare in infancy because of passive maternal antibody. UK GPs report a 10-year mean weekly incidence of herpes simplex of around 6 per 100,000 population. Amongst the general populations of eight European countries there are large inter-country and intra-country differences in HSV-1 and HSV-2 seroprevalence. Age standardised HSV-1 seroprevalence ranged from 52% in Finland to 84% in Bulgaria, while HSV-2 seroprevalence ranged from 24% in Bulgaria to 4% in England and Wales. Generally, seropositivity was greater in females and older age groups. A large proportion of teenagers and young adults are HSV-1 susceptible and this may have implications for transmission and clinical presentation of HSV-1 and HSV-2.

Clinical features

Primary infection produces a painful gingivostomatitis. As a result of autoinoculation, lesions may affect other sites such as the eye and finger (herpetic whitlow). The illness resolves after 10–14 days. Complications include eczema herpeticum, Bell's palsy, encephalitis, meningitis, ocular herpes and erythema multiforme. Following primary infection, HSV persists in the dorsal root ganglia of the trigeminal nerve. A range of trigger factors including upper respiratory tract infections, fatigue, emotional stress, physical trauma, exposure to sun, dental extraction, menstruation and drugs such as corticosteroids may lead to reactivation of the virus leading to herpes labialis (the cold sore). Reactivation may affect 45% of persons who have had a primary infection.

Genital herpes is the most common ulcerative STI in the UK. Characterised by recurrent infections, it causes significant physical and psychological morbidity and is a co-factor in HIV transmission. Between 1999 and 2008,

HSV-1 has increasingly been implicated in genital infections in Europe and North America, possibly because of decline in early acquisition of HSV-1 infection and an increase in oral sex in young adults.

Laboratory confirmation

HSV is a large DNA herpes virus with a typical appearance on electron microscopy. The diagnosis is often made clinically, but PCR for HSV-1 and HSV-2 DNA in vesicle fluid or scrapings has now replaced electron microscopy and viral culture as the preferred method of diagnosis.

Transmission

Humans are the only reservoir of infection and spread is by contact with oral secretions during kissing, skin contact during contact sports (herpes gladiatorum) and during sexual intercourse. Neonates may be infected vertically or at the time of delivery. The virus does not survive for long periods in the environment and cannot penetrate intact skin. HSV is highly infectious, especially in young children and attack rates approach 80% in non-immune subjects.

Acquisition

The incubation period is 2–20 days (mean 6 days). The virus may be shed in saliva for 2–20 days (mean 7 days) in primary infection and 1–4 days in recurrent infection. The longer periods of shedding previously reported are now thought to have been due to reactivation. At any one time, 20% of young children may be shedding virus. HSV infection is lifelong and patients with impaired cellular immunity, skin disorders and burns are at risk of severe and persistent infections.

Prevention

• Health education and attention to personal hygiene may reduce exposure.

• Gloves should be available for health and social care staff in contact with potential infection.
• Patients with HSV infection should avoid contact with infants, burns patients and people with eczema or impaired immunity.
• Sunscreen and oral antivirals may be considered to prevent reactivation.

Response to a case/cluster/ outbreak

• Treatment is symptomatic and supportive.
• Oral antivirals may be considered for primary infection and reactivation particularly when there is severe disease.
• Topical antivirals may be used for reactivation.
• Ocular herpes simplex disease is the most common cause of corneal blindness in high-income countries and should be treated as an ophthalmic emergency.
• Patients with extensive infection should be nursed with source isolation.
• Children with cold sores do not need to be excluded from school.

Suggested case-definition for an outbreak

Characteristic lesions with or without laboratory confirmation by PCR, electron microscopy or viral culture.

3.38 *Haemophilus influenzae* type b

Haemophilus influenzae type b (Hib) is a bacterial infection of young children, which causes meningitis and other bacteraemic diseases including pneumonia, epiglottitis, facial cellulitis and bone and joint infections. Its importance lies in the high rate of disease complications and the availability of a vaccine.

Epidemiology

The disease is most common in children under 5 years. Before vaccination was introduced, Hib was the second most common cause of bacterial meningitis overall, and the most common in young children. In Europe the incidence in children under 5 years was 42 per 100,000, this has dropped to less than 1 per 100,000. The case fatality rate is 4–5% (higher in infants) and up to 30% of survivors have permanent neurological sequelae, including deafness, convulsions and mental impairment. There is a seasonal trend, with more cases reported in winter months.

Between 2000 and 2005 an increase was observed in the UK, in both vaccinated children and unvaccinated adults. The reasons for this increase included reduction in herd immunity, absence of a booster dose and the use of an acellular pertussis-containing combination vaccine causing Hib interference. Following introduction of a booster dose the disease incidence has declined again.

Other serotypes of *H. influenzae* occasionally cause invasive disease and non-encapsulated *H. influenzae* sometimes cause ear infections or acute exacerbations of chronic bronchitis.

Clinical features

Hib meningitis typically has a slower onset than meningococcal meningitis, with symptoms developing over 3–4 days. There is progressive headache, drowsiness and vomiting with intermittent fever. Photophobia may be present. A haemorrhagic rash can be present, but is unusual. In soft tissue, bone and joint infections there is swelling of the affected area. Hib epiglottitis presents with acute respiratory obstruction.

Laboratory confirmation

This is important as the clinical features are variable and non-specific; this is also to ascertain vaccine failures. A positive culture may be obtained from blood or cerebrospinal fluid (CSF). Alternatively, Hib antigen can be demonstrated by latex agglutination or PCR. All strains should be sent to the national reference laboratory for confirmation and typing.

Transmission

Humans are the only reservoir. Transmission is by droplet infection and direct contact with nose and throat secretions. In unvaccinated populations carriage is common in young children; about 4–5% of unvaccinated 3-year-olds are carriers. Vaccination prevents carriage.

Acquisition

The incubation period is not known, but is probably only 2–4 days. Cases are non-infectious within 48 hours of starting effective antibiotic treatment. Disease usually results in lifetime immunity, although repeat infections have been described. Immunity is also derived from carriage, from infection with cross-protective antigens such as *E. coli*, and from vaccination.

Prevention

Routine vaccination of infants with protein-polysaccharide conjugate vaccines has been implemented throughout Europe. Three doses are required in infants; children over

12 months require only a single dose. A booster dose is required in the second year of life.

Surveillance

• Hib meningitis is notifiable in most EU countries; this does not apply to other forms of invasive Hib disease. Hib surveillance in Europe is co-ordinated by the European Centre for Disease Prevention and Control (ECDC) and annual European surveillance data is available on the ECDC website. Notifications should always be based on laboratory reports.
• Report any case in a vaccinated child to the national surveillance unit.

Response to a case

• Laboratory confirmation must be sought.
• Check vaccination status of the case and of household contacts.
• Household contacts do not require chemoprophylaxis if all children in the household have been vaccinated.
• If there are any unvaccinated children under 5 years in the household, they should be vaccinated and all household members (including adults, who may be the source of infection) should be given chemoprophylaxis (Box 3.38.1). The case should also receive chemoprophylaxis and vaccine.
• Warn patients of the adverse effects of rifampicin (red staining of urine, sputum, tears and contact lenses, interference with the oral contraceptive pill).
• Cases should be excluded from school/nursery until antibiotic treatment has started; there is no need to exclude siblings or other close contacts of cases.

Box 3.38.1 Chemoprophylaxis for invasive Hib disease

Rifampicin, orally, 20 mg/kg/day for 4 days (maximum 600 mg/day).

Investigation and control of a cluster

• Give chemoprophylaxis (and vaccine, if unvaccinated) to nursery contacts if there are two or more cases within 120 days.
• In addition to the measures described for a case, there may be a need to conduct a local vaccination programme if coverage is low.

Suggested case-definition of an outbreak

Confirmed: clinically compatible illness with an isolate or antigen detection of Hib from a normally sterile site.
Clinical: meningitis or epiglottitis with no other cause in:
• an unvaccinated child under 5 years of age; *or*
• an unvaccinated individual with links to confirmed case(s).

3.39 HIV

Acquired immune deficiency syndrome (AIDS), first described in 1981, is the result of advanced infection with human immunodeficiency virus (HIV-1). There is a second human immunodeficiency virus, HIV-2, which is endemic in western Africa. It causes a spectrum of disease similar to that produced by HIV-1.

Suggested on-call action

• Most cases do not require an on-call response.
• Advise on the management of HIV-related incidents, particularly exposure incidents (Box 3.39.1).

Box 3.39.1 HIV post-exposure prophylaxis

• Evidence of HIV transmission from healthcare worker (HCW) to patient is limited to three incidents involving transmission to eight patients. HIV transmission from patients to HCWs is more common, with over 100 confirmed cases of occupational spread and many more probable cases. In the UK, confirmed occupational transmission of HIV is becoming less common because of post-exposure prophylaxis (PEP). Since 1997, there has been only one documented HIV seroconversion following a significant occupational exposure.
• The risk of acquiring HIV infection from a patient with HIV infection following a needle-stick injury is 3 per 1000 injuries and less than 1 per 1000 following mucous membrane exposure. Risks are greater with hollow needles, needles that are visibly blood-stained or which have been in an artery or vein, deep injuries and injuries from source patients who are terminally ill. Risk of infection can be reduced by 80% by PEP with antiretroviral drug combinations.
• PEP may also be considered following HIV exposure in non-occupational settings.

Epidemiology

Worldwide, since the beginning of the HIV epidemic, 60 million people have been infected with HIV and 25 million people have died. In 2008, there were an estimated 33.4 million people living with HIV, 2.7 million new infections, 2 million HIV-related deaths and 430,000 children born with HIV. Africa remains the region of the world most affected, with 67% of prevalent cases and 70% of new infections. HIV incidence appears to have peaked in 1996 although prevalence continued to rise because infected people were living longer as a result of antiretroviral therapy (ART). HIV prevalence among adults aged 15–49 years is now stable. Some countries are more affected than others and within countries there are often wide variations between different geographical areas and subsections of the population as a result of uneven distribution of risk factors.

In several Europe countries there is evidence of increasing transmission of HIV. In 2008, there were 51,600 new cases of HIV. The highest rates were reported from Estonia, Latvia, Kazakhstan, Moldova, Portugal, Ukraine and the UK (Table 3.39.1). In Eastern Europe injecting drug use (IDU) is still the main route of transmission, while in Central and Western Europe the two main routes of transmission are sex between men and heterosexual contact. Between 2000 and 2008 the overall European HIV rate increased from 39 to 87 per million population.

In the UK, in 2009, the number of persons newly diagnosed with HIV was 6630 compared with 7298 the previous year. This is the fourth consecutive annual decline in diagnoses and is mainly due to a fall in those infected heterosexually abroad (mostly in sub-Saharan Africa). Fifty four per cent of those diagnosed in 2009 probably acquired their infection through heterosexual contact and 42% through sex between men. UK-acquired heterosexual infections increased slightly from 1030 in 2007 to 1130 in 2009 (43% white, 38% black-African). The number of new HIV diagnoses in men who have sex with men (MSM) remains high (2760 in 2009). A total of 65,319 people were living with diagnosed HIV infection in 2009. An increasing proportion of persons living with HIV are aged 50 years or older because of ART improving survival and continued transmission at older ages. In the UK a range of different sources of surveillance data are available (Table 3.39.2).

Clinical features

The clinical manifestations of HIV infection range from the initial acute retroviral

Table 3.39.1 HIV infections and rates per 100,000 population by country and year of diagnosis (2006–2008), EU and European Economic Area/European Free Trade Association (EEA/EFTA) countries

Country	2008 Total confirmed cases	2008 Notification rate per 100,000 population	2007 Confirmed cases and notification rate — Cases	2007 Rate	2006 Confirmed cases and notification rate — Cases	2006 Rate
Austria[a]	–	–	–	–	–	–
Belgium	1079	10	1052	9.9	995	9.4
Bulgaria	122	1.6	126	1.6	92	1.2
Cyprus	37	4.7	46	5.9	35	4.5
Czech Republic	148	1.4	121	1.2	91	0.9
Denmark	–	–	306	5.6	245	4.5
Estonia	545	41	633	47	668	50
Finland	154	2.9	190	3.6	191	3.6
France	4068	6.4	5592	8.8	5645	8.9
Germany	2806	3.4	2774	3.4	2663	3.2
Greece	543	4.8	536	4.8	482	4.3
Hungary	145	1.4	119	1.2	81	0.8
Ireland	405	9.2	391	9.0	353	8.3
Italy[b]	1958	–	1607	–	1556	–
Latvia	358	16	350	15	299	13
Lithuania	95	2.8	106	3.1	100	3
Luxembourg	47	9.7	38	7.9	44	9.3
Malta	28	6.8	14	3.4	26	6.4
Netherlands[c]	1361	8.3	1300	7.9	1177	7.2
Poland	804	2.1	714	1.9	749	2
Portugal	1124	11	1551	15	1665	16
Romania	179	0.8	185	0.9	217	1
Slovakia	53	1	39	0.7	27	0.5
Slovenia	48	2.4	37	1.8	33	1.6
Spain[d]	1583	–	1498	–	1534	–
Sweden	359	3.9	444	4.9	365	4
UK	7298	12	7495	12	7608	13
EU total[e]	**25,347**	**5.7[e]**	**27,264**	**6.3[e]**	**26,941**	**6.2[e]**
Iceland	10	3.2	13	4.2	11	3.6
Liechtenstein	–	–	–	–	–	–
Norway	299	6.3	248	5.3	276	5.9
Total[e]	**25,656**	**5.7[e]**	**27,525**	**6.3[e]**	**27,228**	**6.2[e]**

Note: The data for some countries may be provisional data.
[a] HIV is not notifiable in Austria.
[b] HIV reporting undertaken in 11 of the 20 Italian regions in 2008, covering 47.6% of the total population.
[c] The Dutch data here reflect reporting year rather than year of diagnosis.
[d] HIV data from 12 autonomous regions of Spain in 2008, covering 44% of the total population.
[e] Rates calculated excluding the Italian and Spanish data.

syndrome to full-blown AIDS (Table 3.39.3). HIV-1 binds to CD4 receptors on lymphocytes or macrophages. The virus is internalised and integrated into the host cell genome leading to permanent infection. Virions may bud from the cell surface to infect another cell or infection may be spread when cells divide. Eventually the infected cells are killed by the virus. The CD4 count is normally 600–1200 cells/mm^3, but in HIV infection it

Table 3.39.2 Main sources of UK surveillance data: HIV and AIDS

Diagnoses of HIV, AIDS and HIV-related deaths	Information is received from laboratories, genitourinary clinics and regional reporting centres. Data on paediatric infections are collected separately and collated to produce the national surveillance tables
SOPHID	SOPHID is a cross-sectional survey of all persons who attend for HIV-related care at an NHS site in England, Wales and Northern Ireland within a calendar year
HIV incidence	STARHS can distinguish between long-standing and recently acquired HIV infections (typically around 6 months)
Laboratory reporting of CD4 counts	Trends in immunosuppression among HIV-infected adults by analysis of CD4 cell counts
Antiretroviral HIV resistance	HIV resistance data from HIV-infected drug-naïve individuals and those already receiving antiretroviral drugs
UAPMP	Monitors the prevalence of HIV infection in selected adult populations (pregnant women, injecting drug users and genitourinary medicine clinic attendees)

SOPHID, Survey of prevalent HIV infections diagnosed; STARHS, Serological Testing Algorithm for Recent HIV Seroconversion; UAPMP, unlinked anonymous HIV prevalence monitoring.

Table 3.39.3 Clinical manifestations of HIV infection

Acute retroviral syndrome	About 1–6 weeks after exposure, fever, sweats, malaise, myalgia, rash HIV (p24) antigen is usually detectable in serum, EIA antibody test is often negative
ARC	ARC includes PGL, ITP, oropharyngeal candidiasis, herpes zoster, chronic diarrhoea, hairy leukoplakia and the constitutional wasting syndrome
AIDS: infections	*Pneumocystis jirovecii* pneumonia
	Oesophageal or bronchial candidiasis
	Cytomegalovirus infection
	Extrapulmonary cryptococcosis
	Mycobacterium avium-intracellulare infection
	Coccidioidomycosis, disseminated
	Cryptosporidiosis of more than 1 month's duration
	Herpes simplex
	Histoplasmosis, disseminated or extrapulmonary
	Isosporiasis, chronic intestinal
	Toxoplasmosis
AIDS: neoplasms	Kaposi's sarcoma
	Non-Hodgkin's lymphoma
	Invasive cervical cancer
	Brain lymphoma
Other conditions	Tuberculosis
	Perianal and genital condyloma acuminata
	Seborrhoeic dermatitis
	Psoriasis
	Molluscum contagiosum
	HIV encephalopathy
	Peripheral neuropathies

ARC, AIDS-related complex; EIA, enzyme immunoassay; ITP, immune thrombocytopenic purpura; PGL, persistent generalized lymphadenopathy.

may fall to less than 200 cells/mm^3 leading to severe immunosuppression which is associated with opportunistic infections, neoplasia and full-blown AIDS. Following exposure to HIV there is a period of viraemia during which the individual is very infectious and may experience fever and rash. Antibodies to HIV develop and the infection may then remain dormant for many years.

Laboratory confirmation

Diagnosis is made with an enzyme-linked immunosorbent assay (ELISA) test that detects both anti-HIV-1 and anti-HIV-2. A positive test should be confirmed by a Western blot test which also detects antibody. Tests for p24 HIV antigen are no longer widely used. Rapid antibody tests are qualitative immunoassays that can be used as point-of-care tests on blood or oral fluid. Nucleic-acid-based tests (NAT) identify certain target sequences located in specific HIV genes and can detect disease soon after infection. They can be used to screen blood donations when, because of expense, 8–24 samples are usually pooled before testing. Quantification of plasma HIV-1 RNA is used to predict disease progression and monitor response to antiviral treatment. Genetic analysis can identify subtypes of HIV suggesting connections between individuals sharing the same strain. Antiviral resistance testing is also available.

Transmission

HIV is spread from person to person as a result of exposure to infected blood or tissues, usually as a result of sexual contact, sharing needles or syringes or transfusion of infected blood or blood components. Normal social or domestic contact carries no risk of transmission. Transmission is especially efficient between MSM in whom receptive anal intercourse and multiple sexual partners are particular risk factors. In countries where heterosexual spread is common, sexually transmitted infections (STIs) causing genital ulceration and multiple partners are associated

with the highest rates of transmission. HIV is present in saliva, tears and urine but transmission as a result of contact with these secretions is uncommon. HIV infection is not thought to be transmitted by biting insects. Between 15% and 30% of infants born to HIV infected mothers are infected with HIV as a result of vertical transmission either before, during or shortly after birth due to breast-feeding.

Acquisition

Following exposure, HIV nucleic acid sequences may be detected in the blood within 1–4 weeks and HIV antibodies can be detected within 4–12 weeks. Untreated, half of those with HIV infection will develop AIDS within 7–10 years and of these 80–90% will die within 3–5 years. ART reduces disease progression. A person with HIV infection will be infectious to others from shortly after the onset of the HIV infection throughout the rest of his/her life. Infectiousness increases with the degree of immunosuppression, viral load and the presence of STIs. Susceptibility to HIV infection is universal.

Prevention

• The development of an effective vaccine is unlikely in the near future.
• Most HIV prevention programmes rely on public health education to reduce activities that carry a risk of HIV transmission, particularly high-risk sexual activity and IDU. The main HIV preventative measures are summarised in Box 3.39.2.

Surveillance

• HIV and AIDS are not statutorily notifiable in the UK, but good voluntary case-based reporting systems are established.
• Surveillance of AIDS and HIV in Europe is variable.

Box 3.39.2 HIV prevention measures

• To reduce sexual transmission: promote sexual abstinence or completely monogamous relationships between two uninfected partners, reduce number of sexual partners and minimise exposure to body fluids during intercourse by using condoms.

• Ensure quality services for diagnosing and treating sexually transmitted infections (STIs).

• HIV counselling and testing should be promoted to ensure early diagnosis, treatment and to reduce further transmission.

• HIV testing should be offered to persons attending genitourinary medicine (GUM) or sexual health clinics, antenatal services, termination of pregnancy services and drugs services and those with TB, hepatitis B, hepatitis C and lymphoma. HIV testing should also be offered as part of routine care to persons with an STI, sexual partners of HIV-infected persons, men who have sex with men (MSM), female sexual contacts of MSM, those who have injected drugs, persons from (and those who have had sexual contact in) countries with HIV prevalence >1%. In addition, HIV testing should be offered to blood donors, dialysis patients, organ transplant donors and recipients and all patients requiring immunosuppressant therapy. In areas where the prevalence of diagnosed HIV infections is 2 per 1000 population or above it may be cost-effective to offer HIV tests to all those aged 15–59 years who present in hospital and primary care settings.

• Ensure that needle exchange and harm reduction programmes are available for injecting drug users.

• Ensure that pregnant women with HIV infection are identified as part of antenatal care and managed with interventions to reduce the risk of vertical transmission from mother to infant including antiviral treatment, caesarean section and advice to refrain from breastfeeding.

• Healthcare workers and others should be advised to take particular care when handling blood or sharp instruments and to adopt infection control measures for the prevention of blood-borne viral infections when caring for any patient with HIV infection. Treatment with antiviral drugs may be appropriate following occupational exposure to HIV-contaminated material (see below).

• Transmission by tissues, blood and blood products can be prevented by serological testing of blood and by heat treatment of blood products. Persons at increased risk of HIV infection should be advised to refrain from donating blood, organs or tissues.

• Improve the quality of surveillance data including data on routes of transmission to monitor effectiveness of interventions and/or developing problems in specific risk groups.

• Sexual health services and health promotion activities should be promoted amongst recognised high-risk behaviour groups including sex-workers, MSM and black African heterosexuals.

• Case-based reporting of cases to local and national surveillance schemes is encouraged in all countries.

Response to a case

• There is no cure for HIV infection, but a large number of antiviral drugs are available that slow the progression of disease. Treatment guidelines and standards are available. Treatment is aimed at reducing the plasma viral load and is started before the immune system is irreversibly damaged. Hospital patients with HIV infection should be nursed with infection control precautions for blood-borne viral (BBV) infections (see Chapter 2.10). Side room isolation is unnecessary unless there is a risk of haemorrhage.

• The person with HIV infection should be offered advice on preventing further spread and should be encouraged to identify sexual and needle sharing contacts so that counselling and HIV testing can be arranged.

Investigation and control of an incident or cluster

• Clusters of cases of HIV infection may be detected when contact tracing is carried out in sexual or drug using networks. Occasionally, a local increase in the incidence of HIV infection may occur. Standard outbreak investigation methods should be adopted. Particular care is needed to preserve patient confidentiality. Colleagues in the local genitourinary medicine (GUM) clinic or drug team should be able to assist with case finding, interviews and blood tests.

• HIV-related incidents occur more commonly and may include: a healthcare worker (HCW) with HIV infection, a percutaneous injury involving exposure to material from an HIV-infected person (Box 3.39.1) or a person with HIV infection who will not reliably follow advice to prevent further spread. Guidelines on how to respond to many of these incidents are available (see Appendix 2). Generally, public health legislation has not proved to be helpful in controlling spread from a person with HIV infection.

Action following an HIV exposure

• Following an exposure, all HCWs should have immediate, 24-hour access to an expert service including a designated doctor. Such a service is best delivered by an occupational health department but out-of-hours cover may be provided in the emergency room. The importance of *preventing* BBV exposure should not be overlooked but healthcare providers must also ensure there are robust post-exposure arrangements including policies, services and staff training.

• Following an exposure, the wound should be washed liberally with soap and water and free bleeding should be encouraged. Exposed mucous membranes including conjunctivae should be irrigated and contact lenses should be removed. The injury should be reported promptly.

• The designated doctor should assess the risk of transmission of HIV (and HBV, HCV) and the need for post-exposure management. The risk assessment is based on the type of body fluid involved and the route and severity of the exposure. Injuries from sharp objects that break the skin, exposure of broken skin and exposure of mucous membranes including the eye are significant injuries. Most body fluids pose a risk of transmission. The exceptions are urine, vomit, faeces and saliva unless visibly blood-stained. Saliva associated with dentistry is considered blood-stained.

• As a routine, the designated doctor or member of the clinical team (not the exposed worker) should approach the source patient (if known) and obtain informed consent, after pre-test discussion, to test for anti-HIV, HBsAg, anti-HCV and HCV RNA. Testing of the source patients should be completed within 8–24 hours.

• If there is an HIV risk, post-exposure prophylaxis (PEP) should be started within 1 hour. Subsequently, PEP may be discontinued if it is established that the source patient is HIV negative.

• Zidovudine is the only drug that has been shown to reduce risk of HIV transmission following occupational exposure but newer, better tolerated drugs are now preferred, although none are licenced for PEP and therefore they must be used off-label. Various PEP regimens have been recommended. In the UK, on the basis of acceptability and shelf life, the following PEP starter packs are used:

(a) One Truvada tablet (245mg tenofovir and 200mg emtricitabine (FTC)) once a day; *plus*

(b) Two Kaletra film-coated tablets (200mg lopinavir and 50mg ritonavir) twice a day.

• PEP should be started within hours and certainly within 48–72 hours of exposure and continued for at least 28 days. If the HCW is pregnant, has an existing medical condition, is taking other medication or if there is the possibility of viral resistance then expert advice should be obtained. The HCW should be followed up weekly during the period of PEP, to monitor treatment side effects and ensure compliance.

• In addition, the hepatitis B virus (HBV) immunity of the HCW should be assessed and if necessary blood should be taken for urgent anti-HBs testing. An accelerated course of vaccine, a booster dose of vaccine and/or hepatitis B immunoglobulin (HBIG) may be given according to published algorithms. For hepatitis C virus (HCV) no immunisation or prophylaxis is available. A baseline blood sample should be obtained from the exposed worker and stored for 2 years. If the source is HIV infected, the worker should be tested for anti-HIV at least 12 weeks after the exposure or after HIV PEP was stopped, whichever is the later. Testing for anti-HIV at 6 weeks and 6 months is no longer recommended. Also, if the source is HCV infected, the worker should be tested for HCV-RNA at 6 and 12 weeks and for anti-HCV at 12 and 24 weeks.

• In the absence of seroconversion, restriction of working practices is not necessary but infection control measures, safer sex practices and avoiding blood donation should be observed during the follow-up period. Generally, management of workers exposed to a potential BBV source whose status is unknown or a source that is unavailable for testing will depend upon a risk assessment and a discussion of the benefits of intervention.

• Of the eight probable occupationally acquired HIV infections reported in the UK, seven were associated with exposure in high-prevalence areas abroad. Employers should consider making starter packs of PEP drugs available to workers and students travelling to countries where ART is not commonly available.

• Exposure outside the healthcare setting including sexual exposure and sharing drug-injecting equipment may give rise to a request for PEP or the need to consider it. A similar process of risk assessment should be followed: guidelines are available but practical issues may be encountered outside the healthcare environment.

Suggested case-definition

HIV infection is defined by positive laboratory tests for HIV. In addition, AIDS is defined by the development of one or more of the specific marker infections or neoplasms.

3.40 Influenza

Influenza virus is a highly infectious cause of acute respiratory infection. It is a major cause of morbidity during epidemics and can be life-threatening in the elderly and chronically unwell. It also has the potential to cause devastating pandemics (see Chapter 4.11).

Suggested on-call action

• Suggest case limits contact with non-vaccinated individuals who are at risk of severe disease.
• If linked to other cases in an institution, activate Outbreak Control Plan.

Epidemiology

Influenza causes annual winter epidemics of varying size and severity, and occasionally more severe pandemics. All age groups are affected, with highest incidence in children, but most hospitalisations and deaths are in the elderly. Between 3,000 and 30,000 excess winter deaths per year are attributed to influenza in the UK, depending on the size of the epidemic. Community outbreaks occur at variable times between November and March and tend to last 6–10 weeks, peaking at around the fourth week of the outbreak.

Influenza A and B viruses may alter gradually by 'antigenic drift': every few years this will result in a significant epidemic with rapid spread and a 10–20% attack rate. Influenza A may also change abruptly by 'antigenic shift' leading to the circulation of a new subtype to which there is little existing population immunity and causing a major pandemic, usually with severe disease in all ages: these have occurred in 1918 (causing 20–40 million deaths worldwide), 1957 and 1968. Despite the huge impact of pandemics, more deaths result from the steady accumulation associated with yearly non-pandemic influenza activity.

Clinical features

About half of cases will have the classic flu picture of a sudden onset of fever, chills, headache, muscle aches, myalgia and anorexia. There may also be a dry cough, sore throat or runny nose. Up to 25% of children may also have nausea, vomiting or diarrhoea if infected by influenza B or A (H1N1). The illness lasts 2–7 days and may include marked prostration. Up to 10% of these cases progress to tracheobronchitis or pneumonia. Those at particular risk of complications are people with underlying chronic chest, heart or kidney disease, diabetes or immunosuppression, smokers and pregnant women.

Some 20% of infections are asymptomatic and 30% have upper respiratory symptoms but no fever. Influenza A may cause more severe disease than influenza B, particularly in the elderly.

Laboratory confirmation

Confirmation of diagnosis is dependent upon laboratory tests, usually by direct immunofluorescence (DIF), virus isolation, rapid antigen testing, PCR or serology. The virus may be detected from nasopharyngeal aspirates, nasal swabs or throat swabs: these must be collected early in the disease and require special transport media. Results can be available in 2–3 days, although 1 week is usual for routine samples. Serology requires two specimens, 10–21 days apart, and is about 80% sensitive: it is useful for retrospective diagno-

sis. In outbreaks, PCR testing (highly sensitive in early infection) or same day DIF or ELISA results may be available, although cultures are still useful for identifying the infecting subtype.

Influenza virus has three types (A, B, C) of which influenza C produces only sporadic infections. Subtyping of influenza A is based on a combination of H antigen (15 subtypes) and N antigen (9 subtypes) e.g. H1N1 or H3N2. All recent common human pathogens are combinations of H1, H2 or H3 with N1 or N2. Strains may be further differentiated by serology and named after the place and year of their identification (e.g. A/Sydney/97): these can be compared with current vaccine strains.

Transmission

Influenza in humans is transmitted via the respiratory secretions of cases, mainly by airborne droplet spread, but also via small particle aerosols. Coughing and sneezing particularly promote spread. Transmission is facilitated by overcrowding and enclosed spaces, particularly by the number of susceptibles sharing the same room as the case. Spread in such circumstances is usually rapid and attack rates high.

Transmission may also occur via direct or indirect contact: this may occasionally cause a slowly evolving outbreak with low attack rates. Many outbreaks have occurred in hospitals.

The reservoir for influenza A is zoonotic, particularly aquatic fowl (Box 3.40.1): transmission to humans is rare but new strains may be spread directly or via intermediaries such as pigs. Influenza B only affects humans.

Acquisition

The incubation period is short, usually 7–67 hours, with a median of 34 hours for type A and 14 hours for type B. The infectious period starts 1 day before onset of symptoms, peaks after 1–2 days of symptoms and then declines, so that infectivity is very low after

---

Box 3.40.1 Avian influenza

In recent years there has been much international concern over reports of human infection with avian influenza strains such as H5N1, H9N2 and H7N7. Some avian viruses cause serious infections in humans (H5N1 disease in Hong Kong in 1997 had 33% mortality) but fortunately they do not spread easily, if at all, between humans. However, influenza viruses have the ability to undergo genetic reassortment and co-infection with both avian and human influenza strains in humans or pigs could produce a new strain with the increased virulence of the avian strain and the ability to spread easily from person to person like human influenza. Transmission of this highly pathogenic virus could then occur to a population with no existing immunity and, as yet, no vaccine to protect them. Although such a virus is most likely to arise in China or South-East Asia, modelling suggests that it would only take 2–4 weeks to spread from Hong Kong to the UK (and presumably the rest of Europe) because of modern patterns of international travel. Rapid containment of incidents where avian strains infect humans is therefore essential to reducing the risk of future pandemics.

Although most containment activities will take place in the source area, European countries can limit the risk to their population by measures aimed at early detection of cases and minimising their contact with others.

European residents may occasionally be exposed to infected birds that have migrated from an infected area or to other birds that have been exposed to them (e.g. at poultry farms). Government animal health agencies will have plans to respond to cases in birds, but the public health professional may have to undertake a risk assessment of those potentially exposed, advise on protective equipment, prophylaxis, measure to prevent co-infection with human strains and surveillance of cases or contacts.

---

7 days in adults. Shedding is higher in children and may be earlier and longer. Immunocompromised and other chronically ill patients may also excrete for a longer period. The infectious dose is low.

Immunity develops and protects against clinical illness with the same strain for many years. Cross-immunity to related strains occurs. It is not clear why outbreaks often cease before exhausting the pool of susceptibles.

Prevention

• Basic personal hygiene to reduce transmission by coughing, sneezing or contaminated hands.
• Immunisation reduces the risk of hospital admissions and death and has a good safety record. Annual immunisation with WHO recommended vaccines should be offered to all those with an increased risk of serious illness from influenza ('at risk'). All European countries recommend vaccination of older adults (most commonly defined as aged 65 years or more) and most recommend vaccination of people with chronic medical conditions, such as chronic respiratory, heart, renal, liver or neurological disease; immunosuppression or diabetes mellitus. Pregnant women are also at higher risk and may be offered vaccination.
• In addition, people in long stay residential care homes should also be vaccinated because of the risk of rapid spread and the potentially severe consequences of infection. As efficacy in elderly people may be lower than the 70–90% in younger adults, indirect protection in this group may also be valuable.
• Immunisation is offered to healthcare workers in most European countries, both to protect patients and maintain staffing levels, and it is recommended that residential care providers should also offer vaccination to their staff.
• Some European countries also immunise household contacts of 'at-risk' individuals (in line with WHO recommendations), children on long-term aspirin and pregnant women. A

few countries recommend vaccination of all children in certain age groups.

- Uptake of immunisation in disease-based risk groups has been poor in some European countries, including the UK. Primary care staff can increase uptake by compiling an at-risk register from chronic disease, computerised patient or prescription records, or as patients are seen during the year. A letter should be sent to each of these patients, preferably from their GP, recommending vaccination. Education on the benefits of vaccination is required both for the target population and for healthcare workers. Local health services should appoint a co-ordinator to lead on improving influenza immunisation uptake locally.
- The antiviral drugs oseltamivir or zanamivir can be prescribed when influenza A or B virus is circulating in the community for the prevention of influenza in those who:

    (a) belong to an 'at-risk' group, and

    (b) have not received an influenza immunisation this season, or who had one within the last 2 weeks, or have had an influenza immunisation but the vaccine did not match the virus circulating in the community, and

    (c) have been in close contact with someone with influenza-like symptoms in the same household or residential setting, and

    (d) can start taking oseltamivir within 48 hours (36 hours for zanamivir) of being in contact with the person with influenza-like symptoms.

- National and local planning prior to occurrence of a pandemic (see Chapter 4.11).

Surveillance

- Influenza activity can be monitored via a combination of clinical surveillance for 'influenza-like illness' and laboratory data.
- At the international level, WHO co-ordinates a global network covering 105 countries and publishes regularly updated information online. Most European countries contribute to European Centre for Disease Prevention and Control (ECDC) co-ordinated

surveillance data, which is published in the online Weekly Influenza Surveillance Overview.

- At the UK national level, data are available from:

    (a) telephone helplines for patients (e.g. NHS Direct diagnostic algorithms);

    (b) GP consultations (e.g. sentinel surveillance systems);

    (c) illness in schoolchildren (e.g. Medical Officers of Schools Association);

    (d) death certification (e.g. Office of National Statistics);

    (e) emergency admissions to hospital (e.g. via NHS systems);

    (f) collaborative studies (e.g. surveillance samples collected from primary care patients with influenza-like illness);

    (g) laboratory surveillance of routine samples. However, these samples are heavily biased in terms of age (particularly children) and severity (hospitalisation).

UK data from these sources are available on the HPA website (www.hpa.org.uk).

- Regional or district monitoring may also be useful. Clinical data can be obtained from computerised GPs or other primary care providers. Participating GPs and local laboratories should ideally co-operate to obtain representative virological surveillance data. Timely local feedback of interpreted data is particularly useful to local health service planners during the winter.
- Some countries set thresholds for clinical activity indices. These vary according to each system (e.g. for the Royal College of General Practitioners (RCGP) system in England there are thresholds for baseline; <30 consultations per week per 100,000 population); normal seasonal activity (30–199); above average (200–399); and epidemic (400+) levels.

Response to a case

- Although spread may occur before diagnosis, symptomatic cases should ideally not attend work or school until recovered.

• Avoid contact with those at increased risk of severe illness. In hospital, isolate during acute illness.

• Handwashing and safe disposal of respiratory secretions. Droplet precautions in hospital.

Response to a cluster

Only of concern if cases have links to institutions containing individuals at increased risk of severe disease and/or rapid spread.

Control of an outbreak

For outbreaks in institutions containing individuals at risk of severe disease:

• If virological diagnosis of outbreak not confirmed, organise rapid testing.

• Organise typing of virus to compare to vaccine.

• Immunise anyone not yet protected.

• Oseltamir or zanamivir prophylaxis for 'at risk' patients for 2 weeks until vaccine induced protection present (influenza A or B).

• Exclude staff and visitors with respiratory illness.

Suggested case-definition

Confirmed: upper or lower respiratory tract infection with laboratory evidence of influenza infection.

Clinical:

• Managing an institutional outbreak: upper or lower respiratory tract infection without other identified cause in person epidemiologically linked to a confirmed case.

• Monitoring a community outbreak: syndrome of fever, muscle ache and cough occurring during a period of high influenza virus activity.

• Isolate or cohort those with acute symptoms.

• Reinforce hygiene measures.

• Treat influenza-like illness in 'at risk' patients (irrespective of vaccine status) with zanamivir or oseltamivir, unless contraindicated or symptoms have been present for over 48 hours (36 hours for zanamivir).

3.41 Japanese B encephalitis

This is a mosquito-borne viral encephalitis caused by a flavivirus. It occurs throughout South-East Asia and the Far East. Most infections are inapparent, although the illness can be severe with high mortality and permanent neurological sequelae in survivors. The reservoir is pigs, and occasionally birds. Transmission to humans is via a mosquito that lives in rice-growing areas. Transmission rates are highest in the rainy season.

Travellers to endemic countries are considered at risk if they spend long periods (more than a month) in rural areas where pig farming and rice growing co-exist. The risk to rural travellers has been estimated to be between 1 in 5000 and 1 in 20,000 per week. A new inactivated vaccine has recently become available which is licensed for adults; the schedule is two doses 28 days apart. The need for booster doses has not yet been established. The usual precautions against mosquito bites should be taken (see Chapter 4.10).

3.42 Kawasaki disease

Kawasaki disease, also known as Kawasaki syndrome or 'mucocutaneous lymph node syndrome', is an acute vasculitis of unknown aetiology. Of untreated children, 20–25% develop coronary artery abnormalities.

Suggested on-call action
None required.

Epidemiology

Kawasaki disease is seen worldwide. Most (80%) cases are less than 5 years old and boys outnumber girls (1.5 : 1). The incidence is greatest in children of Asian ancestry. In Japan, the incidence in children younger than 5 years is approximately 140 per 100,000 per year. Bimodal seasonality with highest rates in January and in June/July has been noted. US data suggests the highest incidence in children of Asian and Pacific Island descent and lowest amongst Caucasians (9 per 100,000). Several regional outbreaks have been reported.

Clinical features

Kawasaki disease is a clinical diagnosis based on the history and physical findings. Features may include conjunctivitis; swollen, fissured lips; strawberry tongue; cervical lymphadenopathy; erythematous rash; and peeling of fingers and toes. Consideration of measles is important; appropriate control measures cannot be taken if measles is misdiagnosed as Kawasaki disease.

Laboratory confirmation

None.

Transmission

Unknown.

Prevention

Initial therapy is directed at preventing the development of coronary arteritis using intravenous immunoglobulin and oral acetylsalicylic acid.

Surveillance

Cases should be reported to any specific Kawasaki disease reporting system. Clusters should be reported to local public health departments.

Response to a case

Report to surveillance system.

Investigation of a cluster or outbreak

Seek specialist advice. A cluster of Kawasaki disease cases should be used as an opportunity for detailed investigation to learn more about the aetiology.

Suggested case-definition for an outbreak
For epidemiological surveillance, Communicable Disease Control (CDC) defines a case as illness in a patient with fever of 5 days or more duration (or fever until the date of administration of intravenous immunoglobulin if it is given before the fifth day of fever), and the presence of at least four of the following five clinical signs: • Rash; • Cervical lymphadenopathy (at least 1.5 cm in diameter); • Bilateral conjuctival injection; • Oral mucosal changes; • Peripheral extremity changes. Patients whose illness does not meet the above Kawasaki disease case definition but who have fever and coronary artery abnormalities are classified as having atypical or incomplete Kawasaki disease.

3.43 Legionellosis

Infection with *Legionella pneumophila* can cause a potentially life-threatening atypical pneumonia (Legionnaires' disease) or a milder febrile illness (Pontiac fever). Its public health importance lies in its ability to cause outbreaks, including large outbreaks in the community and hospital outbreaks with high case fatality in particularly susceptible patients.

Suggested on-call action

- If linked to other cases, consult Outbreak Control Plan.
- If in hospital during incubation period, inform the hospital infection control team.
- Otherwise, organise investigation of the case on the next working day.

Epidemiology

The true incidence of Legionnaires' disease is not known: estimates range from 1 to 20 per 100,000. Legionnaires' disease has been reported to be responsible for 0.5–15% of community-acquired pneumonias, with the proportion increasing with severity of disease. Approximately 5500 cases of Legionnaires' disease are reported in the EU each year, of which about three-quarters are in males and over 80% are in those aged over 45 years (age, sex differences are not obvious in Pontiac fever). Cases peak from June to October.

Travel is a major risk factor for Legionnaires' disease: 40% of reported UK cases are contracted abroad and a further 6% on trips within the UK. Within Europe those travellers most commonly affected are residents of northern European countries visiting southern Europe; the highest number of cases occur in travellers to Italy, France, Spain and Turkey. The highest rate (per traveller) is in visitors to Turkey. About 10% of UK cases are linked to identified local outbreaks (pre-dominantly due to 'wet cooling systems' or hot water systems) and about 4% are hospital acquired. However, many cases are sporadic and often from an unidentified source. Professional drivers may have an increased risk of exposure.

Clinical features

Both Legionnaires' disease and Pontiac fever commence with non-specific flu-like symptoms such as malaise, fever, myalgia, anorexia and headache, often with diarrhoea and confusion. Pontiac fever is self-limiting, but Legionnaires' disease progresses to pneumonia which, in an individual patient, is difficult to differentiate clinically from other causes of atypical pneumonia. In an outbreak, diagnostic clues might be 25–50% of cases with diarrhoea, confusion, high fever, a lack of upper respiratory symptoms and poor response to penicillins or cephalosporins. About 10% of reported Legionnaires' disease cases die, rising to about one-third of nosocomial cases. Many individuals who seroconvert to *Legionella* will be entirely asymptomatic.

Laboratory confirmation

There are 52 species of *Legionella*, comprising over 60 serogroups. Over 90% of legionellosis in immunocompetent individuals is due to *L. pneumophila*, which comprises at least 16 serogroups, of which serogroup 1 is responsible for the large majority of diagnosed infections. Legionellae are not usually identified in routine culture of sputum, although special media can be deployed. Serogroup 1 antibody may be tested for in most laboratories (e.g. by indirect immunofluorescent antibody (IFA) test) but takes 3–6 weeks to rise to diagnostic levels. Serogroup 1 antigen may be detected in urine samples at a much earlier stage of the illness (reference laboratories may also be able to test for the virulent 'mAb2+ve' subgroup in urine samples). Organisms may be detected in lung tissue, sputum and other secretions by direct fluorescence antibody testing, although this is less sensitive. Reference laboratories may be able to diagnose infection due to other serogroups if routine samples are negative in epidemiologically suspected Legionnaires' clusters. Ideally, all suspected cases of Legionnaires' disease should have urine antigen testing (for rapid diagnosis of serogroup 1) *and* culture of appropriate respiratory secretions on selective media to exclude other species (e.g. *L. longbeachae*) and serogroups and to allow subtyping to be performed.

Legionellae are common contaminants of water and so routine environmental testing is not helpful. However, culturing is useful in investigating suspected water sources for identified cases: 5 L of water is necessary for culture. Biofilms are also worth culturing in outbreaks. Although some positive samples can be detected in 2–3 days, it may take 10 days to confirm a sample as negative. If cultures are available from both patient and suspected source, then subtyping is available for comparison of the organisms.

Transmission

The reservoir for the organism is environmental water, in which it occurs in low concentrations. Transmission to humans occurs via inhalation of aerosols or droplet nuclei containing an infective dose of the organism. Legionellae grow at temperatures between 25°C and 45°C (preferably 30–40°C) and so the highest risk occurs with water systems that lead to the aerosolisation of water that has been stored at these temperatures. Such systems include hot water systems (especially showers), wet cooling systems (e.g. cooling towers and evaporative condensers), plastics factories, whirlpool spas, indoor and outdoor fountain/sprinkler systems, humidifiers, respiratory therapy equipment and industrial grinders. Wet cooling systems may contaminate air outside the building up to 0.5–3 km away, depending on conditions.

Legionellae can survive in water stored between 0°C and 60°C. They survive normal levels of chlorination and are aided by sediment accumulation and commensal microflora in the water. Temperatures above 63°C are bactericidal, as are many common disinfectants (e.g. phenol, glutaraldehyde, hypochlorite).

Acquisition

The incubation period for Legionnaires' disease is usually 2–10 days (median 6 days) but may occasionally be longer, and for Pontiac fever is 5–66 hours (average 36 hours). Legionella is not communicable from person-to-person.

The infectious dose is unknown, but certainly low. Attack rates are higher in Pontiac fever (>90%) than Legionnaires' disease (<5%). Risk of disease may be related to amount of time exposed to the source. Cigarette smoking, advanced age, diabetes, chronic lung or kidney disease, haematological malignancy, immunosuppression and excess alcohol intake are risk factors for identified infection.

Prevention

• Design, maintenance and monitoring of water systems: store hot water above 60°C and deliver above 50°C; store and deliver cold water below 20°C. Eliminate stagnant water.
• New air-conditioning systems to be air-cooled.
• Maintenance and hygiene of wet cooling systems in line with national recommendations (e.g. Health and Safety Executive guidance in UK). Drain when not in use.
• Disinfection, regular cleaning and changing of water in indoor fountains and whirlpool spas.
• Use sterile water for respiratory therapy devices.

Surveillance

• Mandatory notifiable in all EU countries.

- Cases of laboratory-confirmed legionellosis should be reported to local public health authorities on the day of diagnosis.
- Clusters of respiratory infection should be reported without waiting for confirmation.
- Confirmed cases should also be reported to the relevant national surveillance scheme.
- Legionellosis should be included in hospital infection surveillance schemes, especially for higher risk patients. Nosocomial pneumonia cases should be tested for *Legionella*.
- Cases associated with travel to other European countries are reported to the European Legionnaires' Disease Surveillance Network (ELDSNet) at ECDC.

Response to a case

- Ensure appropriate laboratory confirmatory tests are undertaken.
- Report to the local public health authority and national surveillance centre.
- Obtain risk factor history for 2–14 days (Legionnaires' disease) or 0–3 days (Pontiac fever) before onset of symptoms: details of places of residence and work; visits for occupational or leisure reasons; exposure to industrial sites, hotels, hospitals, leisure/sport/garden centres; air conditioning, showers, whirlpools/jacuzzis, fountains, humidifiers, nebulisers, etc.
- If a recognised risk factor is identified discuss inspection of the possible source, examination of maintenance records and sampling with environmental health and microbiology colleagues. Enquire about respiratory illness in others exposed to the potential source.
- Report travel outside the district to the relevant public health authority and travel outside the country to the national surveillance centre.
- If the case is likely to have acquired infection in hospital, convene incident control team. A single nosocomial case should lead to an environmental investigation, including the potable water supply. Isolation is unnecessary.
- If no risk factor is identified, consider domestic water system as a possible source. Also consider if possible nosocomial case spent part of incubation period at home.

Investigation of a cluster

- Undertake hypothesis-generation exercise of risk factors as identified for individual cases including day-by-day analysis of movements in 14 days before onset.
- Further case finding: ensure all cases of community or hospital-acquired pneumonia are tested for legionellosis. If serogroup 1 disease, encourage urine antigen testing for rapid diagnosis. Where possible, also encourage culture so that typing may be performed. Alert colleagues in other areas to check whether cases visited your locality.
- Use geographical analysis of home, work and places visited of cases to look for links. Geographical information systems can be used to see if cases have been near each other and can also use weather data.
- If cases have been to same area, identify all potential sources. Consider identification, inspection and sampling of all cooling towers in the area.
- In nosocomial outbreaks, test all water sources (hot and cold) and relevant environmental samples (e.g. showerheads) in suspect wards. Obtain specialist engineering advice on plumbing and heating systems.
- Compare typing results from cases and suspected source.

Control of an outbreak

- Shutdown of suspected source whilst expert engineering advice obtained.
- Drainage, cleaning, disinfection, maintenance and re-evaluation of suspected source. Occasionally, major redesign or closure is necessary.
- Warn clinicians of increase and of appropriate antibiotics.
- Rarely, temporary chemoprophylaxis in high-risk populations during a severe nosocomial outbreak may be considered.

3.44 Leprosy

Leprosy is a chronic inflammatory disease caused by *Mycobacterium leprae*.

Epidemiology

Leprosy occurs in tropical and warm temperate regions. It is associated with overcrowding and becomes less common as living standards rise. Cases in Europe are rare and mostly imported.

Clinical features

The organism has a predilection for the skin and nerves. Nerve involvement results in an area of anaesthesia and or muscle weakness/wasting; tissue damage occurs secondarily to the anaesthesia.

The clinical appearance of the disease depends upon the degree of cell-mediated immunity. In tuberculoid (TT) disease there is a high degree of cell-mediated immunity and disease is localised; in lepromatous (LL) there is little cell-mediated immunity and skin and nerves are heavily infiltrated with bacilli.

Immunologically mediated reactions, which include erythema nodosum leprosum and tender enlarging nerves, may occur as cell-mediated immunity returns during treatment.

Laboratory confirmation

The diagnosis can usually be made following a careful examination. Confirmation is by identifying mycobacteria in slit skin smears or histological preparations. In lepromatous patients nodules should be biopsied and the nasal mucosa scraped. In tuberculoid patients the edge of a lesion should be biopsied.

Transmission

The major source of infection is patients with lepromatous leprosy who shed large numbers of bacilli in their nasal secretions. The portal of entry is probably the respiratory tract.

Acquisition

The incubation period varies from a few months to many years. Lepromatous patients may be infectious for several years.

Prevention

Identification and treatment of lepromatous patients is the mainstay of prevention.

Surveillance

Leprosy is a notifiable disease in most countries. In the UK there is a leprosy register of all cases.

Response to a case

Cases should be referred to a specialist unit for treatment. Lepromatous cases should be isolated until treatment has been initiated.

Investigation of a cluster

A cluster should be investigated for misdiagnosis or laboratory contamination.

Suggested case-definition for an outbreak
A clinically compatible case that is laboratory confirmed by demonstration of acid-fast bacilli in skin or dermal nerve.

3.45 Leptospirosis

Leptospirosis is rare cause of septicaemia caused by the zoonotic genus *Leptospira*, which occurs worldwide.

Suggested on-call action
• Person-to-person spread is very rare so no urgent on-call action is required. • In the event of an apparent outbreak associated with flooding/recreational activity ensure early circulation of guidance to the public.

Epidemiology

Leptospirosis is an occupational hazard to farmers and sewage workers and a recreational hazard of water sports. Epidemics may be seen in areas of poverty. In the UK, the most commonly identified serovars are *Leptospira hardjo* and *Leptospira icterohaemorrhagiae*, associated with cattle and rats, respectively. Incidence varies from 0.1–1 per 100,000 population per year in temperate climates to 10 or more per 100,000 population per year in tropical areas. A total of 832 confirmed cases were reported from 26 EU and EEA/EFTA countries in 2007.

Clinical features

The clinical course is highly variable; infection is often mild or subclinical. When symptomatic the onset is characteristically abrupt with severe headache, myalgia, conjunctival suffusion and fever. After 3–7 days symptoms resolve. In biphasic disease, following a transient remission, meningism, renal and vasculitic manifestations occur. The phases may merge. Leptospirosis with jaundice and uraemia is sometimes known as Weil's disease. The case fatality rate is 1–5% (Weil's disease 20–40%). Death is usually associated with renal failure or may result from myocarditis or massive blood loss.

Treatment is based upon antibiotics and physiological support. Early antibiotic treatment is critical and may not be effective if given late.

Laboratory confirmation

Leptospira interrogans comprises over 200 serovars in 24 serogroups. This classification is being replaced by genotyping. During the first phase organisms may be visualised in (under dark field illumination) and cultured from blood, CSF or urine. The organism may persist in urine. The microscopic agglutination test is the reference method for serological diagnosis. Antibodies may be detected using ELISA.

During the first phase of the illness there may be leukopaenia. Jaundice may be associated with neutrophilia. About one-quarter of cases will have an elevated urea.

Transmission

Infection results from contact with the urine of infected animals or contaminated material (water, soil). The organism probably enters through mucosa or broken skin.

Acquisition

The incubation period is usually 7–13 days (range 2–30 days). Patients excrete leptospires for many months, but person-to-person spread is rare. Contaminated soil can remain infective for 14 days. Previous infection protects against re-infection with the same serovar, but may not protect against other serovars.

Prevention

• Control rodent populations.
• Education to those at risk to avoid contaminated areas and cover broken skin.
• Providing alert/information cards to those likely to be exposed.
• Adequate occupational clothing.
• Immunisation of those with occupational exposure to specific serovars has been tried in some countries.

Surveillance

Leptospirosis is notifiable in many countries. Report cases to authorities so that areas of risk can be identified.

Response to a case

• Treatment with intravenous antibiotics (e.g. benzyl penicillin) in the first 4 days probably reduces the severity of disease.
• Obtain risk factor information.

Investigation of a cluster

Investigate clusters to determine areas of risk – such as water sports locations, so that the public can be informed. Laboratory typing may help identify risk factors.

Control of an outbreak

• Outbreaks usually occur in areas of poverty, particularly following flooding and disasters that have increased the rodent population. Rodent control is the main activity.
• Outbreaks resulting from occupational exposure (e.g. to cattle) should be reported to the veterinary authorities.
• If the outbreak is associated with flooding or recreational exposure, ensure early circulation of guidance to the public to reduce exposure and to professionals to ensure early recognition.
• Antibiotic prophylaxis (e.g. doxycycline) may be considered.
• For more information see Human leptospirosis: Guidance for Diagnosis, Surveillance and control (http://whqlibdoc.who.int/hq/2003/WHO_CDS_CSR_EPH_2002.23.pdf).

Suggested case-definition

Clinical: presence of fever plus at least two clinically compatible features, particularly in the presence of known risk factor(s).
Confirmed: isolation of *Leptospira sp.* from clinical specimen or fourfold or greater rise in antibody titre or demonstration of *Leptospira sp.* in a clinical specimen by immunofluorescence or silver staining.

3.46 Listeria

Infection by *Listeria monocytogenes* is usually food-borne but often presents as septicaemia or meningitis. Although rare, infection in vulnerable groups has high case fatality with fetuses, neonates, the elderly and the immunocompromised particularly at risk.

Suggested on-call action

If you or the reporting clinician/ microbiologist know of associated cases consult the Outbreak Control Plan.

Epidemiology

The incidence of reported cases is Europe is 0.31 per 100,000 population (2008), although the true incidence is likely to be substantially higher. Incidence of reported cases is highest in those over 65 years of age (56% of total cases; 0.94 per 100,000), followed by children under 4 years (0.35 per 100,000). Rates are particularly high in pregnant women and neonates. At the European level, reports are highest from August to October, although this is not apparent for every country or every year. Incidence rates for reported cases are highest in Scandinavian countries.

Clinical features

Listeriosis may present in a variety of ways, including the following:
• Acute gastroenteritis: this often affects previously well, non-pregnant individuals. The most common symptoms are headache, fever, abdominal pain, sleepiness, nausea and diarrhoea. Fatigue, myalgia, arthralgia, vomiting and sore throat may also be reported.
• Systemic illness, which may include septicaemia or meningitis: these manifestations more often affect individuals with immunosuppression or chronic disease and the elderly. Case fatality rates are high in those with underlying disease. Other features include encephalitis, abscess, endocarditis and septic arthritis.
• Infection in pregnancy or neonates: although infection in pregnant women usually causes mild infection in the mother, it may lead to miscarriage, premature delivery or stillbirth or neonatal infection (up to

10 days after delivery), particularly meningitis, with high mortality.
• Asymptomatic infection, with excretion in the stools, may also occur.

Laboratory confirmation

Diagnosis is usually by blood or cerebrospinal fluid (CSF) culture, which usually takes 48 hours, plus another 24 hours for confirmation. In *Listeria* meningitis, less than half of cases have organisms demonstrable on CSF microscopy, which also shows polymorphs or lymphocytes, increased protein and normal or decreased glucose. *Listeria* may also be identified from other sterile sites and in faecal, food and environmental samples, particularly after 'cold enrichment' in the laboratory.

Typing is helpful in the investigation of outbreaks. There are 17 serovars of *L. monocytogenes*, of which 4b, 1/2a and 1/2b cause 90% of clinical cases in Europe. Phage typing is also obtainable on 80% of serovar 4 and 37% of serovar 1/2 strains. Genotyping is available in many countries.

Transmission

L. monocytogenes is widespread in the environment and can be found in soil, surface water, vegetation and a wide range of wild and domestic animals. It is extremely hardy and survives drying and freezing, remaining viable in soil or silage for long periods.

The main route of infection for humans is consumption of contaminated food. The organism can grow at temperatures as low as 0°C (although optimum growth temperature is 30–37°C), is relatively tolerant of salt and nitrates, resulting in an ability to survive in processed, preserved and refrigerated foods. *Listeria* do not 'spoil' or affect the taste of food even at high levels of contamination.

Many foods have been associated with transmission of infection but most have some or all of the following features: highly processed, refrigerated, long shelf life, near-neutral pH and consumed without further cooking. Regularly implicated vehicles include processed meat/fish products, dairy products, especially if unpasteurised, and pre-prepared meals (see Response to a cluster). Some outbreaks have been explained by long-term colonisation of difficult to clean sites in food processing facilities. Infected cattle can contaminate milk.

Other sources of infection include direct transmission from animals, which may cause cutaneous infection often with obvious occupational exposure; direct contact with a contaminated environment; transplacental transmission in pregnant women; exposure to vaginal carriage during birth or hospital cross-infection for late-onset neonatal sepsis; and nosocomial transmission in hospital nurseries and renal transplant units.

Acquisition

Reported incubation periods vary widely from about 10 hours to months. Outbreaks of *Listeria* gastroenteritis and/or flu-like illness have a median incubation period of about 24 hours. Much longer incubations have been reported for severe disease and/or infection in pregnant or immunocompromised individuals.

Human excreters with normal hygiene are unlikely to be an important source of infection, except for neonates. The infectious dose is uncertain (possibly 100–1000/g food) and it is unclear what level is 'safe' for immunocompromised patients or pregnant women, leading many to suggest a 'zero tolerance' policy for food.

In addition to fetuses, neonates and the elderly, those at risk of severe infection include patients with malignancy, chronic disease and impaired immunity. Low gastric acidity increases susceptibility.

Prevention

• Hazard analysis in food processing to reduce the risk of contamination and multiplication.

• Pasteurisation of dairy produce effectively kills *Listeria*. Post-pasteurisation hygiene is also important.
• Limiting the length of storage of at-risk refrigerated food (e.g. cook-chill and ready-to-eat meals).
• Advice to pregnant women and the immunosuppressed to avoid unpasteurised soft cheeses, refrigerated paté and pre-packed salads.
• Thorough reheating of cook-chill/microwave foods, especially if served to vulnerable populations (e.g. hospital patients).
• Pregnant women should avoid contact with pregnant or newborn animals or silage.
• Thoroughly wash raw vegetables, fruit and salad before eating.
• Adequate infection control in delivery rooms and neonatal units.

Surveillance

• Listeriosis should be reported to local public health authorities: compulsory notification in many EU countries.
• Laboratories should report all clinically significant infections to regional and national surveillance: these may detect outbreaks not apparent at local level.
• Consider as a cause of two or more cases of 'late onset' neonatal meningitis/septicaemia.

Response to a case

• Report to local and national/regional public health authorities to aid detection of clusters.
• Collect data on consumption of risk foods in last month.
• No exclusion required, although enteric precautions sensible for hospitalised patients.
• Send isolate to reference laboratory for typing.

Response to a cluster

• Discuss with microbiologist further investigation such as serotyping, phagetyping or genotyping.

• Institute case finding with microbiologists and relevant clinicians to ensure adequate microbiological investigation of meningitis/septicaemia in neonates and the elderly.

• Undertake a hypothesis-generating study to include all foods consumed, particularly those at increased risk of high level *Listeria* contamination: for example, processed meat/fish products, such as paté/rillettes, cold meats, hot dogs and processed fish; dairy products, such as soft cheese, butter and milk, especially if unpasteurised; and pre-prepared meals, such as 'cook-chill' meals, sandwiches and salads. The prolonged incubation will make accurate recall difficult: 'food preference' questions may also be useful as are questions on cafes/restaurants visited, food shops and travel. Consider direct exposure to animals (e.g. farms).

• If cases are predominantly neonatal, look at age in days at onset: could this be nosocomial?

Control of an outbreak

• Product withdrawal of any implicated food.

• Obtain specialist Environmental Health advice to investigate and modify suspect food processes.

Suggested case-definition for an outbreak

Flu-like illness, gastroenteritis, septicaemia or CNS infection, associated with isolate of the outbreak strain of *L. monocytogenes* from blood or CSF.

3.47 Lyme disease

Lyme disease (erythema migrans, borreliosis) is a multisystem illness resulting from exposure to *Ixodes* ticks infected with a spirochaete, *Borrelia burgdorferi, Borrelia afzelii*

or *Borrelia garnii*. It may be called Bannwarth's syndrome in parts of Europe when neurological symptoms are present.

Suggested on-call action

None required.

Epidemiology

Lyme disease is common in North America and Northern and Central Europe in areas of heathland, affecting ramblers and campers. Geographical distribution of disease in Europe is associated with the known range of *Ixodes ricinus*. The true incidence of disease is unknown as reporting is incomplete. Estimates of incidence per 100,000 population are Slovenia 206, Austria 135, Czech Republic 36, Germany 25, France 16, Scotland 1.9, England and Wales 1.1 and Italy 0.02.

Clinical features

Following a tick bite, which may be inapparent, a rash (erythema migrans) develops; the appearance is of an expanding erythematous circle with central clearing. Other manifestations include large joint polyarthritis (usually asymmetrical), aseptic meningitis, peripheral root lesions, radiculopathy, meningoencephalitis and myocarditis. These features may occur without the rash and symptoms may persist over a prolonged period. The clinical manifestations seen in Europe and North America differ, with milder disease often reported in Europe.

Laboratory confirmation

Serological testing early in the disease may be unhelpful although it may be more useful in later disease. Positive or equivocal results on an enzyme-linked immunosorbent assay (ELISA) or indirect immunofluorescent antibody (IFA) assay require confirmatory testing with a Western blot test. Some chronic patients may remain seronegative. PCR tests for *B. burgdorferi* DNA are available in specialist centres.

Transmission

B. burgdorferi is transmitted by the bite of *Ixodes* ticks. Deer are the preferred host for adult ticks in the USA; sheep in Europe. Other mammals (e.g. dogs) can be incidental hosts and may develop Lyme disease. Lyme disease is not transmissible from person to person.

Acquisition

Erythema migrans, the best clinical indicator of Lyme disease, develops between 3 and 32 days after a tick bite.

Prevention

The main method of prevention is avoidance of tick bites through wearing long trousers. Transmission of *B. burgdorferi* does not usually occur until the tick has been in place for 36–48 hours; thus, screening and removing ticks after exposure can help prevent infection (see Chapter 3.82).

Surveillance

Cases should be reported to the public health authorities so that assessments of risk can be made.

Response to a case

No public health response.

Investigation of a cluster and control of an outbreak

Clusters should be investigated to determine areas of high risk, so that those who might be exposed can be informed.

Suggested case-definition
Clinical diagnosis of erythema migrans in a person who has been exposed to ticks.

3.48 Malaria

Malaria is a potentially fatal plasmodial infection. Increasing numbers of patients presenting to healthcare facilities in Europe will have travelled to places where they have been exposed to malaria. There is also a risk of airport and transfusion malaria.

Suggested on-call action
None unless the case is thought to be transfusion related in which case other units from the same donor need to be identified and withdrawn urgently.

Epidemiology

Malaria is endemic in more than 100 countries throughout Africa, Central and South America, Asia and Oceania; more than 2 billion people are exposed to the risk of malaria infection. *Plasmodium falciparum* and *Plasmodium vivax* are the most common species. *P. falciparum* is the predominant species in Africa and Papua New Guinea. *P. vivax* dominates in South America and Asia; *Plasmodium malariae* is widely distributed but is much less common. *Plasmodium ovale* is mainly found in Africa. About 4000 cases a year are reported in Europe (notification rate <1 per 100,000) with a declining trend. In 2007, 70% of the cases were reported by three countries (Germany, Italy and the UK). Patterns of importation reflect travel destinations. The most common source of imported falciparum malaria is West Africa, followed by East and Central Africa.

The case fatality rate in Europe is low (about 0.5% in England and Wales).

Clinical features

Malaria may present with almost any clinical pattern. The most classic symptom is the malarial rigor, the periodic nature of the attacks of fever may give a clue as to the diagnosis. The disease must be considered in anyone who has been exposed to the parasite, by travel, blood transfusion or the rare airport malaria.

Complications are associated with high parasitaemia and are therefore more common in non-immune adults and children. The course may be rapid: delay in diagnosis of *P. falciparum* malaria is associated with increased mortality (e.g. due to cerebral malaria).

Laboratory confirmation

Diagnosis is by demonstrating parasites in the peripheral blood. A minimum of three specimens should be taken at the height of fever. Thick films are of particular value when the parasitaemia is low; the technique requires experience. A thin film enables a parasite count (number of parasites per 100 red blood cells) to be performed and the parasite species to be more clearly identified. Slides should be reviewed by an expert so that a species diagnosis, essential to guide chemotherapy, can be made.

Serology has no part to play in diagnosis of acute malaria. Antigen detection methods for malaria antigen are under development, but as yet do not compare with the sensitivity and specificity of microscopy.

Transmission

Malaria is normally transmitted by the bite of the female anopheline mosquito. Rare cases of 'airport malaria' happen when an infected mosquito introduced to Europe bites a host before dying. There are also rare transmissions through blood donation, needlestick injury or poor hospital infection control.

Acquisition

The incubation period (time from infection to appearance of parasites in blood) varies with infecting species:
P. falciparum : 5–7 days
P. vivax: 6–8 days
P. malariae: 12–16 days
P. ovale: 8–9 days
In transfusion-associated malaria the incubation period is much shorter.

In *P. vivax* and *P. ovale* some parasites remain dormant in the liver (hypnozoites): these can take up to a year before becoming active.

Prevention

• Good advice to those travelling is essential. The risk of those visiting relatives is often underestimated by travellers and those providing advice: pre-existing immunity will probably have waned.
• Prevention of mosquito bites (the mosquitoes bite mainly at night):
   (a) sleep in fully air-conditioned or screened accommodation and use knockdown insecticide in the room each evening;
   (b) if the room cannot be made safe, sleep under bed nets; impregnation with pyrethrum enhances the efficacy of nets;
   (c) electrical pyrethroid vapouriser in the room may also be useful;

(d) wear long-sleeved garments and long trousers between dusk and dawn; and

(e) use mosquito repellents.

• Suppression of the malaria parasite with chemoprophylaxis. Regular antimalarial prophylaxis should generally be taken for 1 week before travel to an endemic area and 6 weeks after return. Changing patterns of resistance mean that specialist advice should be consulted.

• Control of malaria in populations depends on diminishing or eradication of the vector, the *Anopheles* mosquito. Methods include spraying of houses with insecticides and the destruction of larval sites by removing standing water.

Surveillance

• Malaria is notifiable in many countries, including most of Europe.

• Cases should be reported to national authorities so that advice on prophylaxis can be based upon observed patterns of risk.

Response to a case

• A travel history should be taken.

• If there is no travel history, information about transfusions or injections (including drug misuse) and proximity to airports should be sought.

• Patients should be reviewed 28 days after treatment to confirm parasitological and clinical cure. Patients who have splenic enlargement should avoid body contact sports and strenuous exercise due to a risk of splenic rupture.

Investigation of a cluster and control of an outbreak

• If clusters arise from areas where malaria has not previously been recognised, the national authorities should be informed. Travel advice should be reviewed.

• If cases occur in people who have not been abroad, consider blood, nosocomial and airport exposures.

Suggested case-definitions for an outbreak

Clinical: fever and/or compatible illness in person who has travelled to an area in which malaria is endemic.
World Health Organization categories:
Autochthonous:
• *indigenous:* malaria acquired by mosquito transmission in an area where malaria is a regular occurrence;
• *introduced:* malaria acquired by mosquito transmission from an imported case in an area where malaria is not a regular occurrence.
Imported: malaria acquired outside a specific area.
Induced: malaria acquired through artificial means (e.g. blood transfusion, common syringes or malaria therapy).
Relapsing: renewed manifestation (i.e. of clinical symptoms and/or parasitaemia) of malarial infection that is separated from previous manifestations of the same infection by an interval greater than any interval resulting from the normal periodicity of the paroxysms.
Cryptic: an isolated case of malaria that cannot be epidemiologically linked to additional cases.

3.49 Measles

Measles is a systemic viral infection caused by a paramyxovirus. Its main features are fever, rash and respiratory disease. The public health significance of measles is that it is highly infectious but can be prevented by vaccination.

Epidemiology

In the pre-vaccination era, measles circulated widely and most people were infected in childhood. The epidemiology of measles in the post-vaccination era varies across Europe, depending on the evolution of vaccine strategies and vaccine coverage. In countries where coverage has been high for many years, the disease has been virtually eliminated. In 2008, eight European countries reported rates below 1 per million, and five countries (Estonia, Hungary, Slovakia, Slovenia and Iceland) reported zero cases (Table 3.49.1). The highest rates were in the UK (2.4 per 100,000), Italy (2.1 per 100,000) and Austria (1.9 per 100,000). These countries, as well as France and Germany, have reported large outbreaks in recent years. One death (in the UK) and five cases complicated with encephalitis were reported in 2008. Continuing suboptimal vaccine coverage in countries reporting outbreaks means that the World Health Organization target of measles elimination in Europe has not been met.

Clinical features

In an unvaccinated child, there is a prodromal illness with a high fever and a coryzal respiratory infection. There is cough, conjunctivitis and runny nose. Koplik's spots appear during the early part of the illness – these look like grains of salt on a red inflamed background and are found on the mucosa of the cheek next to the upper premolars and molars. The rash of measles starts on day 3 or 4, initially in the hairline, but spreads rapidly to cover the face, trunk and limbs. It is maculapapu-lar but not itchy. Koplik's spots fade as the rash appears. The rash fades over 1 week to 10 days.

In a vaccinated person, the illness is usually mild with a low-grade fever, transient rash and absent respiratory features.

Complications of measles include pneumonitis, secondary bacterial infection, especially acute otitis media and pneumonia, and encephalitis. Complication rates are higher in malnourished or immunosuppressed children. Subacute sclerosing panencephalitis is a late, slow-onset, progressive complication which occurs in about 1 per million cases. It is always fatal.

Laboratory confirmation

The diagnosis can be confirmed by PCR testing of oral fluid (Oracol) throat swabs, nasopharyngeal aspirate (NPA), urine, CSF or tissue or serology (single raised IgM or rise in IgG). Measles IgM can be detected in saliva if the specimen is collected between 1 and 6 weeks after the onset of symptoms.

Transmission

Humans are the only reservoir. Carriers are unknown. Spread is from person to person by direct contact with nose and throat secretions or respiratory droplets; less commonly, indirectly by articles freshly soiled with nose and throat secretions.

Acquisition

The incubation period is 7–18 days, usually about 10 days. The period of communicability starts just before the onset of the prodrome and lasts until 4 days after the rash appears. Measles is highly infectious, with a reproduction rate of 15–17 (i.e. 15–17 secondary cases in a susceptible population for every index case). Natural infection provides lifelong immunity. Vaccine-induced immunity is lower, but is also usually lifelong and

Table 3.49.1 Measles cases and notification rate in Europe in 2008

Country	Total cases	Confirmed cases	Notification rate per 100,000
Austria	446	156	1.9
Belgium	98	98	0.92
Bulgaria	1	1	<0.1
Cyprus	1	1	0.13
Czech Republic	2	2	<0.1
Denmark	14	14	0.26
Estonia	0	0	0.00
Finland	5	5	<0.1
France	604	305	0.48
Germany	916	779	0.95
Greece	1	1	<0.1
Hungary	0	0	0.00
Ireland	55	13	0.30
Italy	5311	1236	2.1
Latvia	3	3	0.13
Lithuania	1	1	<0.1
Luxembourg	1	1	0.21
Malta	1	1	0.24
Netherlands	109	109	0.66
Poland	100	89	0.23
Portugal	1	1	<0.1
Slovakia	0	0	0.00
Slovenia	0	0	0.00
Spain	229	198	0.44
Sweden	25	25	0.27
UK	1462	1442	2.4
EU total	**9400**	**4495**	**0.90**
Iceland	0	0	0.0
Liechtenstein	–	–	–
Norway	4	4	<0.1
Total	**9404**	**4499**	**0.89**

Source of data: European Centre for Disease Prevention and Control (ECDC) Annual Epidemiological Report 2010.

can be boosted by exposure to circulating wild virus. In developed countries, maternal antibody persists for up to 12 months; this period may be shorter when the maternal immunity is vaccine-induced.

Prevention

• Vaccinate with a combined measles/mumps/rubella (MMR) or measles/mumps/rubella/varicella (MMRV) vaccine. Two doses are required: the first at 12–18 months of age;

the timing of the second dose varies from 2 to 13 years of age (for schedules in Europe see www.euvac.net/graphics/vaccination/var.html). The only contraindications to measles vaccine are immunosuppression, allergy to neomycin or kanamycin and a severe reaction to a previous dose. Measles vaccine can be safely given to children with egg anaphylaxis.

• Vaccination should not be given within 3 weeks of another live vaccine (except oral poliovirus vaccine) or within 3 months of an injection of immunoglobulin.

Surveillance

Measles is notifiable throughout Europe, and enhanced surveillance is in place through the EU community network for vaccine-preventable infectious diseases (euvac.net). This surveillance scheme collects the following data for confirmed and probable cases: age group, immunisation status, hospital treatment, whether acute encephalitis occurred, whether the case died and whether infection was imported from another country.

Response to a case

- Obtain laboratory confirmation.
- Determine the source of infection (including travel history).
- Identify vulnerable contacts (immunocompromised, pregnant, infants); assess their exposure risk and susceptibility and give human normal immunoglobulin (HNIG).
- Consider vaccine for other contacts (effective if given within 72 hours of exposure).
- Exclude confirmed and likely cases from school, nursery, college or work until 5 days from the onset of rash.
- Exclude healthcare workers from work who have been contact with a case, if there is no evidence of protection, from the fifth day of exposure, until immunity can be provided (vaccine) or demonstrated (IgG).

Response to a cluster and investigation of an outbreak

As per case investigation, but also convene an outbreak team and consider need for community vaccination programme.

Suggested case-definition for an outbreak

Suspected case:
- Fever (>38°C if measured); *plus*
- Rash; *plus one of*:
- Conjunctivitis, cough, coryza.

Confirmed case:
- Confirmed wild measles virus in any clinical specimen; *or*
- Measles IgM in blood or saliva; *or*
- Fourfold or greater rise in measles IgG in blood.

3.50 Meningococcal infection

Meningococcal infection is the spectrum of disease caused by the bacterium *Neisseria meningitidis*. The infection may present as meningitis, septicaemia, or a combination of both. The public health significance of meningococcal infection lies in the severity of the disease, the absence of effective serogroup B vaccines, the ability of the infection to cause unpredictable clusters and the intense public anxiety that inevitably accompanies a case or cluster.

Suggested on-call action

- Ensure rapid admission to hospital and administration of pre-admission benzyl penicillin.
- Initiate laboratory investigations to confirm diagnosis.
- Arrange chemoprophylaxis for close contacts of confirmed or probable cases.

Epidemiology

The incidence of notified meningococcal infection in Europe in 2008 was 0.9 per 100,000 population and has stabilised in recent years, having decreased by half since 1999 (1.9 per 100,000). The rate varies from <1 to 3.5 per 100,000. Highest rates are in Ireland (3.5 per 100,000) and the UK (2.1 per 100,000). The decrease over the past decade is partly due to the impact of meningococcal

C vaccines in some countries, but also to a general decline in serogroup B disease.

There are 13 serogroups of *Neisseria meningitidis*. In Europe, serogroups B and C account for over 95% of cases. Serogroup B is more common than C.

Children under the age of 5 years are most frequently affected, with a peak incidence at about 6 months of age, which coincides with the loss of maternally derived immunity. There is a second, smaller peak in teenagers.

Most cases arise sporadically, although clusters occur from time to time. These are unpredictable, although they often occur in educational establishments or in the military. Serogroup C disease tends to cause clusters more than serogroup B.

The infection is seasonal, with a higher incidence in the winter months. There are geographical variations in the disease, although these are not consistent over time. Local increases are often associated with the arrival of a strain not previously seen in that community.

There are a number of factors that predispose to meningococcal infection. These include passive smoking, crowding, recent influenza type A infection, absence of a spleen and complement deficiency. Travellers to the meningitis belt of Africa (where outbreaks of serogroup A disease are common) may be at risk of disease. Cases (serogroup A and W135) among pilgrims to the Hajj at Mecca have prompted a requirement for a certificate of meningococcal vaccination from visitors.

Clinical features

The early symptoms are non-specific and are often mistaken for a viral infection. In infants there is fever, floppiness, high-pitched crying and sometimes vomiting. Older children and adults have a fever, malaise, increasing headache, nausea and often vomiting. The illness usually progresses rapidly, although sometimes there is a slower onset, which causes diagnostic difficulty. In infants there is progressive irritability, altered consciousness and sometimes convulsions. Older

children and adults develop photophobia and neck stiffness with a positive Kernig's sign, although these features are sometimes absent.

An important feature is the appearance of a petechial rash, which indicates that there is septicaemia. The rash is not always present, or there may be only a few petechiae, so a careful search for petechiae is important in suspected cases. The 'glass test' (http://www.meningitis-trust.org/meningitis-info/signs-and-symptoms/glass-test/) can be used to distinguish a haemorrhagic rash from other types of rash.

Patients with rapidly advancing disease may develop hypotension, circulatory collapse, pulmonary oedema, confusion and coma. The overall case fatality rate is about 10%, although for patients without septicaemia the outlook is better. Approximately 15% of survivors have permanent sequelae, including deafness, convulsions, mental impairment and limb loss.

Laboratory confirmation

Obtaining laboratory confirmation in suspected cases is essential for public health management. Specimens should be taken as soon as a suspected case is seen in hospital (Box 3.50.1). The single most important specimen is blood for culture and polymerase chain reaction (PCR) diagnosis. There is often reluctance to perform a lumbar puncture because of the risk of coning; however, where a CSF sample has been obtained, this should be submitted for microscopy, culture and PCR. Meningococcal DNA can be found in the cerebrospinal fluid (CSF) up to 96 hours after commencing antibiotics. A throat swab should also be obtained for culture (the yield from cases is about 50% and is unaffected by prior administration of antibiotic). A rash aspirate for microscopy is a further useful specimen. A throat swab from family members before chemoprophylaxis may also help to identify the causative organism, although counselling is advised before swabbing to prevent feelings of guilt should a household member be found to be the source of infection. Acute

> **Box 3.50.1 Suggested laboratory specimens/investigations in suspected meningococcal infection**
>
> - Blood for culture
> - Blood for PCR (EDTA or other unclotted blood specimen)
> - Serum (on admission and 2–6 weeks later)
> - CSF for microscopy, culture, PCR (provided raised intracranial pressure has been ruled out)
> - Aspirate from other sterile sites suspected of being infected (e.g. joints) for microscopy, culture, PCR
> - Nasopharyngeal swab

and convalescent serology can also provide a diagnosis, although the result is often obtained too late to affect either clinical or public health management; however, it may be useful in the investigation of a potential cluster as it provides serogroup information.

It is important to determine the serogroup of the infecting organism, to inform decisions about vaccination. PCR diagnosis is serogroup-specific and a result is available within a few hours. Latex agglutination tests are also available as a rapid screening method when there is a positive culture, although the national reference laboratory should ideally confirm the result. Genotyping methods such as *porA* sequencing, pulsed field gel electrophoresis (PFGE) and multi-locus sequence typing (MLST) provide a much more precise typing than phenotype-based methods.

Transmission

The infection is spread from person to person through respiratory droplets and direct contact with nose and throat secretions. Infectivity is relatively low, and transmission usually requires prolonged close contact such as occurs in the household setting or through 'wet' mouth kissing.

Humans are the only reservoir, and the organism dies quickly outside the host. Approximately 10% of the population carries the organism harmlessly in the nasopharynx. Carriage confers natural immunity. During outbreaks, carriage rates of the outbreak strain may rise sharply, to as high as 50%. How-

ever, there is no consistent relationship between carriage rates and disease, and some outbreaks occur in the absence of normal carriage. Increased rates of carriage have been observed in smokers, in crowded conditions and among military recruits.

The most common setting for transmission to occur is within households, where a member of the household (usually an adult) has recently become a carrier and infects a susceptible household member (usually a child). The absolute risk, in the absence of chemoprophylaxis, of a second case in the same household in the month following an index case is about 1 in 300. In comparison, transmission in other settings is rare; the estimated risks of a second case in the month following an index case in a pre-school group, primary and secondary school are 1 in 1500, 1 in 18,000 and 1 in 33,000, respectively. Transmission from patients to healthcare workers has been documented but is also rare, occurring where there has been direct exposure to nasopharyngeal secretions.

Acquisition

There is no true incubation period, as the organism may be carried in the nasopharynx for a variable time before invasive disease. Investigations of clusters suggest an incubation period of 3–5 days, although it may occasionally be up to 10 days. Patients are usually no longer infectious within 24 hours of starting antibiotic treatment, although it should be noted that some antibiotics used in treatment (e.g. penicillin) will only temporarily suppress carriage. For this reason a chemoprophylactic antibiotic should be given before hospital discharge.

Maternal immunity to meningococcal infection is passed across the placenta to the neonate, but only lasts for a few months. Subsequent carriage of pathogenic and non-pathogenic meningococci confers serogroup-specific natural immunity, which usually develops within 7 days of acquisition. Carriage of pathogenic meningococci is unusual in infancy and early childhood, rises progressively to peak at 25% in 15- to 19-year-olds and then slowly declines through adult life.

Prevention

• Polysaccharide vaccines have been superseded by polysaccharide-protein conjugate vaccines against serogroups A, C, W135 and Y. They induce immunological memory, which is likely to be lifelong. Routine group C vaccination has been introduced in a number of countries in Europe, with dramatic impact. Schedules vary: the first countries to introduce vaccination (e.g. the UK) implemented infant immunisation; more recent programmes have opted for a single dose in the second year of life. The need for subsequent booster doses in older children/ adolescents is under evaluation.
• Serogroup B vaccines have to date performed poorly in clinical trials (particularly in children) and are not yet generally available, although one candidate vaccine appears promising and is likely to be available in Europe soon.

Surveillance

• Both acute meningitis and meningococcal septicaemia are notifiable in most European countries, including the UK.
• Laboratory reports are another important source of data in most countries, although increasing use of pre-admission antibiotics means that there is now greater reliance on non-culture diagnoses for surveillance.

Response to a case

• Public health action is indicated for confirmed or probable cases; it is not indicated for possible cases or infection in non-sterile sites (except for meningococcal conjunctivitis which is an indication for public health action because of the high immediate risk of invasive disease).
• There are four key actions for the public health practitioner:

(a) ensure rapid admission to hospital and that pre-admission benzyl penicillin has been given. Prompt action may reduce the case fatality rate by up to 50%;

(b) ensure that appropriate laboratory investigations are undertaken;

(c) arrange for chemoprophylaxis for close contacts, and vaccine if the infection is due to a vaccine-preventable strain.

The aim of chemoprophylaxis is to eradicate the infecting strain from the network of close contacts, and thus prevent further cases among susceptible close contacts. Chemoprophylaxis should be given as soon as possible. Close contacts are defined as people who have had close prolonged contact with the case in the week before onset. This usually includes household members, girlfriends/boyfriends, regular childminders and sometimes students in a hall of residence. Following a single case classroom, nursery and other social contacts do not need chemoprophylaxis. Chemoprophylaxis for healthcare workers exposed to a case is only recommended for those whose mouth or nose is directly exposed to large particle droplets/secretions from the respiratory tract of a probable or confirmed case of meningococcal disease during acute illness until completed 24 hours of systemic antibiotics.

The aim of vaccination is to prevent late secondary cases. There is less urgency for vaccination, as chemoprophylaxis aims to prevent the early secondary cases. Conjugate vaccine should be offered to all close contacts of serogroup A, C, W135 or Y disease as defined above; the index case should also receive vaccine.

(d) Provide information about meningococcal disease to parents, GPs and educational establishments. The aim here is to improve the outcome of any secondary cases that may occur and to prevent rumours and anxiety.

Investigation of a cluster

• Obtain serotyping or genotyping to see if cases are potentially linked.
• Look for links to educational or other institutions.

Response to an outbreak

• Seek expert advice and establish an outbreak control team.
• Information dissemination is essential.
• Where clusters occur in an educational establishment, the following action is recommended:
(a) two or more possible cases (see case definition): prophylaxis to household or institutional contacts is not recommended;
(b) two confirmed cases caused by different serogroups: only give prophylaxis to household contacts;
(c) two or more confirmed or probable cases that are, or could be, caused by the same strain within a 4-week period: prophylaxis to household contacts and to a defined close contact group within the establishment. This may include, for example, classroom contacts, children who share a common social activity or a group of close friends;
• two or more confirmed or probable cases which are, or could be, caused by the same strain separated by an interval of more than 4 weeks: consider wider prophylaxis, but seek expert advice.
• Where clusters occur in the wider community, age-specific attack rates should be calculated: the numerator is the number of confirmed cases and the denominator is the population within which all the cases reside. This may be difficult to define.
• Vaccination and chemoprophylaxis for the community may be indicated for clusters of serogroup C disease where attack rates are high (e.g. above 40 per 100,000).

Suggested case-definitions

Confirmed case: invasive disease (meningitis, septicaemia, or infection of other normally sterile tissue) confirmed as caused by *Neisseria meningitidis*.

Probable case: clinical diagnosis of invasive meningococcal disease without laboratory confirmation, in which the Consultant in Communicable Disease Control (CCDC), in consultation with the clinician managing the case, considers that meningococcal disease is the likeliest diagnosis. In the absence of an alternative diagnosis a feverish, ill patient with a petechial/purpuric rash should be regarded as a probable case of meningococcal septicaemia.

Possible case: as probable case, but the CCDC, in consultation with the clinician managing the case, considers that diagnoses other than meningococcal disease are at least as likely. This includes cases treated with antibiotics whose probable diagnosis is viral meningitis.

3.51 Molluscum contagiosum

Molluscum contagiosum is a skin infection caused by a poxvirus that replicates in epidermal cells to produce characteristic smooth-surfaced white or translucent papules 2–5 mm in diameter.

Epidemiology

Molluscum contagiosum is more common in boys than in girls. Incidence peaks at age 10–12 years of age and again in young adults due to sexual transmission. It is more common in people who are immunocompromised and prevalence rates of 5–18% have been reported in persons with HIV infection. UK GPs reported a mean weekly incidence in 2009 of 3.5 per 100,000 population which continues a slight downward trend.

Clinical features

Molluscum contagiosum may occur on any part of the body but in adults it often affects the anogenital area. There are usually about 20 lesions but they may be more extensive in HIV infection and atopic eczema. The lesions resolve spontaneously after 6–24 months and treatment is only justified on cosmetic grounds or if there is discomfort. If necessary, diagnosis can be confirmed by the typical appearance of the contents of the lesions on light microscopy or by electron microscopy.

Transmission and acquisition

Transmission is by direct contact, both sexual and non-sexual, from human cases. Indirect spread can occur as a result of contaminated objects and environmental surfaces. Autoinoculation also occurs as a result of scratching. The incubation period is 2–12 weeks and a person will remain infectious as long as the lesions persist. Transmission is thought to be higher in families than in other community settings such as schools.

Response to a case

Normal personal and environmental hygiene should be observed. There is no need for an affected person to stay away from work or school. A child with molluscum contagiosum can take part in most school activities, including swimming.

3.52
Methicillin-resistant *Staphylococcus aureus* (MRSA)

Staphylococcus aureus is a common cause of infection, ranging from minor skin sepsis to life-threatening septicaemia. There are many clones of *S. aureus*, which may be distinguished by molecular genotyping methods. Over 80% of *S. aureus* produce penicillinases and are resistant to benzyl penicillin. Cloxacillin and flucloxacillin are not inactivated by this enzyme and were generally the antibiotics of choice before resistance to these antibiotics became common in the mid-1980s, particularly in hospitals. Laboratory identification of these resistant strains uses methicillin, an antibiotic no longer used therapeutically, and they are referred to as methicillin-resistant *Staphylococcus aureus* (MRSA). The mechanism of methicillin resistance is usually the production of a low-affinity penicillin-binding protein rather than the production of a beta-lactamase. Most MRSA are sensitive to vancomycin but isolates with intermediate-level resistance to vancomycin (VISA) have been reported. Staphylococcal food poisoning is an intoxication rather than an infection (see Chapter 3.73).

> **Suggested on-call action**
>
> • The local health protection team should be prepared to assist the infection control doctor to investigate and control nosocomial outbreaks of MRSA.
> • The public health team may be asked to advise on the management of a cluster of cases of methicillin-sensitive *S. aureus* (MSSA) or MRSA infection in the community.

Epidemiology

In the UK, levels of MRSA in hospitals have risen over the last decade and it has emerged as a major public health problem and source of public and political concern. This rise has been attributed to the appearance of new strains with epidemic potential, hospital patients who are increasingly vulnerable to infections like MRSA, failure to maintain good hospital hygiene including handwashing, more intensive bed usage, greater throughput of patients, more transfer of patients between wards and hospitals and reductions in staffing levels.

Data from the European Antimicrobial Resistance Surveillance System (EARSS) for 2007 indicates that 10 out of 28 countries, mainly Southern European countries, the UK and Ireland reported that the proportion of MRSA bacteraemias was 25% or higher. In Norway, Sweden, Finland, Denmark, Iceland and the Netherlands the proportion remained below 2%. These large variations in MRSA levels in European countries may be due to historical differences in their approaches to MRSA control.

In England and Wales, MRSA as a proportion of total *S. aureus* bacteraemias increased from 2% in 1990 to 42% in the early 2000s but has since declined to 19% in 2009. A mandatory MRSA bacteraemia surveillance scheme for all acute hospitals in England was introduced in April 2001. In the first year of surveillance over 7000 cases were reported and since then cases have declined to 6383 in 2006–2007, 4451 in 2007–2008, 2933 in 2008–2009 and 1898 in 2009–2010. Currently, about half the reported bacteraemias occur 3 days or more after admission to hospital, implying nosocomial rather than community acquisition although many of the community-acquired cases will have healthcare-related risk factors. Risk factors for MRSA bacteraemia include age (mean age 69 years), male gender (65% of patients), pre-existing medical conditions (renal failure, diabetes, immunosuppression) or invasive procedures (surgery, central or peripheral intravenous devices).

In the community methicillin-sensitive *S. aureus* (MSSA) colonisation rates are around 30% while MRSA colonisation rates are 1%. Independent risk factors for MRSA colonisation in one study were age over 75 years, recent hospital admission and diabetes. The prevalence of MRSA among persons without risk factors is 0.24% or lower.

Clinical features

The clinical syndromes associated with *S. aureus* infection are summarised in Table 3.52.1. MRSA causes infection or colonisation in the same way as MSSA. However, because there are fewer antibiotic treatment options MRSA infections are more difficult to treat and morbidity, length of hospital stay and treatment costs may all be increased.

Recently, a new pattern of disease has emerged in the UK caused by strains of *Staphylococcus aureus* that produce Panton–Valentine leukocidin (PVL), a toxin that destroys white blood cells. PVL-SA which currently accounts for 2% of isolates can be either MSSA or MRSA. In the UK, PVL positive MSSA was common in the 1960s causing boils and abscesses in previously healthy individuals. Recently, there has been an increase in infections due to PVL-SA. These are usually mild skin and soft tissues infections (SSTI) but occasionally invasive infections occur including necrotising fasciitis, osteomyelitis, septic arthritis, pyomyositis and necrotising haemorrhagic pneumonia which may follow a influenza-like illness, affecting otherwise healthy young people in the community with high mortality. PVL-SA infections are usually sporadic but there have been clusters and outbreaks in community and healthcare settings. In North America, in recent years, the USA300 clone, a community-associated (CA) MRSA (most isolates of which are PVL positive) has become prevalent in community and hospital settings. It causes clusters of extensive SSTI. Risk factors for CA-MRSA and PVL-SA are similar and include skin lesions, skin-to-skin contact and sharing contaminated items. Settings in which people are

Table 3.52.1 Clinical syndromes associated with *S. aureus*

Infection	Comments
Acute osteomyelitis	Infection is usually haematogenous but may spread from adjacent structures or arise in association with peripheral vascular disease.
Bacteraemia and septicaemia	Often associated with infection in other sites such as pneumonia, cellulitis or wound infection.
Skin infection	Folliculitis, carbuncle, furunculosis (boils), impetigo.
Cellulitis	May follow trauma.
Conjunctivitis	
Septic arthritis	May be due to haematogenous spread from distant site or direct inoculation from a penetrating wound or bite, from adjacent osteomyelitis, prosthetic joint surgery or when intra-articular injections are given. Risk factors include trauma, joint diseases such as rheumatoid arthritis or osteoarthritis, debility, immunosuppressive therapy and intravenous drug abuse.
Staphylococcal pneumonia	Rare but may follow influenza, measles, chronic bronchitis or surgery. May occur in children in the first 8 weeks of life and may be complicated by pleural effusion, empyema or lung abscess.
Staphylococcal scalded skin syndrome	Fever, tender erythematous rash, large bullae and exfoliation of sheets of skin due to certain *S. aureus* phage groups which produce an exotoxin.
Toxic shock syndrome	Due to exotoxins produced by *S. aureus* and comprises fever, hypotension, thrombocytopenia, vomiting and diarrhoea, skin rash with later desquamation, renal, hepatic and CNS dysfunction. Associated with tampon use but can occur with infection at other sites.

in close contact such as households, sports teams, military camps, prisons and gymnasia are particularly likely to be affected.

Laboratory confirmation

The laboratory diagnosis of *S. aureus* infection requires microbiological examination of appropriate clinical specimens. As a minimum, a Gram stain, culture and antibiotic sensitivities should be requested. Historically, biochemical tests and phage typing were the mainstay of diagnosis but advancing laboratory techniques have provided increasing amounts of genotype data and allowed a growing understanding of the molecular basis for virulence, antibiotic resistance and epidemiology. The latest techniques include multi-locus sequence typing (MLST) which allows different genotypes or clones to be identified which have distinct epidemiological features and clinical presentations.

Transmission

The reservoir of *S. aureus* is colonised or infected humans and, rarely, animals. The main sites of colonisation are the anterior nares and skin whilst purulent discharges from wounds and other lesions are the main sources in infected persons. Infection is spread directly on hands and indirectly via skin scales, fomites, equipment and the environment. In about one-third of cases infection is endogenous. Some carriers are more efficient at spreading infection than others. MRSA rarely invades intact skin but can invade pressure sores, surgical wounds and intravascular catheter sites and may then lead to severe infections.

Acquisition

The incubation period is 4–10 days and a person will remain infectious to others as long as the infection or carrier state persists. Risk factors for nosocomial acquisition of MRSA include prolonged hospital stay, intensive care, prolonged antimicrobial therapy and surgical procedures.

Prevention

• Guidelines are available for the control of MRSA and PVL-SA (see Appendix 2).
• In UK hospitals a targeted approach is usually adopted in which the control measures are determined by the type of ward (non-acute, acute, intensive care or high risk), the presence of susceptible patients and the background level of MRSA.
• In addition to basic infection control measures such as handwashing and personal protective equipment, interventions may include isolation, case finding by microbiological screening of patients and staff and clearance of MRSA using topical or systemic antibiotics and antiseptic detergents and dusting powder.
• Movement of patients within and between hospitals should be minimised and appropriate antibiotic prophylaxis should be used during surgery.
• Attention to hospital hygiene, an antibiotic policy, support from senior management and a properly resourced infection control team are further important requirements.

Surveillance

• In the community, specimens for microbiological examination should be collected from cases of suspected staphylococcal infection.
• It is not usually necessary to report individual cases of MRSA in the community but clusters of cases should be reported to the local health protection team. Cases of MRSA bacteraemias may be subject to investigation as a sentinel event or untoward occurrence. Cases of PVL-SA infection should be reported to the local public health team so that risk factors can be considered with a view to identifying, screening and de-colonising contacts of the case.

• In hospitals the infection control team should agree testing protocols. As a minimum all patients with clinical lesions should be sampled. In many hospitals nasal and skin swabs are collected routinely on patients who are admitted to high-risk areas of the hospital such as ICU. Cases of MRSA will then be readily detected by alert organism surveillance.

Response to a case

• Treatment guidelines for cases and carriers in hospitals and the community should be used. Antibiotic treatment should be guided by the results of antibiotic sensitivity testing.
• Discharging lesions should be covered with impermeable dressings if practicable.
• Contact with infants and other susceptible groups should be avoided and school-age children and cases in high-risk occupations should stay at home until no longer infectious.
• Colonisation with MRSA should not prevent a patient being discharged from hospital to their own home or to a nursing home if their general clinical condition allows it. There should be good communication between the hospital infection control team and the nursing home staff.

Investigation of a cluster and control of an outbreak

• Despite the implementation of infection control measures, outbreaks of MRSA and MSSA are reported from hospitals, community nursing homes, military barracks, daycare settings and amongst groups of people participating in contact sports such as wrestling or rugby.
• An outbreak may be defined as an increase in cases of *S. aureus* infection or colonisation or a clustering of new cases due to the transmission of a single strain in a particular setting.
• Outbreaks are investigated in a systematic fashion including search for infected cases and carriers; requesting appropriate

laboratory tests; typing to confirm that cases are caused by the same strain; screening contacts and staff to detect carriers who may be the source of infection; environmental investigation and microbiological sampling; reviewing clinical practice such as wound closure and antibiotic use; and reviewing infection control practice, including hand-washing, cleaning of equipment and care of catheter sites.

• In an MRSA outbreak, additional control measures may be required including restricting or suspending admissions, restricting the movement of staff and patients, limiting the use of temporary staff and ward closure.

Suggested case-definitions for an outbreak

• A patient or staff member who has MRSA isolated for the first time from a clinical sample or screening swab.
  or
• A patient or staff member who is positive for a second or subsequent time having been successfully treated and shown to be microbiologically clear of MRSA.

Cases are classified as infected if any of the signs and symptoms of infection are present otherwise they are classified as colonised.

3.53 Mumps

Mumps is a systemic viral infection characterised by parotitis. It is caused by a paramyxovirus. The public health significance of mumps is that complications are common and it is preventable by vaccination.

Suggested on-call action

None usually required.

Epidemiology

Before vaccination was introduced, mumps caused epidemics every 3 years, with highest attack rates in children aged 5–9 years. Following the introduction of mumps-containing vaccines, the incidence has declined throughout Europe. In 2008 the notification rate was 2.8 per 100,000 and in five countries (Finland, Greece, Netherlands, Slovakia and Iceland) the rate was below 1 per million. Highest rates were reported in Ireland (16 per 100,000), Bulgaria (15 per 100,000), Romania (11 per 100,000), Luxembourg (5.4 per 100,000) and the UK (4.3 per 100,000) (ECDC Annual Epidemiological Report 2010). In recent years, several countries have reported outbreaks in older children and adults; many of whom were previously vaccinated. A number of factors have contributed to these outbreaks, including lack of catch up campaigns when mumps-containing vaccines were implemented, waning immunity after vaccination and possible reduced effectiveness to some strains of wild virus (strains circulating recently in Europe have been genotypes D, F, G and H whereas the commonly used vaccine strains is genotype A).

Deaths from mumps are rare, although meningitis is a relatively common complication: in the pre-vaccine era, mumps was the most common viral cause of meningitis.

Clinical features

Tenderness and swelling of the parotid occur in about 70% of cases. It can be confused with swelling of the cervical lymph nodes. Other common features of mumps include meningitis (which is mild), orchitis (in adult males) and pancreatitis. Rare features are oophoritis, arthritis, mastitis and myocarditis.

Laboratory confirmation

Oral fluid (Oracol), throat swabs, nasopharyngeal aspirate (NPA), urine or CSF may be collected for PCR testing; virus can be found from 7 before up to 9 days after the onset of parotitis. Genotyping is available and may be useful in the investigation of vaccine failures. Serological diagnosis is best achieved either by demonstrating rising IgG antibody (complement fixation, haemaglutination inhibition or ELISA) or IgM antibody by ELISA: blood or saliva (gingival fluid) may be used.

Transmission

Human are the only reservoir. Carriage does not occur. Mumps is moderately infectious, with transmission occurring through droplet spread and direct contact with saliva of a case.

Acquisition

The incubation period is 14–25 days (average 18 days). Cases are infectious for up to a week (normally 2 days) before parotid swelling until several days after.

Prevention

Routine MMR vaccination; two doses required (for schedules in Europe see www.euvac.net/graphics/vaccination/var.html)

Surveillance

Notifiable disease in the majority of EU countries; enhanced surveillance (including laboratory confirmation) is carried out through the EU community network for vaccine preventable infectious diseases (www.euvac.net).

Response to a case

- Exclusion from school for 5 days from onset of parotid swelling.
- Check vaccination status.
- Arrange for laboratory confirmation.

Response to a cluster and control of an outbreak

As for a case, but also consider school, institution or community-wide vaccination if coverage is low or during outbreaks.

Suggested case-definition for an outbreak

Clinical: acute onset of parotid swelling, in the absence of other obvious cause.
Confirmed: positive by PCR, IgM or four-fold rise in IgG. Does not need to meet clinical case-definition.

3.54 *Mycoplasma*

Mycoplasma pneumoniae causes acute respiratory infection and is an important cause of community-acquired pneumonia during its 4-yearly epidemics.

Suggested on-call action

None, unless outbreak is suspected in an institution containing frail individuals (if so, treat symptomatic contacts).

Epidemiology

Most *M. pneumoniae* infection is never diagnosed. Epidemics occur approximately every 3–5 years and last 12–18 months, peaking in winter(s), although this striking pattern has become less evident in recent years. *M. pneumoniae* may be responsible for up to one-third of community-acquired pneumonia during these epidemics. Outside of epidemic periods, as little as 1% of pneumonias may be due to this organism. Incidence rates are highest in school-aged children, with a secondary peak in adults aged 30–39 years. Outbreaks can occur in institutions, particularly amongst military recruits.

Clinical features

Mycoplasma classically presents with fever, malaise and headache with upper respiratory tract symptoms such as coryza, sore throat or unproductive cough. Up to 10% then progress to tracheobronchitis or 'atypical' pneumonia with a more severe cough, although mucopurulent sputum, obvious dyspnoea and true pleuritic pain are rare. Onset is usually insidious, with presentation often delayed 10–14 days. Asymptomatic infection may also occur, particularly in pre-school children. Those with sickle cell anaemia or Down's syndrome may be more severely affected.

Laboratory confirmation

The mainstay of diagnosis has been the demonstration of a fourfold rise in serum-specific IgG antibodies. However, it may take several weeks for such a rise to become apparent. Serology is increasingly being replaced by polymerase chain reaction (PCR) of respiratory samples; lower respiratory samples, such as sputum, are preferred, but nose/throat swabs can be analysed. Other alternatives may be available including culture on special media, detection of serum-specific IgA or IgM (positive after 8–14 days of illness) and antigen detection.

Transmission

Humans are the sole reservoir. Transmission requires relatively close contact. Although school-age children appear to be the main vectors of transmission, they usually only infect family members and close playmates and rarely start school outbreaks. Air-borne spread by inhalation of droplets produced by coughing, direct contact with an infected person (perhaps including asymptomatics) and indirect contact with items contaminated by nasal or throat discharges from cases probably all contribute to transmission.

Acquisition

The incubation period is reported as ranging from 6 to 32 days. Two weeks is a reasonable estimate of the median. The infectious period probably does not start until coryza or cough is evident (the serial interval is usually about 3 weeks). The length of infectiousness is unclear: 3 weeks from onset of illness can be used as a general guideline if coughing has ceased, although excretion may be prolonged despite antibiotics. Immunity does occur post-infection, but later re-infection is recognised. Patients with functional asplenism may be more prone to overwhelming infection.

Prevention

• Avoid overcrowding in closed communities.
• Safe disposal of items likely to be contaminated by respiratory secretions.

Surveillance

• Notifiable in a few countries, including the Netherlands, Finland and Switzerland.
• Report to local public health authorities if associated with an institution.
• Report laboratory confirmed cases to national surveillance systems.

Response to case

• Hygiene advice and care with respiratory secretions.
• Not to attend work or school whilst unwell.

• Avoid contact with those with sickle cell anaemia, Down's syndrome or asplenism, where possible.

Investigation of a cluster

• Look for links to institutions: however, more likely to be links between families via school-age children.
• Although clustering of onset dates may indicate a common exposure, opportunities for active intervention are likely to be limited.

Control of an outbreak

• Re-inforce hygiene and infection control practices, especially relating to respiratory secretions and handwashing.
• Avoid introduction of new susceptibles into affected institutions with frail individuals (e.g. nursing home).
• Warn local clinicians and remind them of appropriate antibiotics for cases with lower respiratory infection (macrolides, tetracyclines or quinolones, i.e. not the usual first choice for pneumonia).
• Consider feasibility of separating coughing residents from asymptomatic ones.
• There is some evidence of the effectiveness of prophylactic antibiotics (e.g. azithromycin 500 mg on day 1 followed by 250 mg for 4 days) to reduce the secondary attack rate for symptomatic infection in vulnerable populations.

Suggested case-definition for an outbreak

Confirmed: serological confirmation of illness (IgM, IgA or fourfold rise in IgG) or demonstration of antigen or PCR in respiratory secretions.
Clinical: pneumonia, bronchitis or pharyngitis without other identified cause in member of affected institution.

3.55 Norovirus

Noroviruses (also known as small round structured viruses, SRSV or Norwalk-like viruses) are the most common cause of gastroenteritis in Europe. Although generally causing mild illness, spread may be rapid, particularly in institutions. Other causes of viral gastroenteritis include other caliciviruses (e.g. sapovirus), rotavirus (see Chapter 3.66), adenovirus and astrovirus.

Suggested on-call action

• If in group at risk for further transmission (Box 2.2.1), exclude from work or nursery.
• If you or the reporting clinician/ microbiologist are aware of related cases, consult local outbreak plan.

Epidemiology

Norovirus causes about 15–20% of all sporadic cases of acute gastroenteritis in Europe and an average of about 60% of all gastrointestinal outbreaks. All age groups are affected and it is the most common cause of gastroenteritis in adults: a survey in England estimated an annual incidence of 12.5 cases per 1000 population, of which about one-sixth consulted medical services and only 1 in 300 were reported to national surveillance. Of those who presented to medical services, rates were highest in those under 2 years of age, followed by those aged 2–4 years. Norovirus is usually more common from January to April, hence its synonym of 'winter vomiting disease'. However, the extent of the winter peak can vary and infections and outbreaks can occur throughout the year. Epidemic strains, associated with a higher incidence of disease worldwide, are not uncommon.

Clinical features

Norovirus infection typically causes any or all of abdominal pain, nausea, vomiting and diarrhoea. Malaise and headache also occur in many cases and fever in a substantial minority. Vomiting may be sudden and forceful, but diarrhoea is usually mild and non-bloody and fever is low grade. Symptoms last from 1 to 5 days, with infants, elderly or previously infirm patients tending to take the longest to recover. About 1% of cases require hospitalisation. Elderly or infirm patients are at increased risk of complications. Death rates in norovirus outbreaks are higher in hospital and elderly care institutions. Asymptomatic infection is common.

Laboratory confirmation

Diagnosis has traditionally been by electron microscopy (EM) of faecal specimens, which should be collected within the first day or two of illness and preferably be unformed. Samples of vomit may also be examined by EM. However, most laboratories now use antigen testing (EIA) or PCR in preference to EM. Genotyping of isolates is possible. Serology (paired samples 3–4 weeks apart) may also be available.

If laboratory confirmation is lacking or awaited, epidemiological criteria can be used to assess the likelihood of an outbreak being due to norovirus (Box 3.55.1).

Transmission

Humans are the only known reservoir of norovirus. Spread is from person to person, either by the faeco-oral or vomitus-oral routes, or indirectly by contamination of the environment, food or water. Norovirus is easily spread by these routes.

• Asymptomatic, pre-symptomatic, symptomatic and post-symptomatic cases have all been shown to excrete norovirus. The risk is highest from onset of symptoms to about 48–72 hours after they cease (co-inciding with the limit reported for detection by EM). Newer, more sensitive tests can demonstrate virus in faeces for up to 3 weeks, but the relevance of this for infectivity in asymptomatic patients with good personal hygiene is not clear. Excretion may be prolonged in chronic illness or immunosuppressed individuals.

• Norovirus is identifiable in vomit and vomiting has been linked to many outbreaks. This can be directly from aerosols created by vomiting or contamination of food or the environment.

Box 3.55.1 Epidemiological criteria for suspecting that an outbreak is due to norovirus

• Stool cultures negative for bacterial pathogens.* (N.B. check that all relevant pathogens have actually been tested for.)
• Incubation period, if known, of 15–50 hours.*
• Vomiting in over 50% of cases.*
• Diarrhoea generally mild without blood or mucus.
• Over half have nausea and abdominal cramps, and over one-fifth have malaise, low-grade fever, myalgia and headache.
• Mean duration of illness is 12–60 hours.*
• High secondary attack rate. Even if originally food-borne, likely to be signs of ongoing person-to-person spread (see Box 2.2.3).
• Staff are also affected.

* 'Kaplan criteria'.

• Environmental contamination in outbreaks has been shown for bathroom surfaces, taps, door handles, light switches and on kitchen surfaces. Transmission of norovirus in faeces to such surfaces can occur via contaminated fingers and cloths. Norovirus may also remain viable on carpets or curtains.

• Norovirus is a commonly reported cause of food-borne outbreaks. This may be via infected food handlers or from the use of already contaminated foods such as oysters and other shellfish and imported soft fruit. More than one norovirus genogroup can occur in the same outbreak, particularly those related to shellfish harvested from waters contaminated by human sewage.

• Drinking water that is inadequately chlorinated or contaminated post-treatment may transmit norovirus, as may swimming in contaminated water.

• Outbreaks are most commonly reported in hospitals, nursing homes and elderly care homes, but also occur in nurseries, schools, restaurants, hotels and cruise ships. The attack rates are usually highest in food-borne outbreaks (about 50%), lower in institutions (about 30%) and lowest in holiday venues (about 9%).

Acquisition

The average incubation period for norovirus is about 32 hours after exposure, with a range of 6–72 hours. The infective dose is extremely low (infection can occur from ingestion of 100 particles) and the high concentration of virus in faeces can lead to high attack rates. Immunity occurs post-infection, but may only last a few months (sufficient to remove recovered cases from the pool of susceptible people in an outbreak). This, plus the existence of several antigenic types, means later re-infection is possible.

Prevention

• Good standards of personal and food hygiene, including adequate handwashing.

• Good standards of infection control in hospitals and residential homes, including adequate cleaning arrangements.
• Cook raw shellfish before consumption and wash fruit.

Surveillance

• Laboratory-confirmed cases should be reported to local and national surveillance systems.
• Cases with links to institutions such as hospitals, care homes, daycare centres or restaurants should be reported to local public health authorities, as should any suspected outbreak.

Response to case

• Exclude cases in groups with risk of further transmission (Box 2.2.1) until 48 hours after resolution of diarrhoea and vomiting.
• Enteric precautions with particular attention to environmental contamination related to vomitus.
• Cases in institutions should be isolated where practicable.
• Treat symptomatic contacts in high-risk groups (Box 2.2.1) as cases.
• Hygiene advice to cases and contacts.
• Collect basic risk factor data.

Investigation of a cluster

• Most recognised clusters are associated with an institution or a social function.
• If an institution, use Box 2.2.3 to help assess likelihood of person-to-person or food-borne source.
• If a social function, consider infected food handler, contaminated premises or contaminated food, especially shellfish.
• If a community outbreak, describe by person, place and time and obtain full food (especially seafood, fruit, salad, sandwiches), occupational, family and social histories including links to hospitals; residential institutions, hotels and restaurants) 6–72 hours before onset

as a hypothesis-generating exercise. Organise further case finding (e.g. requesting faecal samples from cases of gastroenteritis presenting to GPs).

Control of an outbreak

• Report to local public health authorities.
• For outbreaks in institutions, form an outbreak team, which includes a senior manager who has the authority to commit the institution to agreed action.
• Reinforce good infection control (especially handwashing) and food hygiene practices. Ensure toilet facilities are adequate.
• Increase cleaning, particularly of toilet areas and 'contact points' (e.g. taps and door handles). Wear disposable gloves and aprons for cleaning potentially contaminated areas.
• Disinfect contaminated areas with 1000 p.p.m. hypochlorite in addition to detergent. Immediate cleaning of areas contaminated by vomiting.
• Isolate cases where practicable in residential institutions. Cohorting of cases otherwise.
• Exclude cases in non-residential institutions until symptom-free for 48 hours.
• Staff to wear gloves and aprons and to observe enteric precautions when dealing with infected patients.
• Exclude staff with gastrointestinal symptoms until 48 hours after resolution. Nausea and cramps may precede vomiting and diarrhoea; do not wait until they vomit on the premises!
• Do not admit more susceptible individuals into an outbreak area, preferably until 72 hours since last episode of diarrhoea or vomiting. Outbreaks in institutions will normally terminate in 1–2 weeks if new susceptible people are not introduced. There is evidence that the earlier that hospital units or nursing homes are closed, the sooner the outbreak terminates.
• Do not discharge potentially incubating patients into another institution.
• Restrict unnecessary patient and staff movements between wards: the main aim is to prevent transmission to other wards, whilst the outbreak 'burns-out' in the affected ward.
• Staff working in affected wards should not then work in unaffected wards until remaining asymptomatic for 48 hours from last exposure.
• Exclude non-essential personnel from the ward.
• Give advice on norovirus and hand hygiene to adult visitors. Restrict visiting by children if possible.
• Thoroughly clean before re-opening to admissions. Change curtains in hospital.
• The infection control nurse or environmental health practitioner will need to maintain constant supervision to ensure that the agreed actions are fully implemented and maintained.

3.56 Paratyphoid fever

Paratyphoid fever is a potentially severe infection. Although rare in developed countries, it is a potential hazard in travellers to developing countries and can be spread by infected food handlers. Paratyphoid and typhoid (see Chapter 3.82) are both also known as enteric fever.

Suggested on-call action

• Exclude cases and contacts who are food handlers.
• Exclude cases and symptomatic contacts in other risk groups (see below).

Epidemiology

The incidence of enteric fever (includes typhoid and paratyphoid) in the EU, based on reports to surveillance systems, is 0.3 per 100,000. Incidence has fallen over the last decade. Cases are more common in late summer and in spring. Reported cases in Europe are most common in young children.

The majority of cases in Europe are imported. About 200 laboratory reports of paratyphoid are made annually in the UK: about 95% of these cases had travelled abroad, most commonly to the Indian subcontinent.

Clinical features

Paratyphoid may cause gastroenteritis or enteric fever. The most commonly reported symptoms are fever, chills, diarrhoea, abdominal pain and headache. Other symptoms reported are nausea, vomiting, cough, constipation, anorexia and delirium. Examination may reveal splenomegaly, hepatomegaly, rose spots, bradycardia and possibly signs of bronchitis, tonsillitis or tympanitis. Paratyphoid A infection can be as severe as typhoid, although paratyphoid B is often less severe. Complications include hepatitis, perforation and relapse; death may result, but is rare in treated cases. Asymptomatic infection also occurs.

Enteric fever should be considered when patients returning from an endemic or epidemic area develop a febrile illness.

Laboratory confirmation

Paratyphoid fever is caused by *Salmonella enterica* subspecies *enterica* serotype Paratyphi, more usually shortened to *S.* Paratyphi. Of the three serotypes, A is the most common in the UK and C the least common. Organisms initially reported as *S.* Paratyphi B may actually be *S.* Paratyphi B var. Java (*S.* Java), which does not usually cause enteric fever. *S.* Java is common in poultry in the Netherlands and Germany.

Culture for *S.* Paratyphi can be performed on samples of blood, stool, urine, rose spots, bone marrow and gastric or intestinal secretions. Blood, urine and faeces culture are usually the first line: faeces are usually positive after the first week of illness and results should be available in 72 hours. The sensitivity of blood culture can be as high as 80%.

Antibiotics may suppress *Salmonella* below detection levels for several weeks after completion of the course. However, bone marrow culture has 90% sensitivity, even after 5 days of antibiotic therapy. The Widal test may be positive, although sensitivity may be less than for typhoid. Phage typing or molecular typing may be available for unexplained clusters (the most common types in the UK are PT13, 1, 1a, 2 and 4). *S.* Java is differentiated from *S.* Paratyphi B by the dextro-tartrate test.

Transmission

Humans are the main reservoir, although environmental contamination may occur from human faeces. *S.* Paratyphi B occurs rarely in cattle. *S.* Java may be associated with poultry, tropical fish and cattle.

Spread is faeco-oral, most commonly via a food-borne vehicle. Water-borne spread also occurs. Direct person-to-person spread is uncommon. *S.* Paratyphi B infection has been associated with milk and unpasteurised cheese.

Acquisition

The incubation period has a range of 1–17 days, although up to 3 weeks is reported. Most cases occur within 10 days of exposure (median 3–7 days).

Over 10% of cases excrete the organism for weeks (about 6% in children) and about 2% for more than a year. Cases and carriers are infectious whilst they are excreting the organism (carriers commonly excrete 10^7–10^{10}/g stool), but risk, other than through contamination of food or water, is low unless there are poor hygiene practices. Ninety-five per cent of excretors are detected by three consecutive faecal samples; five consecutive negative faecal samples gives reasonable certainty of microbiological clearance. Infection produces partial immunity.

Prevention

- Control depends on sanitation, clean water, handwashing and food hygiene.
- There is no licensed vaccine against paratyphoid. Oral typhoid vaccine may have some cross-protection with paratyphoid B.

Surveillance

- Paratyphoid is a notifiable disease in most countries, including the UK.
- Report to local public health departments on clinical suspicion.
- Laboratory-confirmed cases should be reported to local and national public health agencies. Some countries (e.g. the UK) have enhanced surveillance systems for enteric fever.

Response to a case

- Usually requires antibiotic treatment, but check sensitivity of isolate.
- Advice on good personal and food hygiene to cases, carriers and contacts, especially handwashing.
- Enteric precautions for cases; consider isolation if hospitalised.
- Obtain food and travel history for the 3 weeks prior to onset of illness.
- Cases who have not visited an endemic country in the 3 weeks before onset should be investigated to determine the source of infection.
- Exclude cases who are:
  (a) food handlers (Box 2.2.1: risk group 1): UK recommendations are until six consecutive negative stool specimens taken at 1 week intervals and commencing 3 weeks after completion of antibiotic therapy;
  (b) health/social care workers, children aged under 5 years and cases with poor personal hygiene (risk groups 2–4): UK recommendations are until three consecutive negative faecal samples taken at weekly intervals, commencing 3 weeks after completion of treatment.

- Exclude all other cases until clinically well for 48 hours with formed stools and hygiene advice given.
- Exclude contacts (or others in same travel group) in risk groups 1–4: usually until two negative faecal specimens taken 48 hours apart and hygiene advice given. If any other contacts unwell, exclude from work/school until well for 48 hours.
- Quinolones may reduce the period of carriage in those for whom exclusion is producing social difficulties.
- For *S.* Java, microbiological clearance is less likely to be advised and exclusion is 48 hours from last episode of diarrhoea or vomiting.

Investigation of a cluster

- Clusters should be investigated to ensure that secondary transmission has not occurred within Europe.
- Check each case (and their household contacts) for travel abroad.
- Interview cases to identify the source of infection. This could be contact with a chronic carrier, with faecal material or with contaminated food, milk, water or shellfish. Obtain and compare food histories. Explore family and social links between cases.

Control of an outbreak

- Exclude cases and contacts as above.
- Exclude and test food handlers in any associated institution or food premises. Ensure adequate personal and food hygiene.
- Organise testing and withdrawal of any implicated food. Ensure only pasteurised milk, treated water and cooked shellfish used.

Suggested case-definition for an outbreak

Clinical illness compatible with paratyphoid and isolate from blood, stool or bone marrow.

3.57 Parvovirus B19 (fifth disease)

Parvovirus B19 is the cause of a common childhood infection, erythema infectiosum, also known as fifth disease or slapped cheek syndrome. It is important because of the risk of complications in pregnancy, in those with haemoglobinopathies and the immunocompromised.

Suggested on-call action

If case is a healthcare worker in contact with high-risk patients, consider either exclusion from work or avoiding contact with high-risk patients.

Epidemiology

Infection occurs at all ages, although children aged 5–14 years are at greatest risk. Outbreaks in schools and nurseries are common, usually occurring in early spring. The disease tends occur in 3–4 yearly cycles. By the age of 10, up to 50% of children will have been infected.

Clinical features

The main differential diagnosis is rubella. Fever is the first symptom, which lasts for 2 or 3 days until the rash appears. The rash is maculopapular and is found on the limbs, less commonly the trunk. The cheeks often have a bright red ('slapped cheek') appearance. The 'slapped cheek' rash lasts for 1–4 days. In a healthy person, the illness is usually mild and short-lived, although persistent joint pain with or without swelling sometimes occurs, especially in young women, most commonly in knees, fingers, ankles, wrists and elbows.

Parvovirus infection in the first 20 weeks of pregnancy can cause fetal loss (9%) and hydrops fetalis (3%); however, it is not teratogenic. In patients with haemoglobinopathies it can cause transient aplastic crises, and in immunodeficient patients red cell aplasia and chronic anaemia can occur.

Laboratory confirmation

This is important to distinguish from rubella, especially in pregnant women or their contacts. The diagnosis can be confirmed by testing serum for B19 IgM, which is positive from the day of onset of rash. The virus can also be detected by PCR from blood, saliva and respiratory secretions.

Transmission

Humans are the only reservoir; cat and dog parvoviruses do not infect humans. Transmission is from person to person by droplet infection from the respiratory tract; rarely by contaminated blood products. Long-term carriage does not occur.

Acquisition

Parvovirus is highly infectious. The incubation period ranges from 4 to 20 days, but is usually 13–18 days. The infectious period is from 7 days before the rash appears until the onset of the rash. In aplastic crises infectivity lasts for up to a week after the rash appears, and immunosuppressed people with severe anaemia may be infectious for several months or even years. Immunity is lifelong.

Prevention

• Consider avoiding exposure of patients at risk of complications (see above) to potential cases in outbreak situations.
• Transmission is probably reduced by routine hygiene practices (e.g. handwashing).

Surveillance

• Not notifiable in most European countries.
• May only come to the attention of the public health department as a result of investigation of a case of suspected rubella, or when there is an outbreak of a rash illness in a school.

Response to a case

• Arrange for laboratory confirmation.
• Isolation or school exclusion of cases is of no value as any transmission occurs before the onset of symptoms (however, see below for teachers).
• Consider exclusion of a non-immune healthcare worker (HCW) who has been exposed to a case, if a fever develops, until either the rash appears or for 15 days from the last contact with the case. Alternatively, advise the HCW to avoid contact with high-risk patients (women in the first 20 weeks of pregnancy, those with haemoglobinopathies and the immunocompromised), or to take respiratory precautions until a rash appears or for 15 days. Screening of HCWs may be justified for those who have frequent contact with high-risk patients, or for laboratory workers who work with infectious material known to contain B19 virus.
• If infection is confirmed in a HCW, test high-risk contacts (as above) for immunity and monitor for evidence of infection, as they need specialist care if infected. Consider 400 mg/kg human normal immunoglobulin intravenously for 5–10 days for immunosuppressed contacts (efficacy uncertain).

Investigation and control of an outbreak

In addition to measures described above for a case, it may be worth excluding susceptible teachers who are in the first 20 weeks of pregnancy from a school in which an outbreak is occurring until they are more than 20 weeks pregnant. Consideration should also be given to excluding children with haemoglobinopathies and the immunocompromised.

Suggested case-definition for an outbreak

IgM or PCR positive in presence of clinically compatible illness.

3.58 Plague

Plague is a serious and potentially highly infectious disease caused by *Yersinia pestis*.

Suggested on-call action

• Ensure that cases are isolated.
• Ensure staff monitoring is instituted.
• Ensure samples are handled appropriately.
• Identify those at risk.
• Liaise with rodent and flea control experts if there is a possibility of local acquisition.

Epidemiology

Yersinia pestis is a pathogen of rodents (ground squirrels, gerbils, etc.) in many parts of the world. Plague is still endemic in parts of Africa, Asia, the Americas and the former Soviet Union; in the EU transmission risk is minimal. Humans are infected by the bite of an infected flea associated with the natural host or domestic rats.

Clinical features

Bubonic plague is acquired cutaneously. There is rapid onset of high fever, malaise and delirium. Regional adenopathy and tender buboes draining the site of infection develop. Petechial or purpuric haemorrhages are common. Septic shock develops, with an untreated mortality of 60–90%.

Pneumonic plague, acquired by respiratory spread, is a severe illness with high fever, tachypnoea, restlessness and shortness of breath. Respiratory signs may be absent until frothy blood-tinged sputum is produced as a pre-terminal event; untreated mortality is 100%.

Laboratory confirmation

The organism can be isolated from the blood, sputum and buboes. Smears can be Gram-stained. Serology and antigen detection may also be available. The definitive tests for *Y. pestis* are:

• culture from a clinical specimen with confirmation by phage lysis;
• a significant (fourfold or greater) change in antibody titre to F1 antigen in paired serum samples.

Transmission

Bubonic plague is transmitted by the bite of infected rat fleas. Spread is from the bite site to lymph nodes, rapidly followed by septicaemia and pneumonia. Pneumonic plague is acquired directly by the respiratory route from another case of pneumonic plague.

Acquisition

The incubation period for bubonic plague is 1–6 days and for pneumonic plague is 10–15 hours. Patients are infectious until at least 48 hours of appropriate chemotherapy has been received and a favourable clinical response is seen. Partial immunity results from infection.

Prevention

• Pest control (rats and fleas) is essential.
• Laboratory staff likely to come into contact with the organism should be vaccinated. The organism should be handled only in Class 4 laboratory facilities.

Surveillance

• Notifiable: cases should be reported to national authorities and to the WHO.
• Suspected cases should be reported urgently to local public health departments.

Response to a case

• Streptomycin and tetracyclines or chloramphenicol are the drugs of choice. Treatment after 15 hours may not influence the course of pneumonic plague.
• Patients should be considered highly infectious and should be strictly isolated.
• All care should be taken with specimens.
• Staff should be monitored carefully for fever and treated promptly.
• Household contacts should be offered tetracycline prophylaxis.
• Patients and possessions must be disinfected of fleas.
• If pneumonic plague develops in someone who has not been to an endemic area, consider deliberate release.

Investigation of a cluster and control of an outbreak

• Identify source as a matter of urgency and institute pest control.
• Contacts should be offered prophylaxis.
• Consider deliberate release if two or more suspected cases linked in time and place or if any confirmed case has not been to an endemic area.

<table>
<tr><td>

Suggested case-definition for an outbreak

Suspected case: the diagnosis should be considered if the following clinical presentations occur in previously healthy patients, especially if two or more cases arise that are linked in time and place:
• Sudden onset of severe, unexplained febrile respiratory illness.
• Unexplained death following a short febrile illness.
• Sepsis with Gram-negative cocco-bacilli identified from clinical specimens.
In the event of a known or suspected deliberate release, or among contacts of plague cases, the threshold for making a diagnosis of plague should be lower.
Confirmed case: a case that clinically fits the criteria for suspected plague and, in addition, positive results are obtained on one or more specimens by the Reference Laboratory.

</td></tr>
</table>

Response to a deliberate release

• Report to local and national public health authorities.
• Define exposed zone and identify those exposed (include those who have left the scene).
• Cordon off exposure zone.
• Decontaminate those exposed: remove clothing and possessions, and then shower with soap and water.
• Chemoprophylaxis (currently ciprofloxacin for 7 days) as soon as possible for those exposed.
• Record contact details for all those exposed.
• Some health and emergency workers may also need prophylaxis.
• Police may take environmental samples.

3.59 Pneumococcal infection

Streptococcus pneumoniae ('pneumococcus') is the most common cause of community-acquired pneumonia and a common cause of bacteraemia and meningitis.

<table>
<tr><td>

Suggested on-call action

• If case of meningitis, reassure contacts that no prophylaxis is needed.
• If outbreak in institution suspected, consult local outbreak control plan.

</td></tr>
</table>

Epidemiology

Around 14,000 invasive pneumococcal infections are reported annually in the EU, but true incidence is much higher; pneumococcal pneumonia is estimated to affect 0.1% of adults per annum. All ages are affected, but the distribution is bimodal: with an incidence of 12 per 100,000 population in the over 64 years and 7 per 100,000 population in children below the age of 5 years, while in older children and young adults the incidence is below 2 per 100,000 population. Pneumococcal pneumonia and meningitis are both more common in the winter. Pneumococcal infection is more common in smokers, heavy drinkers and those who live in overcrowded sleeping quarters. Incidence increases during influenza epidemics. An absent or non-functioning spleen increases the risk of invasive disease. Recurrent meningococcal meningitis may occur in association with skull defects, cerebrospinal fluid (CSF) leaks, cochlear implants or skull fractures.

Although the incidence of pneumococcal meningitis is highest in young children, its relative importance is highest in middle-aged and elderly adults, in which it is the most common cause of bacterial meningitis. Most recent (2008) national rates in Europe varied from 0.13 per 100,000 population in Latvia to 17 per 100,000 population in Belgium.

Resistance to antibiotics such as erythromycin (15% in Europe in 2008), penicillin (10%) and cephalosporins has been increasing in most European countries and is particularly high in Southern and Eastern Europe, but generally lower in the Netherlands, Germany and the Scandinavian countries. Resistance is to a large extent observed in the serotypes predominant in young children.

Pneumococcus is the most important bacterial cause of otitis media, which is particularly common in children under 3 years of age.

Clinical features

The clinical spectrum of pneumococcal infections ranges from upper respiratory tract infections (acute otitis media and sinusitis) to pneumonia and invasive pneumococcal diseases (i.e. bacteraemia, meningitis and other focal septic infections). The most common symptoms of pneumococcal pneumonia are cough sputum and fever. Factors that may suggest pneumococcal rather than 'atypical' pneumonia in an outbreak include mucopurulent or blood-stained sputum, pleuritic chest pain and prominent physical signs. Respiratory symptoms may be less obvious in the elderly. Many cases have predisposing illnesses such as chronic respiratory, cardiac, renal or liver disease, immunosuppression or diabetes. Bacteraemia may occasionally lead to meningitis. The case fatality rate for bacteraemia or meningitis is 20% and for pneumonia is about 10% (higher in the elderly).

Laboratory confirmation

Gram staining and culture of good quality sputum specimens are the mainstay of diagnosis of pneumococcal pneumonia, although they are only 60% sensitive and 90% specific. Twenty-five per cent of cases of pneumonia will also have a positive blood culture, which can be useful confirmation that the pneumococcus is a pathogen rather than a co-incidental commensal. Antigen detection in sputum or urine may be available in some laboratories. Gram-positive diplococci in CSF suggest pneumococcal meningitis. Serology may be available for retrospective clinical diagnosis.

Serotyping of strains is performed for epidemiological purposes in some laboratories. There are over 90 serotypes of varying pathogenicity. The 10 most common serotypes in young children with invasive pneumococcal disease in Europe are 14, 6B, 19F, 23F, 18C, 19A, 1, 6A, 9V and 4, accounting for more than 80% of these infections.

Transmission

Pneumococci find their ecological niche by colonising the human nasopharynx, especially in young children. Carriage is common, ranging from about 10% in adults to 50% in children in daycare centres, and is high in winter. Transmission requires extensive close contact with cases or carriers and is usually by droplet spread, but may also be via direct oral contact or article soiled by respiratory discharges. Elderly patients are mostly infected through contacts with children. In hospitals, spread is usually to patients in the next one or two beds. Staff may also become colonised. Cases of pneumococcal meningitis are viewed as sporadic.

Acquisition

After acquisition of a new serotype, clinical infection typically occurs within a few days. As nasopharyngeal carriage can be prolonged (mean carriage time 7 weeks), endogenously acquired invasive disease in asymptomatic carriers may rarely occur at a late stage, giving an 'incubation period' of weeks.

The infectious period probably lasts as long as there are viable bacteria in nasal, oral or respiratory discharges. Even though penicillin does not eradicate nasopharyngeal bacteria, treatment still renders patients with susceptible organisms non-infectious in 48 hours.

Type-specific immunity follows infection and is long-lasting. Colonisation may also lead to immunity: one study estimated that two-thirds of those who became colonised developed antibody within 30 days. Risk of infection is higher in those with splenic dysfunction (including sickle cell and coeliac disease) and immunodeficiency (e.g. due to chemotherapy, diabetes and HIV).

Prevention

• A single-dose polysaccharide vaccine with 50–70% efficacy for bacteraemia in those over 2 years of age is available (effectiveness for pneumonia, otitis media and exacerbations of chronic bronchitis remain unproven). In most European countries the vaccine is recommended to all those in whom pneumococcal infection is likely to be more common and/or dangerous. This includes all those aged over 65 years of age and those with chronic renal, heart, lung or liver disease, splenic dysfunction, immunosuppression, diabetes, cochlear implants or CSF shunts. The present vaccine covers 23 serotypes that are responsible for more than 95% of invasive infections, including all common antibiotic-resistant strains.

• Three pneumococcal conjugate vaccines, covering 7, 10 and 13 common serotypes, respectively, have been introduced since 2000. The 7-valent vaccine (PCV7) covers 72% of serotypes in invasive pneumococcal infections in children in Europe, and is included in the childhood immunisation programmes from the age of 2 months in many European countries. The newer 10-valent and 13-valent vaccines cover 80% and 88% of these infections, respectively (with variations between the countries). The conjugate vaccines reduce the risk of pneumococcal meningitis, bacteraemia, pneumonia and otitis media in vaccinated children (direct effect), but also provides an indirect 'herd effect' in elderly contacts to the children. The conjugate vaccine also decreases nasopharyngeal carriage, and has a serotype composition covering the vast majority of penicillin non-susceptible and most erythromycin-resistant strains.

• Avoid overcrowding in institutions such as hospitals, daycare centres, military camps, prisons and homeless shelters.

Surveillance

• Invasive pneumococcal infections are reportable in 20 EU countries.

• Possible outbreaks of pneumococcal infection should be reported to local public health authorities.

• Isolates from blood, CSF or other normally sterile sites should be reported to national surveillance systems. Isolates from sputum are not usually reported because of their uncertain clinical significance. Antibiotic susceptibility (especially penicillin and erythromycin) should be given for all reported cases.

Response to a case

• Safe disposal of discharges from nose and throat.

• Antibiotic therapy as appropriate to clinical condition and sensitivity will reduce infectivity.

• There may be some value in separating patients from others with an increased risk of serious disease until 48 hours of appropriate antibiotics have been received.

• Immunisation of children under 5 years of age who have suffered pneumococcal meningitis or bacteraemia.

Investigation of a cluster

• Organise serotyping of strains.

• Check for links via institutions. Otherwise no action is usually necessary.

Control of an outbreak

- Immunise all contacts that are at higher risk of serious infection: polysaccharide vaccine usually protects more quickly than conjugate.
- Check antibiotic susceptibility and serotype of isolates.
- If outbreaks in institution/ward, vaccinate all residents (unless known to be strain not in vaccine). Institute case finding and early treatment of symptomatics for at least 7–10 days.
- Ensure adequate environmental decontamination.

Suggested case-definitions for an outbreak

Confirmed: clinically compatible illness with isolate from normally sterile site (e.g. blood or CSF).
Probable: clinically compatible illness with either:
(a) Isolate of outbreak serotype from non-sterile site (e.g. sputum); or
(b) Antigen positive from normally sterile site (e.g. urine).

3.60 Poliomyelitis

Poliomyelitis is an acute viral infection of the nervous system caused by poliovirus types 1, 2 and 3. Its public health importance lies in the ability of polioviruses to cause permanent paralysis and sometimes death. It is readily transmitted, causing both endemic and epidemic disease.

Suggested on-call action

- Arrange for urgent laboratory confirmation.
- Obtain vaccination and travel history.
- Notify national surveillance unit.

Epidemiology

Poliomyelitis has been eliminated from most developed countries by vaccination. The WHO European Region (which includes 53 countries) was certified as polio-free in 2002. Imported cases occur occasionally, from countries where endemic transmission still occurs (India, Pakistan, Nigeria and Afghanistan). Vaccine-associated polio, a complication of live oral polio vaccine (OPV), occurs at a rate of two cases per million doses.

Global eradication of polio has not yet been achieved, and there have been recent outbreaks in non-endemic countries (Tajikistan, Congo). An outbreak of over 400 cases in Tajikistan, with cases in the Russian Federation, Turkmenistan and Kazakhstan in 2010 suggests that public health officials will need to remain alert. The latest WHO target for cessation of all wild polioviruses transmission is the end of 2012.

Clinical features

Most cases of polio are asymptomatic or present with a sore throat or diarrhoea. A few cases develop meningitis that is indistinguishable from other causes of viral meningitis. Paralysis is relatively rare: the proportion of paralytic cases increases with age from about 1 in 1000 in infants to 1 in 10 in adults.

Poliomyelitis should be considered in any patient with acute flaccid paralysis particularly if there is a history of recent travel to an endemic area. Vaccine-associated polio should be considered in an individual with acute flaccid paralysis recently vaccinated with OPV (particularly after the first dose) or in a close contact with a recently vaccinated individual. The main differential diagnosis is Guillain–Barré syndrome. The paralysis in polio is usually asymmetric and there is always residual paralysis in polio whereas in Guillain–Barré syndrome the paralysis is usually symmetrical and recovery is complete.

Laboratory confirmation

The most important diagnostic specimen is a stool sample, which should be sent for viral culture. Poliovirus can be recovered from faeces for up to 6 weeks and in nasopharyngeal secretions for up to 1 week from onset of paralysis. At least two stool samples, 24 hours apart, should be obtained within 7 days of the onset of paralysis. Absence of virus does not, however, rule out the possibility of poliomyelitis; where available, molecular diagnosis by polymerase chain reaction (PCR) is the technique of choice. All cases of acute flaccid paralysis should be investigated to exclude polio. The diagnosis can also be made serologically or by cerebrospinal fluid (CSF) examination.

Transmission

Polio is spread by the faeco-oral route. Humans are the only reservoir and there is no carrier state (except rarely in immunodeficiency). The virus can survive in sewage, soil and infected water for a few weeks. Poor hygiene favours spread.

Acquisition

The usual incubation period is 7–14 days for wild cases and vaccine-associated (recipient) cases, although it may be as long as 35 days. For vaccine-associated (contact) cases the incubation period may be up to 60 days. Immunodeficiency is a risk factor for vaccine-associated paralysis, and immunodeficient patients with either vaccine-associated or wild polio may excrete virus for many months.

Prevention

• Two types of vaccine: oral poliovaccine (OPV) and inactivated poliovirus vaccine (IPV) are available. Most countries in Europe now use IPV. Three doses are given at 2, 3 and 4 months of age, with boosters at 3–5 years and 15–19 years (see Box 4.7.1).
• Boosters are required at 10-yearly intervals for travel to endemic areas.

Surveillance

Notifiable in all EU countries. Report on clinical suspicion.

Response to a case or cluster

• Immediate notification to the public health department. Request urgent stool virology.
• Treat a single case of indigenous wild polio as a national public health emergency; ECDC and WHO should be notified.
• If confirmed, mass vaccination with OPV would be required, possibly at the national or subnational level.
• For an imported case, notify national surveillance unit and WHO.
• For vaccine-associated cases, no specific action is required, although it may be an opportunity to review vaccine coverage locally.

Suggested case-definitions for an outbreak

Possible: acute flaccid paralysis without other apparent cause.
Probable: acute onset of flaccid paralysis with decreased/absent tendon reflexes, without other identified cause, and without sensory or cognitive loss.
Confirmed: serological evidence or positive virus culture or PCR, together with clinically compatible illness.

3.61 Q fever

Q fever is a zoonotic disease caused by the rickettsia *Coxiella burnetii*. It causes an acute febrile illness, which may occur as outbreaks or, more rarely, a serious chronic infection.

Epidemiology

The true incidence of infection is not known because of under-reporting, partly due to the high proportion of asymptomatic or mild cases. The incidence of reported cases in Europe is about 0.2 per 100,000. The Netherlands has had a higher level in recent years due to outbreak-related cases.

Most cases are reported in adults, with a peak in those aged 40–64 years. Reported cases in children are rare, probably because of an increased likelihood of infection being asymptomatic, and males are more than twice as likely to be reported with Q fever than females, mainly due to occupational exposure. Cases are usually reported to peak in spring although this is less obvious in some countries.

Occupationally acquired disease occurs in those who work with animals or animal products, including farmers, abattoir workers, veterinarians and laboratory staff.

Clinical features

Infection with *C. burnetii* may be asymptomatic, a mild febrile illness or a more severe illness with pneumonia, hepatitis, myocarditis or neurological symptoms.

The most common symptoms reported in acute infection are fever, headache, myalgia and cough. Other symptoms include fatigue, chills/rigors/night sweats, anorexia/weight loss, arthralgia and nausea/vomiting. Some symptoms, such as fatigue, can be long-lasting. Severe disease has been reported in the fetus and newborn.

Chronic Q fever can follow clinically apparent or subclinical infection, possibly after a latent period of years. It is estimated to oc-

cur in about 1–2% of cases. The most common presentation is a culture-negative endocarditis, although hepatitis and osteomyelitis may also occur. Previously abnormal heart valves predispose to endocarditis. Case fatality rates can be as high as 10%, even with appropriate treatment.

Laboratory confirmation

The diagnosis of Q fever is usually confirmed by the demonstration of a fourfold rise in serum antibodies: this usually takes 14–20 days to become apparent (range 7 days to 6 weeks). IgM may be detected earlier than IgG (7–10 days) and usually persists for 6 months, although a single high titre is non-diagnostic of an acute event. 'Phase II' antibody generally occurs in acute infection and 'Phase I' in chronic. Culture of this organism is potentially hazardous. PCR may be available. Strain typing is not routinely available.

Transmission

The natural reservoir for *C. burnetii* is a number of animal species, particularly sheep, goats, cattle, cats, dogs, wild rodents, birds and ticks. Most infected animals are asymptomatic, although abortions may occur. In mammals such as sheep and cats, the infection localises to the endometrium and mammary glands and is reactivated during pregnancy to be aerosolised during parturition. These aerosols may be inhaled directly or may contaminate the environment for many months (*C. burnetii* spores are resistant to heat and drying), leading to the creation of secondary aerosols. Animal excreta or carcasses may also contaminate the environment with *C. burnetii*. Human infection is usually via inhalation from close exposure to animals, wind-borne aerosols (usually within 5 km, although longer distances are reported) or contaminated fomites such as wool, straw and contaminated clothing. Infection via raw milk and via blood and marrow transfusion are described, but rare. Necropsy and laboratory animals (especially pregnant sheep) have also been reported as sources of infection.

Acquisition

The incubation period for Q fever is mostly within 9–33 days of exposure, with an average of about 20 days, although shorter and longer incubations have been reported. The incubation period varies with the size of the infecting dose. Although person-to-person spread has been reported it is rare and, in practice, human cases can be viewed as non-infectious under normal circumstances. The infective dose is low, perhaps only 1–5 organisms: 1 g of placenta from an infected sheep may contain 10^{10} infective doses. Immunity from previous illness is probably lifelong. Children may be less susceptible to clinical disease than adults, females possibly less susceptible than males, and the immunocompromised and cigarette smokers are more susceptible than the general population.

Prevention

• Adequate hygiene practices in premises dealing with animals, particularly sheep, cattle and goats.
• Pasteurisation of milk.
• An effective vaccine does exist, but also has potential side-effects in those previously exposed to *Coxiella*. It is not commercially available for the general public in most countries, but may be given to individuals in high-risk occupations.
• Chemoprophylaxis with oxytetracycline late during the incubation period (8–12 days after exposure) has been reported to prevent the onset of clinical disease. Doxycycline can be used for a probable *C. burnetii* exposure.

Surveillance

• Report laboratory-confirmed cases to local and national surveillance centres. Q fever reporting is compulsory in many countries (e.g. Germany, Ireland, the Netherlands and Sweden).
• Potential clusters or linked cases should be reported to local public health authorities.

Response to a case

• Check for exposure to animals.
• No exclusion/isolation is necessary, although avoid blood/tissue donation.
• Universal precautions in hospitals, including care with body fluids and at autopsy.

Investigations of a cluster

Undertake hypothesis-generating study to cover 6 weeks before onset, including:
• Full occupational history.
• Full travel history.
• Exposure to sheep, cattle, goats and other farm animals or farm equipment, clothing, etc.?
• Exposure to pets, especially cats, or pet owners/household after parturition? Visit to pet-shop?
• Exposure to potentially contaminated fomites including straw, hay, peat, manure and wool?
• General outdoor exposure. Check local veterinary and meteorological data for clues (e.g. sheep abortions, wind conditions).
• Consider possibility of bioterrorism incident (see Chapter 4.15).

Control of an outbreak

• Plot dates of onset as an epidemic curve: is there ongoing exposure?
• Remove any continuing source.
• Treat human cases.
• In large outbreaks, consider whether case finding to ensure acute cases are treated and/or surveillance of blood/tissue donors is warranted.

Suggested case-definition for an outbreak

• Fourfold rise in serum antibodies to *C. burnetii*. No need to demonstrate symptoms; *or*
• Acute febrile or pneumatic illness with single high convalescent IgM and no other cause identified.

3.62 Rabies

Rabies is an infection of the central nervous system caused by a lyssavirus (a genus of rhabdovirus). The public health significance of rabies is that there are many animal hosts, the disease is always fatal and both human and animal vaccines are available.

Suggested on-call action

Possible exposure:
• Advise cleansing of wound if recent.
• Assess need for post-exposure prophylaxis. If in doubt, seek expert advice.
Possible case:
• Seek history of animal bite, travel and vaccination status.
• Contact virus reference laboratory to arrange laboratory confirmation.
• Arrange admission to specialist unit.
• Prepare list of close contacts and contacts with possible source.
• Inform national public health institute.
• Inform state veterinary service.

Epidemiology

Rabies exists in animal populations in many countries of Europe, although human cases are rare (less than 5 a year in the EU). The risk of rabies from an animal bite varies in different countries; most of Western Europe is rabies-free. However, bats are a potential source of infection even in those countries considered rabies-free such as Spain and the UK.

Clinical features

The early features of human rabies are often mistaken for hysteria, with altered personality and agitation. Pain or numbness at the site of an animal bite is a useful early clue. Painful spasms of the face induced by attempts to drink ('hydrophobia') are the classic feature. The case fatality is 100%.

Laboratory diagnosis

This is only possible after the onset of symptoms. The national virus reference laboratory must be involved. Serum antibodies appear after 6 days. Rabies virus can be isolated from saliva, brain, CSF and urine, or demonstrated by immunofluorescent antibody staining of impression smears of skin, cornea or other material. PCR is available for saliva specimens.

Transmission

Animal reservoirs in Europe include dogs, cats, foxes, wolves, racoons and bats. Transmission is from the bite or scratch of an infected animal, or a lick on a mucosal surface such a conjunctiva. Air-borne spread has been demonstrated in bat caves, but this is unusual. Rare cases have occurred in recipients of corneal grafts from patients who died of undiagnosed rabies.

Acquisition

The incubation period is usually 3–8 weeks, but may be as short as 9 days or as long as 7 years, depending on the amount of virus introduced, the severity of the wound and its proximity to the brain.

Prevention

• Control rabies in domestic animals by vaccination before travel to infected countries and implantation of a microchip device.
• Oral vaccination of foxes (using baits), the principal reservoir in Europe.
• Vaccinate high-risk travellers to endemic areas and those at occupational risk such as some laboratory workers and animal handlers (including bat handlers, although immunisation may not protect against some bat lyssaviruses). The primary course is three doses at days 0, 7 and 28, given in the deltoid (NB the response may be reduced if vaccine is given in the buttock) with a booster at 6–12 months.
• Give post-exposure prophylaxis with vaccine (and rabies-specific immunoglobulin for high-risk exposures) following a bite (or cat scratch) in an endemic area. For appropriate schedule seek advice from the national reference unit. Cleanse the wound thoroughly as soon after injury as possible: as a minimum with soap or detergent under running water for at least 5 minutes; antiseptics should also be used if available. Obtain as much information on the exposure as possible (place, species, bite/scratch, behaviour, owned/stray), including name and address of owner of the animal so it can be observed for the next 10 days for abnormal behaviour. All bat bites (some of which are not immediately obvious), including those in rabies-free countries such as the UK should be given post-exposure prophylaxis with vaccine. Expert advice should be sought as to whether immunoglobulin is also indicated.

Surveillance

• Notifiable throughout Europe.
• Inform national public health institute immediately.

Response to a case

• Isolation in a specialist unit for the duration of the illness.

• Healthcare workers attending the case should wear masks, gloves and gowns.
• Vaccination and immunoglobulin for contacts that have open wound or mucous membrane exposure to the patient's saliva (according to the schedule above).
• Investigate source of infection.
• Disinfect articles soiled with the patient's saliva.
• Identify others that may have been exposed to the source.

Investigation of a cluster and control of an outbreak

A cluster of human cases from an indigenous source is unlikely in Europe. Refer to national plan for control of animal rabies.

Suggested case-definition for an outbreak

Clinical: acute encephalomyelitis in an exposed individual.
Confirmed: clinically compatible case confirmed by vial antigen, isolate or rabies neutralising antibody (pre-vaccination).

3.63 Relapsing fever

Louse-borne relapsing fever is a systemic disease due to *Borrelia recurrentis*. Tick-borne disease may be caused by a number of different *Borrelia* species.

Suggested on-call action

None required unless ongoing transmission suspected because of presence of lice, in which case institute delousing procedures.

Epidemiology

Louse-borne fever is found in Africa, especially highland areas of East Africa, and South America. Endemic (tick-borne) disease is widespread, including foci in Spain.

Clinical features

The illness is characterised by periods of high fever lasting up to 9 days, which are interspersed with afebrile periods of 2–4 days.

Laboratory confirmation

Definitive diagnosis is by visualising spirochetes in peripheral blood smear. Multiple smears may need to be examined (thick and thin, Wright and Giemsa stains).

Transmission

Relapsing fever is vector-borne; there is no person-to-person spread. The disease is classically epidemic when spread by lice and endemic when spread by ticks.

Acquisition

The incubation period is 5–11 days. There is no person-to-person spread.

Prevention

Maintenance of personal hygiene and by impregnation of clothes with repellents and permethrin in endemic areas.

Surveillance

Relapsing fever is a notifiable disease in many countries, including the UK.

Response to a case

The case does not need isolation once deloused. The immediate environment should also be deloused. Treatment of choice is with tetracycline, doxycycline, erythromycin or chloramphenicol.

Investigation of a cluster and control of an outbreak

Vector control.

3.64 Respiratory syncytial virus

Respiratory syncytial virus (RSV) causes bronchiolitis in infants and upper and lower respiratory tract infection at all ages. It may cause serious nosocomial outbreaks in children, the elderly and the immunocompromised.

Suggested on-call action
• Suggest case limits contact with infants, frail elderly and the immunocompromised. • If linked cases in an institution suspected, activate Outbreak Control Plan.

Epidemiology

RSV epidemics occur every winter, peaking from November to January. Almost all children who have lived through two epidemics in urban areas will have become infected, causing 20,000 hospital admissions a year in the UK. Most cases are not specifically diagnosed, but 80% of cases of bronchiolitis and 20% of pneumonia in young children are caused by RSV. Re-infections occur throughout life. About 5% of elderly people suffer RSV infection each year, and it is a significant cause of infection and outbreaks in nursing homes, day units and hospitals, particularly neonatal units. Male gender; age under 6 months; birth during first half of RSV season; crowding and/or siblings; daycare exposure; tobacco exposure and lack of breastfeeding are potential risk factors for RSV infection.

Clinical features

The most common presentation is upper respiratory tract infection with rhinitis, cough and possibly fever. Children may also develop otitis media or pharyngitis. Bronchiolitis (wheeze, dyspnoea, poor feeding), pneumonia or croup may develop after a few days. Infants with congenital heart disease or chronic lung disease risk severe disease as do those under 6 weeks of age and premature infants. In adults, RSV infection is usually confined to the upper respiratory tract but it may cause exacerbations of asthma or chronic bronchitis, or, particularly in the elderly, acute bronchitis or pneumonia. Few infections are asymptomatic. Case fatality is particularly high in the immunocompromised.

Laboratory confirmation

Nasopharyngeal aspirates (NPAs) taken early in the illness may be positive for RSV by antigen detection, which can provide immediate results, or viral culture, which takes 3–7 days but is slightly more sensitive. NPAs may not be obtainable from elderly patients: nose or throat swabs are less sensitive and, as the elderly do not shed the organism for as long as infants and often present later in the illness, the diagnosis rate is low in this group. More sensitive PCR tests are now available and may be particularly useful for these patients. Serology is available for retrospective diagnosis.

Transmission

Humans are the only known reservoir of RSV. Spread occurs from respiratory secretions either directly, through large droplet spread, or indirectly via contaminated hands, handkerchiefs, eating utensils or other objects or surfaces. RSV may survive for 24 hours on contaminated surfaces and 1 hour on hospital gowns, paper towels and skin. Infection results from contact of the virus with mucous membranes of the eye, mouth or nose. Hospital staff and visitors are thought to be important vectors in hospital outbreaks and in the relatively common transmission of sporadic nosocomial infection.

Acquisition

The incubation period is 2–8 days with a median of 4.4 days. The infectious period lasts from shortly before to (usually) 1 week after commencement of symptoms. Some infants and the immunosuppressed may shed RSV for many weeks. Immunity is incomplete and short-lived, although re-infections are usually milder. Those with defective cellular immunity are at increased risk of more severe disease.

Prevention

• Personal hygiene, particularly handwashing and sanitary disposal of nasal and oral discharges.
• Good infection control in hospitals (especially important in paediatric wards), nursing homes and day units. Avoid overcrowding.
• Avoid young infants, frail elderly and the immunocompromised coming into contact with individuals with respiratory infection.
• Consider use of monoclonal antibody (palivizumab) prophylaxis for certain high-risk groups during RSV season. Consult local guidance for details, but groups to consider include:

   (a) infants born before 35 weeks' gestation, who have chronic lung or heart disease and are aged under 9 months at the onset of the RSV season;

(b) children aged under 2 years who have severe combined immunodeficiency or are on long-term ventilation.

Surveillance

• RSV cases associated with institutions should be reported to local public health authorities.
• Laboratory-confirmed cases should be reported to national surveillance system.
• Hospitals should include RSV in nosocomial surveillance programmes.

Response to a case

• Contact isolation for hospital patients.
• Avoid contact with infants, frail elderly and the immunocompromised until well.
• Exclude from nursery, work, school or non-residential institution until well.
• Sanitary disposal of nasal and oral discharges.

Investigation of a cluster

• Rarely investigated unless a link to an institution is thought likely. Undertake case finding at any institution containing infants, elderly or the immunosuppressed, if linked to a case.
• Antigenic and genomic fingerprinting may be useful in investigating hospital clusters, but beware that more than one strain may be involved (i.e. there may be more than one source).

Control of an outbreak

• Contact isolation and cohorting of suspected cases in hospitals. Closest feasible equivalent in nursing and residential homes.
• Reinforce hygiene and infection control measures, particularly handwashing, sanitary

disposal of nasal and oral discharges and cleaning of potentially contaminated surfaces.
• Exclude staff and day attenders at institutions with respiratory infection until well. Restrict visiting.
• Active surveillance of new and existing patients in hospital for respiratory infection with rapid testing for RSV.
• Cancel non-urgent admissions.
• Consider other measures to limit the transfer of RSV by hospital staff (e.g. use of eye–nose goggles, gloves and perhaps gowns and masks).
• Maintaining adequate compliance with the above recommendations will require constant monitoring and reinforcement.
• Consider use of RSV-specific prophylaxis in high-risk individuals.

Suggested case-definition in an outbreak

Upper or lower respiratory tract infection and antigen or culture positive for RSV.

3.65 Ringworm

The dermatophytoses, tinea and ringworm, are synonymous terms that refer to fungal infections of the skin and other keratinised tissues such as hair and nails. These infections are common throughout the world. They are caused by various species of the genera *Trichophyton*, *Epidermophyton* and *Microsporum*, and are classified according to the area of the body that is affected: corporis (body), faciei (face), cruris (groin), pedis (foot), manuum (hand), capitis (scalp), barbae (beard area) and unguium (nail).

Suggested on-call action

Advise on laboratory diagnosis and treatment.

Epidemiology

Dermatophyte infections are mainly found in pre-pubertal children. Although surveillance by UK GPs indicates that the mean weekly incidence of ringworm has been stable at around 25 per 100,000 population in 2000–2009, in Europe and the USA the pattern of tinea capitis has changed over this period of time, with a significant rise in cases of tinea capitis infection due to *Trichophyton tonsurans* (Table 3.65.1).

Clinical features

For clinical features see Table 3.65.2.

Laboratory confirmation

Hairs infected with *Microsporum* species fluoresce green under filtered ultraviolet (Wood's) light. Hairs infected with most *Trichophyton* species do not fluoresce. Fungal spores and hyphae can be detected by microscopic examination of the hair after preparation in potassium hydroxide. Definitive diagnosis requires culture of the infecting fungus. Specimens for culture are collected by scraping the affected area with a scalpel or glass slide held at right-angles to the skin. Specimens for culture can be obtained using a suitable brush. The brush should be passed through the hair firmly in an affected area several times and then pressed into the surface of an agar-coated Petri dish, which is then incubated for up to 3 weeks. A culture taken from an infected child will usually produce a fungal colony from each of the inoculation points, whereas one taken from a carrier will produce fewer colonies. Identification of the fungus helps determine the source of infection (either an animal or another child) and allows appropriate treatment and control measures.

Transmission

The reservoir of some dermatophyte species such as *Trichophyton rubrum* and *Trichophyton tonsurans* is exclusively human (anthropophilic). Others species have animal reservoirs (zoophilic) including cats, dogs and cattle. Soil (geophilic) species are less common causes of human infection. Transmission is by direct skin-to-skin contact with an infected person or animal, or by indirect contact with fomites (seat backs, combs and brushes) or environmental surfaces (showers,

Table 3.65.1 Epidemiology of ringworm

Tinea capitis Anthropophilic: *Trichophyton tonsurans, T. violaceum, T. soudanense, Microsporum audouinii, T. schoenleinii* Zoophilic: *Microsporum canis* (cat, dog), *Trichophyton verrucosum* (cattle)	Prevalence has increased recently due to anthropophilic *Trichophyton tonsurans* which particularly affects children of Afro-Caribbean ethnic origin. Spread occurs in families and at school and asymptomatic infection is common. Risk factors may include overcrowding within households or schools, exposure in hairdressing salons, use of shared combs, particular hair styles and ethnicity. *T. tonsurans* has also recently been reported in West and East Africa. In other countries *Microsporum canis* is the most common cause.
Tinea corporis, tinea cruris, tinea barbae, tinea pedis *M. canis, T. tonsurans, T. rubrum, T. mentagrophytes, Epidermophyton floccosum*	In Northern Europe since the 1950s, *T. rubrum* has replaced *M. audouinii* and *E. floccosum* as the most frequently isolated dermatophytes. In Southern Europe and the Middle East zoophilic dermatophytes, such as *M. canis* and *T. verrucosum*, are the most frequent.
Tinea unguium (onychomycosis) *T. rubrum, T. mentagrophytes*	*T. rubrum* and *T. mentagrophytes* account for 90% of onychomycoses. Increasing age, diabetes, AIDS and peripheral arterial disease are risk factors and there is a familial pattern.

Table 3.65.2 Clinical features of ringworm

Tinea capitis	The clinical presentation comprises generalised diffuse scaling of the scalp, patchy hair loss, broken-off hair stubs, scattered pustules, lymphadenopathy, boggy tumour (kerion) and favus (hair loss caused by *Trichophyton schoenleinii*, largely confined to Eastern Europe and Asia). Infection with *T. tonsurans* an endothrix dermatophyte whose growth and spore production are confined chiefly within the hair shaft may cause lightly flaky areas, indistinguishable from dandruff or small patches of hair loss. Asymptomatic infection occurs with *T. tonsurans* and a carrier state may exist in which fungus is present in the absence of any hair or skin abnormalities.
Tinea corporis, tinea cruris	Lesions are found on the trunk or legs and have a prominent red margin with a central scaly area.
Tinea barbae, barber's itch	Infection of the beard area of the face and neck with both superficial lesions and deeper lesions involving the hair follicles.
Tinea pedis, athlete's foot	Affects the feet particularly the toes, toe webs, and soles.
Tinea unguium (onychomycosis)	Infection of the nails, usually associated with infection of the adjacent skin. There is thickening and discoloration of the nail.

changing-rooms) contaminated with hair or skin scales. The risk of spread is low in schools but higher with prolonged exposure in families and particularly where there is broken skin.

Acquisition

The incubation period varies with the site of infection but is typically 2–6 weeks. The infectious period lasts for as long as infection is present, which may be from months to years if untreated. Persons who are immunosuppressed, including those with HIV infection, are at increased risk of dermatophyte infection. Certain occupations, such as veterinary surgeons, are at risk of infections of animal origin.

Prevention

• Early recognition of animal and human cases and carriers and prompt effective treatment.
• Maintain high levels of personal and environmental hygiene with attention to handwashing, care of pets, regular cleaning and maintenance of floors and surfaces at home, in schools and in swimming pools and communal changing rooms.

Surveillance

• Cases of scalp and body ringworm in school-aged children should be reported to the school nurse.
• Clusters of cases should be discussed with the local health protection team.
• Fungal culture results for tinea capitis should be collected from a number of sentinel diagnostic laboratories in order to monitor the spread of *T. tonsurans*.

Response to a case

• Anthrophilic dermatophytes can be spread between children at school, but exclusion of an infected pupil from school is unnecessary once treatment has started. However, activities involving physical contact or undressing, which may lead to exposure of others, should be restricted.
• Confirm diagnosis and identity of infecting fungus with skin, nail or hair samples for microscopy and culture.

• Start effective treatment. Most cases of dermatophyte infections respond readily to topical agents used for 2–4 weeks but oral treatment is required for nail and scalp infection. Treatment guidelines have been published. Topical treatment may reduce the risk of transmission to others before oral treatment is established. Selenium sulphide shampoo, used twice weekly, reduces the carriage of viable spores and may also reduce infectivity. It is not recommended for use in children under the age of 5 years, for whom an alternative antifungal lotion may be used.

• If cultures show that the infecting fungus is of human rather than animal or soil origin, a search should be made for other cases. Signs of infection in others may be minimal and so samples should be requested for culture. Those with mycological evidence of carriage may be offered treatment.

• If the source is an animal, family pets should be screened by a veterinary surgeon.

Investigation of a cluster

• Clusters of cases of scalp or body ringworm may be reported from schools or nurseries.

• Spread is well recognised amongst members of wrestling teams (tinea corporis gladiatorum).

• Nosocomial spread has also been documented from patients to nursing staff.

Control of an outbreak

• Confirmation of the diagnosis is important and all contacts should be examined to identify cases and carriers. Samples should be requested for culture.

• The local health protection team should be available to give advice and practical assistance.

• Prompt effective treatment should be offered to cases and carriers (see above).

• Exclusion from school is not normally necessary once treatment has started, but may be considered if control proves difficult.

• An environmental investigation should be carried out to ensure a high standard of hygiene, particularly in communal changing rooms. Additional cleaning may be recommended. Possible animal sources should be investigated.

• In hospitals and nursing homes, cases should be nursed with source isolation precautions, and gloves and aprons should be used.

Suggested case-definition for cluster investigation

Characteristic lesions reported amongst household or other close contacts, with or without laboratory confirmation by microscopy or culture.

3.66 Rotavirus

Rotaviruses are the most common cause of childhood diarrhoea. The public health significance of rotavirus diarrhoea is the high level of morbidity and the potential for control by vaccines.

Suggested on-call action

• Exclude cases in risk groups (Box 2.2.1) until 48 hours after last episode of diarrhoea or vomiting.

• If linked to other cases in an institution, consult outbreak control plan.

Epidemiology

Rotavirus is the main cause of gastroenteritis in children under 2 years, in both developed and developing countries. Laboratory-confirmed cases represent only a small fraction of the total disease burden; it has been estimated that one-third of hospital admissions for childhood diarrhoea are due to rotavirus.

The peak incidence is between 6 months and 2 years of age; clinical infection is unusual above 5 years, although subclinical infection is probably common. In Europe, most cases occur in winter and spring, with a peak in March. Mortality is low in developed countries, although there are an estimated 0.5 million deaths each year in developing countries. Many outbreaks are reported every year, mostly in residential institutions, nurseries or hospitals.

Clinical features

There is sudden onset of diarrhoea and vomiting, often with a mild fever and dehydration. Occasionally there is blood in the stools. The illness usually lasts for a few days only.

Laboratory confirmation

This is needed to differentiate rotavirus infection from other viral infections of the gastrointestinal tract. Rotavirus particles can usually be demonstrated in diarrhoea stools by electron microscopy. PCR and ELISA are available. There are three serogroups, of which group A is by far the most common; rotavirus positive samples can also be characterised by genotyping.

Transmission

There are both animal and human rotaviruses, although animal-to-human transmission does not occur. Person-to-person transmission is mainly by the faeco-oral route, although there may also be spread from respiratory secretions and sometimes via contaminated water. Long-term carriage does not occur. Outbreaks may occur in nurseries, and nosocomial spread may occur in paediatric and occasionally geriatric units, where the virus may contaminate the environment. Attack rates in close child contacts are usually high. It is resistant to many disinfectants, but is inactivated by chlorine.

Acquisition

The incubation period is 2–4 days. Cases are infectious during the acute stage of the illness and for a short time afterwards; this is usually for less than a week in a healthy child, but may be as long as a month in an immunocompromised patient. Re-infection may occur after some months.

Prevention

- No specific preventive measures.
- General enteric precautions may help limit spread in households, nurseries and hospitals. In nurseries, children should have clothing to cover their nappies.
- Two live oral vaccines are now available. They are not widely used in Europe but have been introduced in many countries of Latin America, the USA and in parts of Africa.

Surveillance

- Must be based on laboratory reports. This significantly underestimates the true incidence, as only hospitalised cases are likely to be investigated.
- European-wide surveillance, with strain genotyping, has been established (www.eurorota.net).
- Gastroenteritis is notifiable in some EU countries.

Response to a case

- Isolate cases with enteric precautions in hospital.
- Give hygiene advice to the family in the community.
- Exclude from nursery or school (or risk occupation; see Table 2.2.1) until 48 hours after the last episode of diarrhoea or vomiting.

Investigation of a cluster

• Not often reported, unless linked to an institution.
• Consider also the possibility of a common source (e.g. contaminated water supply).

Control of an outbreak

• Remind the local population of the importance of good hygiene (although this will probably not have an important role in controlling the outbreak).
• In institutions with cases, ensure adequacy of hygiene and toilet facilities.

Suggested case-definition for an outbreak

Confirmed: diarrhoea or vomiting with laboratory confirmation.
Clinical: diarrhoea or vomiting in a person linked to a confirmed case.

3.67 Rubella

Rubella (German measles) is a systemic virus infection characterised by a rash and fever. Rubella virus is a member of the Togaviridae. The public health importance of rubella is the consequences of infection in pregnancy and the availability of a vaccine.

Suggested on-call action

Advise limiting contact with those known to be pregnant.

Epidemiology

Rubella is now uncommon in most of Europe, where immunisation programmes have been in place for many years. In 2008 only 1921 rubella cases were confirmed in Europe. Before immunisation, epidemics occurred at 6-yearly intervals, affecting mainly children in primary school but also adolescents and some adults. During epidemics, up to 5% of susceptible pregnant women caught the disease, leading to congenital rubella syndrome and rubella-associated terminations of pregnancy.

In the post-immunisation era, rubella outbreaks still occur among susceptible young adult males who are too old to have been immunised. Congenital rubella syndrome is now very rare (e.g. in the UK there are less than 10 cases a year).

Clinical features

The main differential diagnosis is parvovirus, which is now more common than rubella. In rubella, there is sore throat, conjunctivitis and mild fever for 2–3 days before the macular rash appears. The lymph nodes of the neck are often swollen. Recovery is usually rapid and complete, although, as in parvovirus infection, persistent joint infection sometimes occurs, especially in adults.

The features of congenital rubella syndrome range from mild sensorineural deafness to multiple defects of several organ systems.

Laboratory confirmation

This is particularly important in pregnancy. The simplest method is by IgM detection or a rising IgG antibody titre in serum or saliva. Polymerase chain reaction (PCR) testing of oral fluid (Oracol), throat swabs, nasopharyngeal aspirate (NPA), urine, cerebrospinal fluid (CSF), amniotic fluid, placenta or fetal tissue is available and may be helpful, particularly in the diagnosis of congenital rubella syndrome.

Transmission

Humans are the only reservoir. Transmission is by direct person-to-person contact by respiratory droplets. There are no carriers.

Acquisition

Rubella is moderately infectious, although not as infectious as parvovirus or measles. The incubation period is 13–20 days. Infectivity is from 1 week before the onset of rash to about 5 days after onset.

The risk of congenital rubella syndrome in a susceptible pregnant woman infected in the first trimester is greater than 90%. This risk declines to about 50% in the second trimester and is zero near term.

Prevention

• Vaccinate all children with combined measles/mumps/rubella (MMR) vaccine. Two doses are required to ensure seroconversion and maintain herd immunity. The only contraindications are immunosuppression and pregnancy, although women accidentally vaccinated in pregnancy can be reassured that the risk of fetal damage is minimal.
• Screen all women in early pregnancy and vaccinate postpartum if found to be susceptible.
• Vaccinate healthcare workers, as they are likely to be in contact with pregnant women.

Surveillance

Notifiable in all European countries, although in some the surveillance system is not national. The clinical diagnosis is unreliable and surveillance should be based on obtaining laboratory confirmation (e.g. by salivary IgM).

Response to a case

• Seek laboratory confirmation (e.g. saliva test), especially in pregnancy or if the case has been in contact with a pregnant woman.
• Check immunisation status of the case and arrange for vaccination if non-immune.
• Exclude children from school for 5 days from the onset of rash.

• Test pregnant women who have been in contact with a case, particularly during the first trimester, for susceptibility or evidence of early infection (IgM antibody) (see Chapter 2.4). Vaccinate susceptible women postpartum; offer infected women termination. In later pregnancy there is a balance between the risk of fetal damage and the desirability of termination.

Investigation of a cluster and control of an outbreak

Laboratory confirmation is essential. In addition to the measures described above for all cases, consider a community-wide immunisation programme if coverage is low.

Suggested case-definitions for an outbreak

Confirmed:
• Presence of IgM in blood, urine or saliva; *or*
• Fourfold or greater rise in haemagglutination inhibition antibody in serum; *or*
• Positive PCR in relevant clinical specimen.
Suspected (for investigation): generalised maculopapular rash, fever and one of cervical lymphadenopathy, arthralgia or conjunctivitis.

3.68 Salmonellosis

Salmonella infection is a common cause of gastroenteritis that can result in large outbreaks, particularly due to food-borne transmission, and severe infection in the elderly, immunosuppressed and pregnant women.

Most microbiologists use a system of nomenclature for *Salmonella* organisms, based on DNA relatedness, which suggests that all salmonellae probably belong to a single species, *enterica,* which has seven sub-groups. Most human pathogens belong to a subgroup also called *enterica,* further divided into serovars; for example, *S. enterica* sub-group *enterica* serovar Enteritidis or *S.* Enteritidis for short. For *S.* Paratyphi and *S.* Typhi see Chapters 3.56 and 3.82, respectively.

Suggested on-call action

• Exclude cases in risk groups for onward transmission (see Box 2.2.1) until formed stools for 48 hours.
• If you or reporting laboratory/clinician are aware of other potentially linked cases, consult local outbreak plan.

Epidemiology

Salmonella infections occur worldwide and are one of the most commonly reported gastro-intestinal infections in Europe. The incidence has fallen from its peak in the early 1990s, particularly infections caused by *Salmonella* Enteritidis PT4. All ages are affected, but re-ported cases are highest in young children. Cases peak from July to September. Travel abroad is a risk factor, and is a substantial con-tributor in lower incidence countries, such as those in Scandinavia. In 2008, the incidence of non-typhoidal salmonellosis in the EU was 30 cases per 100,000, with very large varia-tions between countries. These variations are to a large extent due to differences in detec-tion and case finding.

Clinical features

It is difficult to differentiate salmonellosis from other causes of gastroenteritis on clin-ical grounds for individual cases. The sever-ity of the illness is variable but in most cases stools are loose, of moderate volume and do not contain blood or mucus. Diarrhoea usually lasts 3–7 days and may be accom-panied by fever, abdominal pain, myalgia

and headache. Other symptoms, particularly nausea, may precede diarrhoea, and malaise and weakness may continue after resolution of the gastroenteritis. Rare complications in-clude septicaemia and abscess formation. Fac-tors that may suggest salmonellosis as the cause of a cluster of cases of gastroenteritis in-clude fever in most cases, headache and myal-gia in a significant minority and severe disease in a few. With some serovars (e.g. *S.* Dublin, *S.* Choleraesuis and, to a lesser extent, *S.* Vir-chow) septicaemia and extra-intestinal infec-tion are more common.

Laboratory confirmation

Diagnosis is usually confirmed by culture of a stool specimen, rectal swab or blood culture. Using a stool sample rather than a rectal swab, collecting 5 g of faecal material and, espe-cially when looking for asymptomatic excre-tors, collecting two or more specimens over several days all increase sensitivity. Excretion usually persists for several days or weeks be-yond the acute phase of the illness. Refrigera-tion and/or a suitable transport medium may be necessary if there will be a delay in process-ing specimens, especially in warm weather.

The laboratory may be able to issue a pro-visional report within 48 hours of receiving the specimen (further confirmatory tests will be necessary), although a further day is often required. Serotyping (e.g. 'Typhimurium') is available for all salmonellae and phage typ-ing ('PT' or 'DT') is available for *S.* Agona, *S.* Enteritidis, *S.* Hadar, *S.* Java, *S.* Pullorum, *S.* Thompson, *S.* Typhimurium and S. Vir-chow, usually via reference laboratories. These tests are often useful in detecting and controlling outbreaks of rarer salmonellae. However, for *S.* Enteritidis PT4 or *S.* Ty-phimurium DT104, further more discrimi-natory tests may be required: pulsed field gel electrophoresis (PFGE) and multiple-locus variable-number tandem repeat analy-sis (MLVA) 'fingerprinting' has already been shown to be useful and antibiograms may be a useful marker for case finding in an out-break.

Transmission

Salmonella infection is acquired by ingestion of the organisms. In most cases this is through the consumption of a contaminated food.

• *Salmonella* infection or carriage affects many animals (Table 3.68.1) leading to contamination of foodstuffs before their arrival in the kitchen. If such foods are eaten raw or undercooked then illness can result. Such food sources include undercooked poultry or meat, raw or undercooked eggs (often used in mayonnaise, sweets such as mousse or tiramisu, and 'egg nog' drinks) and raw or inadequately pasteurised milk. Contaminated foodstuffs, particularly raw poultry or meat, may be the source of cross-contamination to other foods that may not be cooked before eating (e.g. salad). This cross-contamination may also occur via food surfaces or utensils. Contamination of food by an infected food handler may occur but is thought to be uncommon in the absence of diarrhoea. Salmonellae can multiply at temperatures ranging from 7°C to 46°C; thus, inadequate temperature control will allow a small number of contaminating organisms to develop into an infective dose. Heating to at least 70°C for at least 2 minutes is required to kill the organism.

• Imported foods (e.g. salad, halva, peanuts) may be contaminated before their arrival in Europe. *Salmonella* is also a risk to travellers abroad.

• Person-to-person spread via the faeco-oral route may occur without food as an intermediary. The risk is highest during the acute diarrhoeal phase of the illness. Person-to-person spread due to inadequate infection control practices may prolong food-borne outbreaks in institutions. Children and faecally incontinent adults pose a particular risk of person-to-person spread.

• Other, rarer, causes of salmonellosis include direct contact with animals, including exotic

Table 3.68.1 Frequency and some possible sources of common *Salmonella* serovars

Serovar	Number of human cases in the EU 2008 (Source: ECDC)	Animal reservoirs (DT/PT)	Some additional vehicles found in outbreaks
S. Enteritidis	70,091	Chickens, other poultry, cattle (PT8)	Egg (PT14b in Spanish eggs), dairy produce, Chinese meals
S. Typhimurium	26,423	Cattle (104, U302, RDNC) Pigs (193, 104, U308a, U302, 170) Poultry (104), Sheep (104)	Halva (from Turkey), manure, salad
S. Infantis	1317	Calves, pigs, poultry	Chicken drumsticks
S. Virchow	860	Chickens	Eggs
S. Newport	787	Poultry, cattle	Peanuts (from China), lettuce, horsemeat, mango
S. Agona	636	Turkeys, chickens	Kosher snack
S. Derby	624	Pigs, sheep, cattle	
S. Stanley	529		Peanuts (from China), alfalfa sprouts, soft cheese
S. Bovismorbificans	501	Pigs, ruminants	Alfalfa sprouts, lettuce
S. Kentucky	497	Pigs, cattle	

Rarer serovars associated with particular animals include *S.* Arizonae (sheep), *S.* Binza (gamebirds), *S.* Braenderup (poultry, cattle), *S.* Dublin (cattle), *S.* Indiana (ducks), *S.* Goldcoast (cattle), *S.* Hadar (chickens, other poultry), *S.* Java (poultry, tropical fish, terrapins), *S.* Livingstone (chicken, ducks, pigs), *S.* Mbandaka (chicken) and *S.* Seftenberg (chicken).

pets; contamination of non-chlorinated water; nosocomially via endoscopes, breast milk, blood transfusion and soiled bedclothes; and contamination of bedding, toys and clothing by excreta.

Acquisition

The incubation period may range from 4 hours to 5 days or occasionally longer and is affected by the number of organisms ingested. Most cases occur within 12–48 hours of ingestion. The infectious period varies enormously; most cases excrete the organism for a few days to a few months with a median duration of 5 weeks. Approximately 1% of adults and 5% of children under 5 years of age will excrete the organism for at least a year.

In most cases the infective dose for salmonellae is 10^3–10^5 organisms but certain food vehicles are thought to protect the organism against gastric acid, reducing the infective dose to only a few organisms. High-fat foods such as chocolate and cheese may be examples. Immunity to *Salmonella* infections is partial, with re-infection possible, if milder. Those at increased risk include patients with low gastric acidity (including antacid therapy), immunosuppression, debilitation or on broad spectrum antibiotics and the young and the elderly.

Prevention

Prevention of food-borne salmonellosis is a classic case of the need for a 'farm to fork' strategy:
• At the farm, action is required to reduce infection and carriage in food animals, particularly poultry to reduce contaminated meat and eggs. Vaccination of poultry flocks is recommended. Slaughter and processing practices for poultry require attention to reduce cross-contamination. The Scandinavian experience suggests that *Salmonella*-free poultry can be achieved.

• Commercial food processing should be subject to the Hazard Analysis Critical Control Point (HACCP) system to identify, control and monitor potential hazards to food safety. Specific measures for *Salmonella* include use of only pasteurised eggs and milk; adequate cooking of meat and poultry; practices to avoid cross-contamination; exclusion of food handlers with diarrhoea; and adequate temperature control. This is particularly important in establishments serving food to vulnerable groups (the very young, the very old and the immunocompromised).
• In the home, routine food and personal hygiene measures need to be supplemented by particular care with raw poultry and eggs. The public need to be made aware that all poultry should be viewed as contaminated and how to prevent cross-contamination from it. Consumption of raw or undercooked eggs should be avoided: date stamped eggs from vaccinated flocks are preferable.

Surveillance

• Salmonellosis is mandatorily notifiable in most EU countries.
• Laboratory isolates of *Salmonella* should be reported to local and the national surveillance systems. Isolates should be sent for further typing to aid epidemiological investigation.

Response to a case

• Hygiene advice, particularly on handwashing, should be given to all cases. Ideally, the case should not attend work or school until he/she has normal stools (preferably for 24 hours).
• Occupational details should be sought. Cases in risk groups 1–4 (Box 2.2.1) should be excluded until 48 hours after the first normal stool.
• Enquiry for symptoms in household contacts (or others exposed to the same putative source) should be made: those with

symptoms, particularly diarrhoea, should be treated as cases.

• Enteric precautions for those admitted to hospital (especially for handling faeces or soiled bedding or clothing) should be followed.

• Asymptomatic excretors rarely require exclusion, provided adequate personal hygiene precautions are followed. This requires adequate knowledge and co-operation of the individual (or a responsible adult) and adequate facilities.

• If illness has been acquired in hospital, inform hospital control of infection team.

Investigation of a cluster

• Arrange with local and reference laboratories for serotyping and phage typing of strains to check if similar organisms.

• Some salmonellae are particularly associated with specific animal hosts (Table 3.68.1): the national reference laboratory can advise on this.

• Although some clues may be obtained by analysis of person/place/time variables, administration of a hypothesis-generating questionnaire is usually necessary (see Chapter 4.3). A general semi-structured questionnaire for investigating clusters of food-borne illness should be routinely available: this can be modified in light of the epidemiology of the specific pathogen (e.g. known animal reservoirs or vehicles associated with previous outbreaks) and outbreak specific factors (e.g. most cases in children).

Control of an outbreak

• In food-borne outbreaks, microbiological examination of faeces from infected patients and food can reveal the organism responsible and a cohort or case–control study may reveal the vehicle of infection. However, in order to prevent recurrence the question 'How did the food consumed come to contain an infective dose of the organism?' needs to be answered.

Particular factors to bear in mind in a food-borne outbreak of salmonellosis are:

(a) Were any potentially contaminated foods consumed raw or inadequately cooked? In the case of *S*. Enteritidis PT4, was poultry inadequately cooked or were raw eggs used in any recipes? Can the raw food be checked for the organisms?

(b) Are food preparation procedures and hygiene practices adequate to prevent cross-contamination, particularly from raw meat or poultry?

(c) Did any food handlers have symptoms of gastrointestinal infection? All food handlers should provide faecal samples for analysis, but remember that they may also have eaten the vehicle of infection and so be victims of the outbreak rather than the cause.

(d) What happened to the food after cooking? Was there scope for contamination? Was it refrigerated until just before eating? Was it adequately reheated?

• Many outbreaks require more than one problem to occur in food preparation. An example is a sandwich tea made for a sports match that used raw egg mayonnaise and then was stored in the boot of a car on a hot summer day until consumed.

• Secondary spread is common in outbreaks of *Salmonella* infection. Outbreak cases should receive intervention as outlined earlier for sporadic cases. Plotting of an epidemic curve may help identify the contribution of person-to-person spread (see Box 2.2.3 for other clues).

• Outbreaks in hospitals or care homes require particular care because of the vulnerable nature of the residents.

Suggested case-definition for analytical study of a *Salmonella* outbreak

---

Clinical: diarrhoea or any two from abdominal pain/fever/nausea with onset 4–120 hours after exposure.
Confirmed: clinical case with isolate of outbreak strain.

3.69 Severe acute respiratory syndrome (SARS)

Severe acute respiratory syndrome (SARS) is a severe viral respiratory illness caused by SARS-associated coronavirus (SARS-CoV).

Suggested on-call action

- Assess whether case fits current case-definition. If so, inform National Surveillance Centre.
- Samples should be taken urgently for laboratory diagnosis.
- Patient(s) should be immediately isolated and respiratory transmission-based precautions instituted.
- The response to the following groups should be considered: cases, potential cases, contacts of cases, the worried well.
- Contacts of persons under investigation for SARS should be traced and placed under observation for 10 days or until SARS has been ruled out. Close contacts are those who have cared for, lived with or have had direct contact with the respiratory secretions, body fluids and/or excretions (e.g. faeces) of SARS cases.
- Individuals at high risk of exposure to a person or persons in a SARS cluster (e.g. healthcare workers) should be managed as contacts until SARS has been ruled out.
- Contacts within the healthcare setting should be managed as follows:
   (a) Inpatients should be isolated or co-horted and transmission-based precautions instituted (respiratory, body fluids and faecal). They should be placed on fever surveillance.
   (b) Exposed staff should be placed on active fever surveillance, and either co-horted to care for exposed patients (as above) or placed under home quarantine.
- Community contacts should be:

   (a) given information on the clinical picture, transmission, etc., of SARS;
   (b) placed under active surveillance for 10 days and voluntary home quarantine recommended;
   (c) visited or telephoned daily by a member of the public healthcare team;
   (d) temperature recorded daily.
- If the contact develops disease symptoms, they should be investigated locally at an appropriate healthcare facility prepared for triage.

Epidemiology

An unusual respiratory illness emerged in southern China in November 2002; the outbreak spread outside China in February 2003 and ended in July 2003. For cases of SARS to reappear, the virus has to re-emerge (from a possible animal source, a laboratory accident or undetected transmission in humans). Since 5 July 2003 the only confirmed SARS-CoV infections resulted from laboratory accidents (Singapore and Taiwan), from exposure to animal sources or environmental contamination (China); none of these cases has been fatal nor resulted in secondary transmission. According to the World Health Organization (WHO), a total of 8098 people (21% healthcare workers) worldwide were notified as having had SARS during the 2003 outbreak. Of these, 774 died. Healthcare workers and close (e.g. household or face-to-face) contacts of cases are at particular risk. The case fatality rate s about 10% and increases with age.

Clinical features

In general, SARS begins with high-grade fever (temperature greater than 38.0°C (100.4°F)). Other symptoms may include headache, chills, rigor, dry cough, malaise and body aches. The symptoms are unspecific. Pulmonary symptoms including dry cough and later breathlessness are the most common primary manifestation during the early phase. Some 20–25% of cases develop severe respiratory failure requiring ICU treatment. About 10–20% of patients have diarrhoea, which is the second most common manifestation. Most patients develop pneumonia and the majority of cases have an abnormal chest radiograph at some stage.

Laboratory confirmation

The most accurate diagnostic tests are reverse transcription polmerase chain reaction (RT-PCR) or real-time PCR of genomic fragments or cultured virus. RT-PCR can be used to make a relatively early diagnosis. A positive RT-PCR test should be repeated by the national reference laboratory using a second, unopened aliquot. Respiratory, serum, stool and urine specimens should be taken for virus isolation and for acute phase serology. Sensitivity can be increased if multiple specimens/multiple body sites are tested. Respiratory samples should include nasopharyngeal aspirates, provided full infection control procedures are in place to protect staff and other patients. Respiratory and stool specimens should be routinely collected for virus isolation or detection of viral genome utilising RT-PCR during the first and second weeks. Serum specimens should also be collected for serology in the second and third weeks to detect a rising titre by testing acute and convalescent sera in parallel.

Clinical samples should be separated into three aliquots at the time of collection. One should be used by the local diagnostic laboratory; the second aliquot, received unopened, should only be used by the national reference laboratory; and the third should be retained for use by the WHO SARS Reference and Verification Laboratory, should verification be necessary.

Transmission

SARS is mainly spread by respiratory droplets, SARS-CoV is also shed in faeces; faecal shedding is more prolonged than respiratory. The number of new cases (R_0) arising from each case of SARS in the absence of interventions is about three, public health interventions can reduce R_0 to below 1 and control the disease. Risk of transmission is greatest during the second week of illness.

Transmission is greatly reduced if the case is isolated within 3 days of onset. Mild cases are less infectious than more severely ill patients. Super spreading events occur but are not understood or predictable. Hospitals act as amplification sites for SARS. Asymptomatic patients are not infectious and cases are no longer infectious 10 days after fever resolution. Children are very rarely affected.

Acquisition

The mean incubation period is 5 days (range 2–10 days), although incubation periods of up to 14 days have been reported. Serial interval is 8.4 days.

Available information suggests that persons with SARS are likely to be infectious only when symptomatic. Patients are most contagious during the second week of illness. Current advice is that recovering patients limit their interactions outside the home for 10 days after they are afebrile and respiratory symptom free.

Prevention

SARS can be controlled by identifying and isolating all cases as early in the illness as possible, rigorous infection control at all stages with monitoring the health of close contacts, so that any infected cases are identified and isolated before they become infectious. This includes the following:
• Isolation and contact tracing to break chains of transmission.
• Care in laboratory handling of specimens (biosafety containment level 3).
• Good hospital infection control.
• WHO recommendations are that patients with probable SARS should be isolated and

accommodated as follows in descending order of preference:

(a) negative pressure rooms with the door closed;

(b) single rooms with their own bathroom facilities; and

(c) cohort placement in an area with an independent air supply and exhaust system. Turning off air conditioning and opening windows for good ventilation is recommended if an independent air supply is unfeasible. Wherever possible, patients under investigation for SARS should be separated from those diagnosed with the syndrome.

Surveillance

• Report urgently to local and national public health authorities.

• National public health authorities should report every laboratory confirmed case of SARS to WHO (see below).

Response to a case

See Suggested on-call action box.

Investigation of a cluster

• Look for a history of travel abroad, contact with a case or recent exposure to a healthcare setting.

• If none of the above explains cases, undertake full hypothesis-generating study.

Control of an outbreak

• Deal with individual case as above.

• Set up dedicated triage area with adequate infection control arrangements. Patients under investigation for SARS should be separated from the probable cases.

• Provide suspected patients with a face mask to wear, preferably one that provides filtration of their expired air.

• Provide triage staff with a face mask, and eye protection.

• Ensure good infection control/handwashing procedures in place.

• Disinfectants, such as fresh bleach solutions, should be widely available in appropriate concentrations.

• Guidance for clinical and laboratory management, and case-definitions available on WHO and Health Protection Agency websites.

Suggested case-definition for an outbreak

Clinical: the following clinical case-definition has been developed for public health purposes.

• A person with a history of fever ($\geq 38°C$); *and*

• One or more symptoms of lower respiratory tract illness (cough, difficulty breathing, shortness of breath); *and*

• Radiographic evidence of lung infiltrates consistent with pneumonia or respiratory distress syndrome (RDS) *or* autopsy findings consistent with the pathology of pneumonia or RDS without an identifiable cause; *and*

• No alternative diagnosis can fully explain the illness; *and*

• In Europe, a history of travel to an area with reported cases or exposure to a case would normally be required for the case-definition.

Laboratory: a person with symptoms and signs that are clinically suggestive of SARS *and* with positive laboratory findings for SARS-CoV based on one or more of the following diagnostic criteria:

• PCR positive for SARS-CoV using a validated method from:

(a) at least two different clinical specimens (e.g. nasopharyngeal and stool); *or*

(b) the same clinical specimen collected on two or more occasions during the course of the illness (e.g. sequential nasopharyngeal aspirates); *or*

(c) two different assays or repeat PCR using a new RNA extract from the original clinical sample on each occasion of testing.

- Seroconversion by ELISA or IFA:
  (a) negative antibody test on acute serum followed by positive antibody test on convalescent phase serum tested in parallel; *or*
  (b) fourfold or greater rise in antibody titre between acute and convalescent phase sera tested in parallel.
- Virus isolation:
  (a) isolation in cell culture of SARS-CoV from any specimen; *and*
  (b) PCR confirmation using a validated method.

3.70 Scabies

Scabies is an inflammatory disease of the skin caused by the mite *Sarcoptes scabiei* var. *hominis*.

Suggested on-call action

Advise on treatment and recommend immediate control measures.

Epidemiology

Scabies is reported to be common, with an estimated 300 million prevalent cases in the world. Although it can affect people of all socio-economic classes, it is particularly prevalent in low income countries where it is associated with overcrowding and poor living conditions. In middle and high income countries, scabies is associated with clusters in hospitals, nursing homes and other similar institutions. It is more prevalent in children and young adults, in urban areas and in winter. Scabies shows a cyclical pattern with a periodicity of 7–30 years. There is anecdotal evidence that in the UK scabies increased in the 1990s in institutional settings, but surveillance by UK GPs indicates that the mean weekly incidence has declined steadily from 9 per 100,000 population in 2000 to 1.7 per 100,000 population in 2009, although this is probably an underestimate.

Clinical features

There may be no sign of infection for 4–6 weeks after exposure, when an allergy develops to mite excretions and an itchy symmetrical rash appears. The time period between exposure and onset of symptoms may be shorter in persons who have been sensitised by prior exposure. The rash comprises small, red papules and is seen anywhere on the body. If the person has had scabies before, the rash may appear within a few days of re-exposure. The itching is intense, particularly at night. Burrows are the only lesions caused directly by the mite and may be seen in the webs of the fingers and on wrists and elbows. In infants, young children, the elderly and the immunocompromised, mites can also infect the face, neck, scalp and ears. Usually, only about 12 mites are present on an affected person at any one time but if there is impaired immunity or altered skin sensation large numbers of mites may be present and the skin is thickened and scaly. This condition is known as atypical, crusted or Norwegian scabies. Scabies is often misdiagnosed, but skin scrapings can be examined under the microscope for mites, eggs or faeces.

Transmission and acquisition

The pregnant female, which is about 0.3 mm long, burrows in the epidermis and lay 2–3 eggs each day before dying after about 3 weeks. The eggs hatch after 2–4 days into larvae which dig burrows and moult twice before developing into adults after 10–14 days. Mating takes place, the male mite dies and the female embeds in a new burrow within 1 hour.

Classic scabies is transmitted via direct skin-to-skin contact so that the risk of transmission is higher amongst family members. In crusted scabies transmission can also occur via skin scales on bedding, clothes and upholstery. It is therefore more infectious. Scabies remains infectious until treated. Animal scabies is called mange or scab. It can be passed to humans but only causes a temporary problem because the mites cannot multiply and soon die out.

Prevention

Prevention of scabies depends on early recognition of cases and prompt effective treatment. This in turn depends on public and professional education and a high level of awareness and diagnostic suspicion.

Surveillance

Scabies is not notifiable; however, clusters of cases of scabies in residential and daycare settings should be reported to the local public health team.

Response to a case

• Topical permethrin should be applied to the whole body, including the scalp, neck, face, ears, between the fingers and toes and under the nails. Earlier guidance only recommended application from the neck down for most healthy adults. A hot bath prior to application should be discouraged as it increases systemic absorption. Ideally, the scabicide should be left on for 24 hours and should be re-applied if the hands are washed during that time. The patient should then have a bath or shower, dress in clean clothes and change bed sheets. A second application after 7 days will kill any larvae that hatch from eggs that survived the first application. Itching may continue for 2–3 weeks after successful treatment and may require treatment with antipruritics.
• All household, close and sexual contacts should receive simultaneous treatment even if symptom free.

• Clothing and bedding should be laundered on a hot washing machine cycle. Any items that cannot be washed in this way should be set aside and not used for 7 days. Under these conditions mites will become dehydrated and die. Normal hygiene and vacuum cleaning of chairs, beds and soft furnishings will minimise environmental contamination with skin scales.
• In crusted scabies, more intensive treatment is necessary, which may be continued for some time. Oral ivermectin (as a single oral dose of 200 μg/kg or two doses 1 week apart) has been shown to be effective in difficult cases and in those with HIV infection. Cases can return to school or work after the first application of scabicide.

Control of an outbreak

• Clusters of cases of scabies may be reported from hospitals, nursing homes or other residential health or social care settings. Confirmation of the diagnosis is important in these settings. All patients and residents may need to be examined in an attempt to identify the index case who is often someone with an unrecognised case of crusted scabies. The GP of the patient, client or service user should be asked to advise. He/she may ask for a second opinion from a consultant dermatologist. A high level of diagnostic suspicion should be maintained. Atypical scabies can spread from patients to nurses and others who provide close care. Use of standard precautions including gloves and aprons will minimise this.
• Outbreaks of scabies in a community setting should be referred to the local public health team (Table 3.70.1).
• The cases, whether members of staff or residents, should be promptly treated (see above).
• Staff can return to work once treatment has been completed.
• If practicable, while affected residents are undergoing treatment they should be separated from other residents.

Table 3.70.1 Responsibilities in control of scabies

LHPT (CCDC and CICN in England)	Receive reports of scabies in community settings
	Advise on management
	Involve district nurses, health visitors, school health nurses, GPs, managers and owners of residential and nursing homes
	Make available information on scabies for the public and professionals
GPs	Maintain a high level of diagnostic suspicion
	Diagnose, treat and follow up cases of scabies amongst their patients and contacts
	Make referrals and request second opinions as appropriate
	Discuss with LHPT whenever an outbreak of scabies is suspected in a residential or nursing home
	Co-operate with the LHPT in dealing with such an outbreak
Residential and nursing home managers, owners and staff	Remain vigilant to the possible diagnosis of scabies
	Involve the GP in diagnosing, treating, referral and follow-up
	Recognise outbreaks and alert the LHPT
	Cooperate with the LHPT in dealing with such an outbreak
Families of those with scabies	Ensure treatment is carried out correctly
	Inform all close contacts, particularly those in a daycare or nursing setting if scabies is suspected
	Follow advice from their GP or the LHPT, particularly relating to treatment and exclusion from work or school

CCDC, Consultant in Communicable Disease Control; CICN, Community Infection Control Nurse; LHPT, local health protection team.

- If the case is a member of staff, treatment is recommended for his/her close household contacts.
- If the case is a resident it may not be practicable to treat everyone else in the residential setting but if there are several cases and the situation appears to be out of control then it may be necessary to treat all residents, staff and their families simultaneously on an agreed treatment date.
- A skin monitoring record form should be used for each person following treatment so that apparent treatment failures and recurrences can be assessed.
- If itching persists for 2–3 weeks after treatment and close monitoring of skin condition shows no improvement then misdiagnosis, treatment failure or re-infection should be suspected. The patient should be re-examined to confirm the diagnosis, further coordinated applications of scabicide correctly applied may be advised and a search should be made for an unrecognised source case of crusted scabies.

Suggested case-definition for an outbreak

A rash of typical appearance and itching, particularly at night. Often with other similar cases reported amongst household and other close contacts.

3.71 Shigella

Shigellae cause intestinal infection including 'bacillary dysentery'. *Shigella sonnei* is the most common species in Western Europe and causes relatively mild illness. Most *Shigella flexneri* and all *Shigella boydii* and *Shigella dysenteriae* are imported and are more severe. *S. dysenteriae* type 1 may cause very severe illness due to production of an exotoxin.

Suggested on-call action

• If case is in a risk group for further transmission, advise exclusion as suggested below (see Response to a case).
• If you or reporting clinician/microbiologist are aware of other linked cases, activate Local Outbreak Plan.
• If infection with *S. dysenteriae*, obtain details of household and ensure symptomatic contacts excluded as suggested below.
• If *S. dysenteriae*, ensure symptomatic contacts receive medical assessment.

Epidemiology

The annual incidence of *Shigella* infection is reported to be about 30 cases per 100,000 population, although only about 2 per 100,000 cases are reported to public health authorities in Europe. The reported rate in Europe has decreased in the last decade. There have recently been about 1200 laboratory-reported cases per year in the UK, of which 62% were *S. sonnei*, 24% *S. flexneri*, 9% *S. boydii* and 4% *S. dysenteriae*. Infection occurs most frequently in late summer and has been reported as peaking 40 days after a peak in ambient temperature.

Shigellosis is primarily a disease of children, with the highest rates reported in those less than 5 years of age followed by those aged 5–14 years. Risk groups for infection include daycare attenders, travellers abroad (particularly for non-*sonnei*) and men who have sex with men. Outbreaks occur mostly in daycare centres and schools, but are also reported from residential institutions, restaurants, camps, religious communities, microbiology laboratories and hospitals.

Clinical diagnosis

The most common symptoms of *S. sonnei* infection are diarrhoea, abdominal pain/cramps and fever. Between 10% and 50% also develop bloody diarrhoea. Nausea and/or vomiting, anorexia, headache or malaise may also occur. Illness lasts from 1 day to 2 weeks (average 4–5 days). Approximately 3% require hospitalisation.

S. flexneri also causes diarrhoea, abdominal pain/cramps and fever, but it is often more severe than *S. sonnei* infection. Dysentery is common, illness can be prolonged and hospitalisation rates may be much higher. Abdominal cramps and fever may precede the onset of diarrhoea. Reactive arthritis and Reiter's syndrome may be a late complication.

S. boydii causes diarrhoeal diseases of varying severity, broadly in line with that produced by *S. flexneri*.

S. dysenteriae type 1 infection is more severe than that from other shigellae. Dysentery occurs in most cases and there is an appreciable death rate. Complications of infection include toxic megacolon, haemolytic uraemic syndrome (HUS), disseminated intravascular coagulation (DIC) and sepsis.

Laboratory confirmation

Diagnostic testing from faecal specimens is routine in most laboratories. Provisional results are usually available within 48 hours. Speciation should always be carried out as control measures vary between species. Serotyping based on 'O' antigens is also available if epidemiologically indicated; for example, any case of *S. dysenteriae* (15 serotypes), possible clusters of *S. boydii* (20 serotypes) or *S. flexneri* (six serotypes, and two variants (e.g. 'type 2a')). *S. sonnei* is antigenically homogeneous, but phage typing or colicin typing may be available from reference laboratories.

Transmission

Humans are the only significant reservoir of infection. Transmission to other humans is via the faeco-oral route either directly or by contamination of food, water or the environment.

Direct person-to-person spread is extremely common in households and institutions, particularly those with young children: 30–50% of household or nursery contacts became infected. Cases with diarrhoea are a much greater risk than asymptomatic excretors, with inadequate handwashing after defaecation the main cause. Such individuals may also contaminate food. Young children may act as a transmission link between households.

Shigellae, particularly S. sonnei, may also survive for up to 20 days in favourable environmental conditions (i.e. cool, damp and dark). This may lead to transmission via lavatory seats, towels and any other vehicle that could become contaminated by faeces, either directly or via unclean hands. Flies may also transfer the organism from faeces to food.

Food and water-borne outbreaks are relatively uncommon but do occur. Food-borne outbreaks are often caused by an infected food handler and salad items are the most common vehicles of infection. Water-borne infection can be via drinking water or recreational water.

Acquisition

The incubation period is between 12 hours and 4 days (usually 1–3 days; median 2 days), but may be up to 1 week for S. dysenteriae type 1. The infectious period is primarily during the diarrhoeal illness: however, cases maintain a low level of infectivity for as long as the organism is excreted in the stool, which is 2–4 weeks on average (although prolonged excretion is documented). The infective dose is very low: the mean infectious dose is about 1000 organisms, but infection may follow ingestion of as few as 10 organisms of S. dysenteriae type 1. Immunity post-infection does occur and lasts for several years, at least for the same serotype. Longer term immunity does not appear to be important.

Prevention

- Adequate personal hygiene, particularly handwashing after defaecation.
- Adequate toilet facilities in nurseries and schools. Supervised handwashing in nursery and infant schools. Regular and frequent cleaning of nurseries and schools, particularly for toilet areas.
- Safe disposal of faeces and treatment of drinking and swimming water.
- Care with food and water for travellers to developing countries.
- Routine cooking kills shigellae.

Surveillance

All clinical cases of dysentery should be reported to public health authorities and Shigella infection is statutorily notifiable in most EU countries.

Response to a case

- Hygiene advice to case and contacts.
- Enteric precautions for case and symptomatic contacts. In institutions, isolate if possible.
- If case or symptomatic contact, exclude from work or school until well.
- For higher risk groups (see Box 2.2.1) with S. sonnei, exclude until 48 hours after first normal stool and hygiene advice given.
- For higher risk groups (see Box 2.2.1) with non-sonnei shigellae, exclude until two consecutive negative faecal specimens taken at least 24 hours apart. This policy may also be adopted for children over 5 years with S. dysenteriae.
- Contacts of cases with non-sonnei shigellae should be screened microbiologically if in a higher risk group. If positive or symptomatic, treat as case.
- Obtain details of any nursery or infant school attended. Check to see if other cases and reinforce hygiene measures. Check that adequate toilet facilities and supervision are available.

• For species other than *S. sonnei*, check if case has been abroad in the 4 days before onset (7 days for *S. dysenteriae* type 1) or has been in contact with another case who was ill abroad or on return. If no link abroad, obtain details of contacts and full food history for 4 days before onset (7 days for *S. dysenteriae*).

• Mild cases will recover without antibiotics. Where needed, quinolones, ceftriaxone, azithromycin, cefixime and co-trimoxazole have all been shown to be effective, but antibiotic resistance is increasing. Antimotility drugs are usually to be avoided.

Investigation of a cluster

• Liaise with microbiologist to organise typing of isolates (may be more than one type in an outbreak).

• Does epidemic curve suggest point source (plus secondary cases) or continuing exposure?

• Does age/sex/ethnic/geographical analysis of cases suggest common factor?

• Look for links via institutions such as nurseries, schools, social clubs, care facilities and links between affected families via child networks. Administer hypothesis-generating food questionnaire for 4 days before onset. Ask about water consumption, hobbies, swimming, social functions and occupation. For non-*sonnei* species, look for social networks that include travellers to developing countries.

Control of an outbreak

• For outbreaks in institutions, public health staff should satisfy themselves of the adequacy of hygiene and toilet facility arrangements. Handwashing by children should be supervised in nurseries and primary schools. Intensive and frequent cleaning and adequate disinfection, especially of 'touch points' is required.

• Exclusion of cases as above, with hygiene advice to families to limit spread within the household, is recommended.

• Further measures in outbreaks need to be appropriate to the situation. Exclusion of all cases of shigellosis until microbiologically negative is one option. Antibiotic treatment of cases can be undertaken, either as an adjunct or an alternative. Cohorting of convalescent cases can be considered instead of exclusion in prolonged outbreaks, if facilities and staffing are adequate to effectively implement this, although the effectiveness of this policy is not proven. Closure of the institution may even be necessary.

Suggested case-definition for an outbreak

Confirmed: diarrhoea *or* abdominal pain with fever with *Shigella* species of outbreak strain identified in faeces.

Clinical: diarrhoea *or* abdominal pain with fever in member of population of affected institution, without alternative explanation.

3.72 Smallpox

Smallpox is an acute contagious disease caused by the variola virus, a DNA virus member of the orthopox genus. Naturally occurring infection has been eradicated worldwide, so its public health importance now lies in the potential of a deliberate release in a bioterrorist attack and the consequent need to re-consider vaccination and other control strategies.

Suggested on-call action

If diagnosis is likely, isolate at the point of contact and notify national surveillance unit urgently. Refer to Response to a case section below.

Epidemiology

The World Health Organization confirmed the global eradication of smallpox in 1980. There are concerns that the virus may exist outside the two official WHO designated laboratories.

Clinical features

There are two clinical forms of the disease: variola major (severe) and variola minor (mild). In variola major there is typically a rapid onset of flu-like symptoms – fever, headache, malaise and aching head and back. The distinctive vesicular rash then appears over the next 1–2 days, eventually covering the whole body. Vesicles are most concentrated peripherally – on the face, arms and leg, also the mouth and throat (unlike chickenpox, which is most common on the trunk). The vesicles develop into pustules over the next week; these crust and fall off over the next 3 – 4 weeks, leaving permanent pitted scars. The case fatality rate in a non-immune person is 30%. There is no specific effective treatment, although vaccination early in the incubation period can modify the course of the disease and reduce mortality. In malignant smallpox, the most severe form, the rash is haemorrhagic and the case fatality rate is over 90%. Variola minor has a much less severe course and most patients recover.

Smallpox may be confused with chickenpox: diagnostic clues are given in Table 3.72.1. Other differential diagnoses include disseminated herpes simplex infection, and (rarely) cowpox and monkeypox.

Laboratory confirmation

This is by electron microscopy (EM) identification of orthopox virus from vesicular fluid, scrapings from the base of lesions, scabs or vesicle crusts. This must be confirmed by polymerase chain reaction (PCR) and viral isolation from culture. Confirmation can only be carried out in a specialised containment level 4 laboratory. Varicella and herpes simplex viruses are easily distinguished from parvovirus on EM. Parapox particles (e.g. from orf) should also be distinguishable from orthopox viruses (such as smallpox). If an orthopox virus is found on routine EM, a clinical history will be required.

Transmission

There is no known animal reservoir or vector. The virus spreads from person to person by droplet nuclei or aerosols expelled from the orophayrynx of an infectious case. Close contact (e.g. household, hospital ward) is

Table 3.72.1 Distinguishing smallpox from chickenpox in a well, non-immune person

	Smallpox	Chickenpox
Overall illness	Almost always severe	Usually mild
Initial signs	Headache, back pain	Mild malaise
First spots	Forehead, face, scalp, neck, hands and wrist	Trunk
'Cropping'	Pocks in one area (e.g. face) appear all at once	Generalised
Limb distribution of spots	More on hands and wrists than upper arms; similarly more on feet and ankles than the thighs	More on upper arms than hands and wrists, more on thighs than feet and ankles
Hands and feet	Circular flattened grey vesicles are characteristic	Such vesicles never seen in chickenpox
Itchiness	Not in first few days of rash	Common in the first few days of the rash and then continuing

normally required; however, air-borne transmission via drafts and air conditioning can occur, also from contaminated clothing and bedding. Under normal conditions, the virus is unlikely to survive more than 48 hours in the environment, although prolonged survival is possible in dry scabs.

Acquisition

The incubation period is usually 10–14 days (range 7–19 days). Patients are infectious from the onset of fever until the last scabs fall off. Immunity following natural infection is lifelong. Past vaccination offers some degree of protection.

Prevention

• Smallpox vaccine is a live vaccine produced from vaccinia virus. It is delivered by multiple skin puncture with a bifurcated needle; a 'take' is successful when a pustule develops, which progressively crusts. Serious vaccine complications occasionally occur (encephalitis, eczema vaccinatum). Re-vaccination is recommended after 3 years for those at continuing risk; after re-vaccination, protection lasts for about 10 years.
• Vaccination should be considered for laboratory workers working with closely related viruses and for frontline workers who might have to care for cases in the event of a deliberate release.

Surveillance

• Any suspected case must be reported immediately to the national surveillance unit.
• Notifiable throughout the EU.
• All suspected cases must be reported to WHO; a number are investigated every year and usually turn out to be another poxvirus infection such as monkeypox.

Response to a case

• Isolate any probable or confirmed case at point of diagnosis, pending transfer to a high-security unit with negative-pressure isolation. Patients should be isolated until all crusts have fallen off.
• Confirm the diagnosis (with appropriate precautions).
• Decontaminate all waste before disposal by autoclaving.
• Vaccination of contacts in the first 4 days of the incubation period reduces mortality by 50%. Antiviral drugs may also be considered.
• Any confirmed case should be assumed to be a deliberate release.

Investigation and management of a cluster

Assume deliberate release and implement control plan (see below). Many health and emergency planning agencies would be involved with central government coordination.

Response to an overt deliberate release

• Define exposed zone and identify exposed people.
• Decontaminate exposed people: remove clothing, shower and wash hair.
• Vaccinate all those exposed.
• Trace those who have left the scene for decontamination and vaccination.
• Isolate exposed zone to allow natural decontamination: formal decontamination is unnecessary.
• Full biological protective equipment for those who enter exposed zone.
• Vaccination of frontline workers.

Suggested case-definition for an outbreak

Clinical: acute onset of fever >38°C, which is persistent, followed by a vesicular or pustular rash with lesions all at the same stage of development without obvious cause and with a centrifugal distribution

Confirmed: identification of orthopox particles by EM and PCR; in an outbreak EM alone is adequate for cases with epidemiological links with others.

3.73 Staphylococcal food poisoning

Staphylococcal food poisoning (SFP) is an uncommon food-borne disease caused by heat-stable enterotoxins produced when certain strains of *Staphylococcus aureus* multiply in food.

Suggested on-call action

If you or the reporting clinician/microbiologist know of associated cases, consult outbreak control plan.

Epidemiology

SFP occurs throughout the world but is now rarely reported in Western Europe and the UK. In England and Wales, there were 38 outbreaks of SFP between 1992 and 2009; however, many people with SFP do not seek medical attention.

Clinical features

There is sudden onset of nausea, cramps, vomiting, diarrhoea, hypotension and prostration. The illness lasts 1–2 days; serious sequelae are uncommon, but admission to hospital may occur because of the intensity of symptoms.

Laboratory confirmation

Gram-positive cocci may be seen on Gram staining of food vehicles. *S. aureus* may be cultured from unheated food at levels of 10^5–10^6

organisms per gram or from the vomit or faeces of cases. Enterotoxin may be detected in food samples. The same strain of *S. aureus* may be found in the implicated food vehicle and on the skin or lesions of food handlers.

Transmission

Food handlers colonised with *S. aureus* or with infected skin lesions contaminate foods such as cooked meats, sandwiches and pastries. These are stored with inadequate refrigeration, allowing the organism to multiply and produce toxin before being eaten. Two hours at room temperature may be long enough to produce a significant amount of toxin. Even with further cooking or heating the toxin may not be destroyed. Outbreaks have followed contamination of dairy products as a result of staphylococcal mastitis in cattle.

Acquisition

The incubation period of SFP is 0.5–8 hours (usually 2–4 hours) but it is not communicable from person to person.

Prevention

SFP can be prevented by:
• Strict food hygiene including kitchen cleaning and handwashing.
• Minimising food handling.
• Safe food storage in particular temperature control above 60°C or below 10°C.
• Excluding food handlers with purulent lesions. Nasal carriers do not need to be excluded.

Surveillance

Cases and outbreaks should be reported to local public health departments (food poisoning is formally notifiable in UK). Outbreaks should be reported to national surveillance centres.

Response to a case

• Enquire about food consumed in the 24 hours before onset of symptoms.
• Exclude risk groups (see Box 2.2.1) with diarrhoea or vomiting.

Investigation of a cluster

• Discuss further microbiological investigation (e.g. genotyping) with microbiologist.
• Undertake hypothesis-generating study covering food histories particularly restaurants, social functions and other mass catering arrangements.
• Investigate the origin and preparation methods of any food items implicated in the outbreak. Submit any leftover food for laboratory analysis.
• Search for food handlers with purulent lesions.

Control of an outbreak

• Identify and rectify faults with temperature control in food preparation processes.
• Exclude any implicated food handler.

Suggested case-definition for an outbreak

Vomiting occurring 1–7 hours after exposure to potential source with appropriate laboratory confirmation.

3.74 Streptococcal infections

Streptococci are part of the normal flora and colonise the respiratory, gastrointestinal and genitourinary tracts. Several species cause disease, including the following:
• Group A streptococci (beta-haemolytic streptococci, *Streptococcus pyogenes*) cause sore throat and skin infection (impetigo, cellulitis,

pyoderma), scarlet fever, necrotising fasciitis, streptococcal toxic shock syndrome, wound infections, pneumonia and puerperal fever.
• Group A organisms may also cause post-infectious syndromes, such as rheumatic fever, glomerulonephritis; and Sydenham's chorea.
• Group B streptococci (GBS) cause neonatal meningitis and septicaemia.
• Group C and G streptococci can cause upper respiratory infections such as tonsillitis.
• Viridans streptococci are a common cause of bacterial endocarditis.

Suggested on-call action

Not usually necessary unless outbreak is suspected.

Epidemiology

Streptococcal sore throat and scarlet fever are found worldwide, although less commonly in the tropics. Up to 20% of individuals may have asymptomatic pharyngeal colonisation with group A streptococci. Particular 'M types' are associated with various sequelae (e.g. 1, 3, 4, 12 with glomerulonephritis). The incidence of sequelae depends upon the circulating M types. Acute rheumatic fever has become rare in most developed countries, although occasional cases and outbreaks are seen. It is associated with poor living conditions and is most common in those aged 3–15 years.

Impetigo is most commonly seen in younger children. The M types associated with nephritis following skin infection are different from those associated with nephritis following upper respiratory infection.

Asymptomatic carriage of GBS is common in pregnant women.

Clinical features

• *Sore throat*: it can be difficult to differentiate streptococcal from viral sore throat; various scoring systems have been proposed but they lack predictive power.

- *Skin infection*: streptococcal skin infection commonly presents as acute cellulitis or impetigo.
- *Scarlet fever*: this may accompany pharyngeal or skin infection and is characterised by a skin rash, classically a fine punctate erythema, sparing the face, but with facial flushing and circumoral pallor. During convalescence, desquamation of the finger and toe tips may occur.
- *Puerperal infection*: puerperal fever occurs in the postpartum or post-abortion patient and is usually accompanied by signs of septicaemia.
- *Necrotizing fasciitis*: this involves the superficial and/or deep fascia; group A streptococci are implicated in about 60% of cases.

Laboratory confirmation

Streptococci are classified by a number of systems including haemolytic type, Lancefield group and species name.

Group A streptococcal antigen can be identified in pharyngeal secretions using rapid antigen detection; negative tests require confirmation. Detection of antibody to streptococcal extracellular toxins may be useful in the diagnosis of necrotising fasciitis.

Confirmation is by culture on blood agar, the production of a zone of haemolysis and showing inhibition with bacitracin.

A rise in antistreptolysin O, anti-DNAase or antihyaluronidase antibodies between acute and convalescent sera may be helpful in retrospective diagnosis.

Transmission

Streptococcal infection is commonly acquired by contact with patients or carriers, particularly nasal carriers. Transmission via contaminated foodstuffs, particularly unpasteurised milk and milk products is recognised.

Group B disease is acquired by the newborn as (s)he passes through the genital tract of the mother.

Acquisition

Group A streptococcal pharyngitis

The incubation period is 1–5 days for acute infection (mean 2 days). The mean time for appearance of immunological sequelae is 10 days for acute glomerulonephritis; 19 days (1–5 weeks) for acute rheumatic fever; and several months for Sydenham's chorea. The infectious period is commonly 2–3 weeks for untreated sore throat. Purulent discharges are infectious. Penicillin treatment usually terminates transmissibility within 48 hours.

Group B infection in infants

Early-onset infection occurs at a mean age of 20 hours. Late-onset infection occurs in infants with a mean age of 3–4 weeks, range 1 week to 3 months.

Immunity develops to specific M types and appears to be long-lasting. Repeated episodes due to other M types occur.

Prevention

Primary

- Personal hygiene.
- Avoid unpasteurised milk.
- Reduce need for illegal abortions.

Secondary

- Prevention of immune-mediated sequelae.
- Prompt recognition, confirmation and treatment of streptococcal infection.
- Those with a history of rheumatic fever should be offered antibiotic prophylaxis to prevent cumulative heart valve damage. Prophylaxis should be for at least 10 years; for patients with established heart disease it should be at least until 40 years of age.

Prevention of group B streptococcal infection

- Intrapartum antibiotic treatment of women colonised with GBS appears to reduce neonatal infection and should be considered particularly if risk factors are present (prematurity, prolonged rupture of membranes, previous baby with neonatal GBS disease). The drug of choice is intravenous penicillin G; intravenous clindamycin is an alternative for those allergic to penicillin.

• Routine screening to detect maternal colonisation is recommended in some countries (USA, Australia), but not in Europe at the present time.

Surveillance

Scarlet fever and/or puerperal fever are notifiable in some EU countries.

Response to a case

• Report acute cases of scarlet fever, puerperal fever and post-streptococcal syndromes to local health authorities.

• Careful handling of secretions and drainage fluids until after 24 hours of penicillin treatment.

• Personal hygiene advice to case and contacts.

• Consider school/nursery exclusion until 48 hours after start of antibiotic treatment.

• Antibiotic chemoprophylaxis is not routinely indicated for close contacts of a case of group A disease. Only administer antibiotics to mother and baby if either develops invasive disease in the neonatal period or to close contacts if they develop symptoms of localised group A disease. Oral penicillin V is the first line drug; azithromycin is a suitable alternative for those allergic to penicillin.

Investigation of a cluster

• Does epidemic curve suggest point source, ongoing transmission (or both) or continuing source?

• Determine mode of transmission, exclude food-borne source, and particularly milk, urgently.

• Search for and treat carriers if considered a potential source of infection.

Control of an outbreak

• Activate outbreak plan.
• Identify and treat carriers.
• Antibiotic chemoprophylaxis for household contacts of invasive group A disease is indicated when there are two or more cases within 30 days, or as a control measure in a community cluster or outbreak.
• Identify and remove contaminated food sources.

3.75 Tetanus

Tetanus is an acute illness caused by the toxin of the tetanus bacillus, *Clostridium tetani*. Its public health significance is the severity of the disease and its preventability by vaccination.

Suggested on-call action
None required for the public health team.

Epidemiology

Tetanus is rare in Europe, although there is probably significant under ascertainment of mild cases. In 2008 there were 103 confirmed cases of which 53 were reported in Italy. Most cases are in unvaccinated people over 65 years of age, although there has been a recent outbreak in young adult injecting drug users (IDU). The case fatality is about 10%.

Clinical features

In classic tetanus there are painful muscular contractions, especially of the neck and jaw muscles (hence the name 'lockjaw'), muscular rigidity and painful spasms. The symptoms can be mild in a vaccinated person. There is often a history of a tetanus-prone wound, although not always.

Laboratory confirmation

This is infrequently obtained and unnecessary in typical cases. It is sometimes possible to culture the organism from the site of the original wound.

Transmission

The reservoir is the intestine of horses and other animals, including humans. Tetanus spores are found in soil contaminated with animal faeces. Transmission occurs when spores are introduced into the body through a dirty wound, through IDU, and occasionally during abdominal surgery. The illness is caused by a toxin. Person-to-person spread does not occur.

Acquisition

The incubation period is 3–21 days, depending on the site of the wound and the extent of contamination; occasionally it may be up to several months. Natural immunity may not follow an attack of tetanus.

Prevention

• Vaccination with tetanus toxoid. Three doses in infancy with two additional boosters (timing varies between different countries in Europe). Further boosters may be required at the time of injury. In a fully vaccinated individual, routine boosters are not justified, other than at the time of injury.
• Give tetanus vaccine (and tetanus immunoglobulin for tetanus-prone wounds) at the time of injury where more than 10 years have elapsed since the last dose of vaccine. The dose of tetanus immunoglobulin is 250 IU by intramuscular injection; 500 IU if more than 24 hours have elapsed since the time of injury.
• Promote safe techniques in IDU (see Chapter 2.12)

Surveillance

Notifiable in most European countries.

Response to case

Seek injury history, ascertain vaccination status and arrange for primary course or booster, depending on history.

Response to a cluster or outbreak

Outbreaks of tetanus are rare. Look for a common source (e.g. surgery, IDU). IDU outbreak – liaise with drug services to promote safer drug use and with clinicians to promote early diagnosis and treatment.

Suggested case-definition for an outbreak
Physician's diagnosis of tetanus.

3.76 Threadworms

Suggested on-call action
None.

Epidemiology

Threadworm (pinworm) infection is an intestinal infection with *Enterobius vermicularis,* a nematode of the family Oxyuridae. It is widespread in temperate regions, particularly amongst children. Clusters of cases may occur in household and residential settings. In England in 2009, GPs reported a mean weekly incidence of threadworm infection of 2 per 100,000 population, similar to previous years but undoubtedly this underestimates the true incidence.

Clinical features

In symptomatic infections there is perianal itching and sleep disturbance. Appendicitis and chronic salpingitis are rare complications of worm migration. The diagnosis can be confirmed by the presence of eggs on a strip of transparent adhesive tape that has been pressed on to the anal region and then examined under a microscope. Adult worms may be seen in faeces or on perianal skin. Adult worms live in the caecum. Female worms are 8–12 mm in length.

Transmission and acquisition

Mature female worms migrate through the anus and lay thousands of eggs on the perianal skin. Infective embryos develop within 5–6 hours and these are transferred to the mouth on fingers as a result of scratching. Larvae emerge from the eggs in the small intestine and develop into sexually mature worms. Re-infection is common and infectious eggs are also spread to others directly on fingers or indirectly on bedding, clothing and in environmental dust. Eggs can survive in moist conditions for up to 3 weeks. Adult worms do not live for longer than 6 weeks. Retro-infection may occur as a result of hatched larvae migrating back through the anus from the perianal region.

Prevention

Control is by prompt recognition and treatment of cases and their household contacts, health education and attention to personal and environmental hygiene, particularly handwashing. The perianal area may be washed each morning to remove eggs and bedding and nightclothes should be changed regularly. Exclusion from school is unnecessary.

Response to a case, cluster and outbreak

- Anti-helminthics such as mebendazole or piperazine are effective against adult worms but must be combined with hygienic measures to break the cycle of auto-infection.
- All household members should be treated.

- An initial course of treatment should be followed by a second course 2 weeks later to kill worms that have matured in the intervening time period.

3.77 Tick-borne encephalitis

Tick-borne encephalitis is a flavivirus infection of the central nervous system (CNS), characterised by a biphasic meningo-encephalitis.

Epidemiology

It has a focal distribution throughout forested areas of countries in Central and Eastern Europe and parts of Scandinavia. The annual incidence ranges from <1 to >20 per 100,000. Related infections occur in Russia (but more severe), and North America. The disease is most common in early summer and autumn. Cases have not been reported in the UK, although louping ill, a related infection, occurs occasionally in Scotland and Ireland.

Clinical features

Diagnosis should be considered in a patient with neurological symptoms with a history of a tick bite in an endemic area.

Laboratory confirmation

Laboratory confirmation is by serology or virus isolation from blood (only in a specialist laboratory). Other tick-borne flaviviruses including louping ill, langat virus and Powassan virus produce a similar encephalitis.

Transmission

Ixodes ricinus, the woodland tick, is the principal reservoir in Central and Northern Europe; in Eastern Europe and Russia it is *Ixodes persulcatus*. Sheep and deer are also hosts for louping ill.

Acquisition

The incubation period is 7–14 days (range 2–28 days). Person-to-person transmission does not occur.

Prevention

• Wear protective clothing against tick bites in endemic areas.
• Use insect repellent (e.g. DEET-containing).
• Inspect skin frequently and remove any attached ticks.
• Killed vaccines are available and are recommended for at-risk travellers and residents, particularly those in occupations such as forestry and farming.

Response to a case

Post-exposure prophylaxis with a specific immunoglobulin is available in some countries.

3.78 *Toxocara*

Toxocara canis is an ascarid parasite of dogs which occasionally infects humans.

Suggested on-call action
None required.

Epidemiology

Infection is found worldwide and is more common in young children.

Clinical features

Infection may be asymptomatic. Covert toxocariasis is the most common presentation with abdominal pain, cough and headache.

Visceral larva migrans occurs in association with pica, and features fever, abdominal pain, eosinophilia and bronchospasm and an urticarial rash. Ocular larva migrans features disturbed vision and irritation of the eyes.

Laboratory confirmation

Diagnosis is based on detecting antibodies to *T. canis* larvae using an ELISA test.

Transmission

The larvae can remain dormant in dogs for long periods, migrate transplacentally and through bitches' milk to infect the pups. Most pups are infected at the time of whelping; the adult worms produce eggs until the majority are expelled when the pups are 6 months old. The eggs, which are the source of human infection, survive in the environment for many years.

Prevention

• Regular worming of dogs.
• Hygienic disposal of dog faeces.

Response to a case

No public health response is usually needed in response to cases.

3.79 Toxoplasmosis

Toxoplasma gondii is a protozoan parasite that causes a spectrum of disease from asymptomatic lymphadenopathy to congenital mental retardation, chorioretinitis and encephalitis in the immunocompromised.

Suggested on-call action
None required unless outbreak suspected.

Epidemiology

Human exposure to toxoplasmosis is worldwide and common. Rates vary widely between countries; seropositivity of adults is about 80% in France, 20% in the UK, 10% in the USA and 5% in South Korea.

Clinical features

There are a number of clinical presentations. Infection is usually asymptomatic, but may produce a mononucleosis-like illness. Congenital infection may follow acute infection during pregnancy and is characterised by fetal hepatosplenomegaly, chorioretinitis and mental retardation. Immunocompromise may result in cerebral reactivation of toxoplasmosis, with presentation as an encephalitis.

Laboratory confirmation

Acute toxoplasmosis may be diagnosed serologically. Specific IgM antibodies appear during the first 2 weeks, peak within 4–8 weeks, and then typically become undetectable within several months. IgG antibodies rise more slowly, peak in 1–2 months, and may remain high for years.

Congenital infection requires the demonstration of IgM in neonatal blood; evidence of acute infection during pregnancy indicates the need for fetal blood sampling at 18 weeks and cord blood at delivery.

Serology is not useful for diagnosis of toxoplasmosis in patients with AIDS. Cerebral toxoplasmosis is usually diagnosed on the basis of clinical features, a positive agglutination test and computed tomography/magnetic resonance imaging (CT/MRI) scan appearance. Polymerase chain reaction (PCR) on fluid or tissue may be helpful in cerebral, ocular and congenital disease.

Transmission

Infected rats and mice are less fearful of cats and therefore more likely to be caught. The cat is the definitive host and oocysts are shed in cat faeces. Hand-to-mouth transmission occurs through contact with oocysts from pets, soil or sandpits; oocysts can survive in the environment for over a year. Alternatively, infection is through contact with, or ingestion of undercooked infected meat. Congenital infection usually occurs following primary infection in a pregnant woman, it occurs in about 3 per 100,000 births.

Acquisition

• Incubation period: 10–25 days.
• Transmissibility: no   person-to-person spread.

Prevention

• Pregnant women in particular should avoid raw or undercooked meat. Contact with soil or food possibly contaminated with cat faeces should be avoided.
• Chemoprophylaxis has been recommended for AIDS patients with positive IgG serology once CD4 cells are low.
• Protect sandpits and play areas from cats.

Surveillance

Report to local public health authorities. Some countries have surveillance of congenital cases.

Response to a case

Investigate likely exposure to cat faeces and raw or undercooked meat.

Investigation of a cluster and control of an outbreak

As for response to a case.

Suggested case-definition for an outbreak

Confirmed: isolate or IgM antibody confirmed.

Clinical: acute fever and lymphadenopathy in a person linked epidemiologically to a confirmed case.

3.80 Tuberculosis

Tuberculosis (TB) is an infection of the lungs and/or other organs, usually by *Mycobacterium tuberculosis*, but occasionally by other species such as *Mycobacterium bovis* or *Mycobacterium africanum*. TB has a long incubation period, produces chronic infection with risk of reactivation and, without treatment, is often fatal.

Suggested on-call action

If the case is a healthcare worker, teacher or other person in contact with particularly susceptible individuals, consult the Outbreak Control Plan. However, action can usually wait until the next working day.

Table 3.80.1 Estimated TB rate in European countries, 2008

Country	Rate per 100,000
Iceland	2
Switzerland	5
Germany	5
Cyprus	6
Sweden	6
Norway	6
France	6
Greece	6
Italy	7
Netherlands	7
Finland	7
Denmark	7
Luxembourg	9
Czech Republic	9
Ireland	9
Belgium	9
Austria	11
UK	12
Slovenia	12
Slovakia	12
Malta	14
Hungary	16
Spain	17
Poland	25
Portugal	30
Estonia	34
Bulgaria	43
Latvia	50
Lithuania	71
Romania	130

Source: WHO.

Epidemiology

TB incidence rates vary significantly across the EU (Table 3.80.1). The incidence has generally fallen consistently in Western Europe over the last 100 years. However, some countries (e.g. the UK) have seen a rise during the last 10–30 years, linked to increased immigration from higher prevalence countries. Rates are substantially higher in South Asia and are extremely high in much of sub-Saharan Africa. High rates of drug-resistant TB are reported from countries of the former Soviet Union.

Marked ethnic differences are apparent. In the UK, about 80% of cases are now in non-white groups, with rates highest in black Africans and South Asians. Rates are higher in those born abroad, with a median time from entry (to the UK) to development of disease of 4 years (inter-quartile range (IQR) 1–13 years). Rates, at least in whites, are higher in deprived communities. Other risk factors for TB include HIV infection, other causes of immunosuppression, chronic alcohol misuse and socially marginalised groups such as the homeless, refugees, drug users and prisoners. Exposure to infectious TB cases in institutions such as hospitals, schools and prisons are regular public health incidents.

Reported levels of HIV co-infection in European countries are in the range from 0–15% (UK 7%) and multidrug-resistant TB levels range from 0–21% (UK 1.2%), with an average of 7% of the being extensively resistant cases. The overall TB mortality rate (in the UK) is around 0.6 per 100,000 population per year.

Clinical features

TB is a biphasic disease. Only about 5% of whose who have primary infection develop clinically apparent primary disease, either from local progression in the lungs or haematogenous or lymphatic spread to other sites. Such spread may lead to serious forms of the disease such as meningitis or milary TB occurring within a few months of the initial infection.

In the remaining 95%, the primary TB lesion heals without intervention, although in at least half of patients, bacilli survive in a latent form which may then reactivate in later life. Five per cent of those originally infected will develop post-primary disease. The risk of reactivation increases with advanced age, chronic disease and immunosuppression (e.g. AIDS). Reactivated TB is often pulmonary and, without treatment, carries a high mortality. The risk of reactivation is lifelong, but half of cases occur within 5 years of the original infection.

Two-thirds of TB in the UK is pulmonary disease, which is initially asymptomatic, although it may be detected on chest X-ray. Early symptoms may be constitutional, such as fatigue, fever, night sweats and weight loss, and often insidious in onset. Chest symptoms often occur in later disease, including cough (usually productive), haemoptysis and chest pain. Hoarseness and difficulty swallowing may occur in laryngeal TB. Symptomatic screening for cases is highly sensitive (most cases have symptoms on enquiry) but not very specific (many other diseases also cause similar symptoms). Chest X-ray has high sensitivity and medium specificity. Specificity is high for sputum smear and very high for sputum culture, but both are of only moderate sensitivity.

Non-pulmonary TB is more common in children, ethnic minorities and those with impaired immunity. The most commonly affected sites are lymph nodes, pleura, genitourinary system, and bones and joints. Constitutional or local systems may be reported. Diagnosis may be supported by tuberculin test (Table 3.80.2) and biopsy results: over 90% of non-AIDS cases are tuberculin test positive. Interferon-gamma release assays (IGRA), which use whole blood to measure T-cell interferon-gamma release in response to TB antigens, have become available and are now widely used in a variety of circumstances including diagnosis of latent TB infection, managing contacts following exposure to

Table 3.80.2 Typical action in response to tuberculin testing

Test result		Interpretation and action	
Heaf grade	Mantoux* (100 units/mL)	Scar from previous BCG	No BCG scar
0/1	0–5 mm	Negative No action[†]	Negative Give BCG[†]
2	6–14 mm	Positive No action[‡]	Positive Investigate?[‡]
3/4	15 mm plus	Strongly positive Investigate	Strongly positive Investigate

* Source: Joint Committee on Vaccination and Immunisation, 2010.
[†] Unless contact of case (may need repeat test).
[‡] Will vary with reason for test, size of reaction and patient circumstances.

infectious TB, diagnosing extrapulmonary TB before starting immunosuppressive treatment and screening of migrants and healthcare workers. IGRA offer advantages over tuberculin testing, particularly in vaccinated populations or in areas with high exposure to environmental mycobacteria.

Laboratory confirmation

Rapid presumptive diagnosis of infectious cases can be achieved by microscopy of sputum (preferably early morning) samples: *M. tuberculosis, M. bovis* and *M. africanum* all stain poorly with Gram stain, but staining with Ziehl–Neelson stain reveals acid-fast (and alcohol-fast) bacilli (AFB). In most laboratories, mycobacteria are detected by auramine fluorescent staining, and the results are available within one working day. As a general rule, sufficient bacilli in the sputum to be detectable by standard methods equates to sufficient to be infectious and three consecutive negative sputum smears is usually assumed to represent non-infectiousness. Although this test is usually sufficient to begin treatment and contact tracing, follow-up culture (preferably liquid culture) is essential as AFBs may occasionally be other species of mycobacteria (Box 3.80.1), culture also increases the sensitivity of diagnosis for cases of lower infectivity and allows antibiotic sensitivities to be checked.

Specimens should be cultured using rapid automated liquid culture and by conventional solid culture. *M. tuberculosis* is usually detected and identified within 7–21 days depending upon biomass. Laboratories may also offer molecular amplification tests such as polymerase chain reaction (PCR) which are less sensitive but faster than culture. Positive samples or isolates should be submitted to a reference laboratory where identification normally includes DNA analysis. Drug sensitivity testing should be performed and results are usually available in 14 days.

Genotyping is useful in identifying and investigating clusters of cases. Prospective typing of all isolates of *M. tuberculosis* complex is carried out in some reference laboratories.

Transmission

Almost all TB in Europe is contracted by inhalation of *M. tuberculosis* bacilli in droplet nuclei. These nuclei derive from humans with pulmonary or laryngeal TB, predominantly by coughing, although sneezing, singing and prolonged talking may contribute. Such nuclei may remain suspended in air for long periods. The risk of transmission depends upon the amount of bacilli in the sputum, the nature of the cough, the closeness and duration of the interaction and the susceptibility of the contact (Box 3.80.2). Without treatment, an average case of pulmonary TB would infect 10–15 people per year.

Bovine TB may be contracted by ingestion of raw milk from infected cows and occasionally via the air-borne route. Although

---

Box 3.80.1 Mycobacteria other than tuberculosis (MOTT)

• Also known as atypical, environmental, anonymous, non-tuberculous, tuberculoid or opportunistic.

• Includes *M. avium, M. intracellulare* and *M. scrofulaceum* (collectively known as *M. avium* complex). Also includes *M. kansasii, M. malmoense, M. marinum, M. xenopi, M. fortuitum, M. chelonae, M. abscessus, M. haemophilium, M. marinum, M. paratuberculosis, M. simiae* and *M. ulcerans.*

• Common environmental contaminants. Occasionally found in water supplies, swimming pools or milk. Some cause nosocomial infections. Person-to-person spread is rare.

• Rarely causes disease in immunocompetent individuals. *M. avium* complex and some others may cause disseminated disease in those with AIDS.

Box 3.80.2 How to assess the likelihood of transmission of TB

1 *How infectous is the source case?*
- Sputum smear positive: infectious to any close contact.
- Smear negative, culture positive: possibly infectious to highly susceptible contacts.
- Sputum negative, bronchial washing positive: possibly infectious to highly susceptible contacts.
- Three consecutive sputum negatives: not infectious.
- Two weeks *appropriate* treatment: not infectious.
- Non-pulmonary/laryngeal disease: not infectious.
- Children, even if smear positive, are less infectious than adults.

2 *How great is the exposure?*
- Exposure to coughing is the most important risk, but sneezing, singing and long (more than 5 minutes) conversation can also produce many infectious droplets.
- Prolonged or multiple indoor exposure usually needed to infect most contacts. Eight hours is often taken as a proxy (e.g. for exposure on aircraft).
- Aerosols may persist after case leaves room.
- Dishes, laundry, etc. not infectious.
- Estimates of risk from specific exposures to infectious case in one review (although there may be reporting bias inflating some of these figures):
  (a) household: 1 in 3
  (b) dormitory: 1 in 5
  (c) bar or social club: up to 1 in 10
  (d) nursing home: 1 in 20
  (e) school or workplace: 1 in 50 to 1 in 3
- Casual social contact: 1 in 100,000
- Background rate: 1 in 100,000

3 *How susceptible is the contact to infection and disease?*
- Susceptibility by age: neonates, very high; age under 3 years, high.
- BCG reduces risk by 50–80% in developed countries.
- Immunosuppressed at very high risk: includes AIDS, lymphoma, leukaemia, cancer chemotherapy and oral corticosteroids (equivalent to 15 mg/day prednisolone).
- Severe malnutrition leads to increased risk. Post-gastrectomy or jejunal-ileal bypass patients at risk if underweight.
- Silicosis or drug misuse increases risk.
- Diabetics and those with chronic renal failure have increased risk of reactivation of latent disease.

M. bovis has increased in cattle in the UK and some other European countries in recent years, most human cases probably represent reactivation of infection acquired before routine treatment of milk supplies and testing of cattle.

Direct transmission, either through cuts in the skin or traumatic inoculation (e.g. prosector's wart), is now rare. Droplet aerosols may be generated in healthcare settings from surgical dressing of skin lesions, autopsy, bronchoscopy and intubation.

Acquisition

The incubation period, as defined by reaction to a tuberculin test, is usually 3–8 weeks (occasionally up to 12 weeks). The latent period may be many decades.

The infectious period is for as long as there are viable organisms in the sputum: cases are usually considered infectious if organisms are demonstrable on sputum smear. Appropriate chemotherapy renders most patients non-infectious in 2 weeks.

Acquisition of an infective dose usually requires prolonged exposure and/or multiple aerosol inoculae, although some strains appear to be more infectious.

Immunity usually occurs after primary infection and involves several responses, including delayed-type hypersensitivity, the basis of the tuberculin test. Conditions such as AIDS, which affect cellular immunity, increase the risk of disease. Other risks are given in Box 3.80.2.

Prevention

Control of TB in developed countries has a number of components:
• Limitation of infectiousness by targeted case-finding and early treatment.
• Limitation of antimicrobial resistance by multidrug therapy (e.g. British Thoracic Society guidelines) and measures to maximise compliance, such as directly observed therapy (DOTS) and patient-centred case management, particularly in socially marginalised groups and those already identified as having drug-resistant infection. Tuberculosis outcome surveillance is important to assess the effectiveness of control services.
• Identification and treatment of further cases is by contact tracing in response to notifications of TB (see Chapter 4.9). Up to 10% of clinical cases in the UK are found by this method. In addition, potentially latently infected individuals can be identified and non-immune contacts offered bacille Calmette–Guérin (BCG) immunisation.
• Those contacts with evidence of infection without active disease (latent infection) can be protected by chemoprophylaxis to prevent later disease developing (either isoniazid + rifampicin for 3 months, or isoniazid for 6 months). Prophylaxis may also recom-

mended for young children or those with HIV who are contacts of an infectious case of TB, even if tuberculin negative.
• BCG vaccine of infants reduces the risk of TB disease and death. Immunisation of previously unvaccinated school children has an efficacy against TB of about 77%, lasting at least 15 years. A similar effect would be expected against drug-resistant strains. Vaccination is recommended in the UK (provided the individual has no previous BCG, is tuberculin test negative and has no other contraindications) for the following:
   (a) all infants living in areas where the annual incidence is 40 per 100,000 or greater;
   (b) children with a parent or grandparent born in a country where the annual incidence is 40 per 100,000 or greater (tuberculin test first for those aged 6–16 years);
   (c) children under 16 years who are contacts of cases of respiratory TB;
   (d) children under 16 years who were born in *or* have lived for 3 months in *or* are travelling to a country where the annual incidence is 40 per 100,000 or greater;
   (e) people in occupations with increased risk of coming into contact with TB (if under 35 years old) in certain roles in healthcare, laboratory, prison, care home and hostel settings.
• BCG is not recommended in many European countries.
• Screening of immigrants and refugees from high prevalence countries for active disease, latent infection and lack of immunity may be offered as part of a total health package in their new district of residence. Such individuals can be identified from a combination of Port Health forms, GP registers, school registers, refugee hostels and community groups.
• Case finding amongst homeless people.
• Infection control and occupational health services in hospitals to reduce exposure of patients to infected healthcare workers or potentially infectious patients, with particular care in units dealing with immunocompromised patients and units likely to admit patients with TB.

Surveillance

• All forms of clinical TB are notifiable in almost every European country, including the UK.
• The two main sources of surveillance data are notifications of clinical cases from clinicians (such as respiratory physicians) and positive reports from microbiology laboratories. Other potential sources are pathologists (histology and autopsy), surgeons and pharmacists. Reliance on only one source will lead to incomplete ascertainment.
• District TB registers are useful and may include data on the following:
   (a) age, sex, ethnicity, country of birth, place of residence;
   (b) type of disease, sputum status, antibiotic sensitivities; and
   (c) treatment outcome.
• Enhanced surveillance of TB has been introduced into a number of EU countries, including the UK, where district co-ordinators collect a standardised dataset on all new cases which is forwarded to regional and national databases.
• The joint ECDC/WHO surveillance programme collects data on TB from national centres throughout Europe. However, reporting systems differ substantially between contributing countries, making comparisons difficult.

Response to a case

• All TB cases should be notified to local public health departments.
• Investigate whether infectious by three early morning sputum samples for microscopy and culture.
• Ensure isolate tested for drug resistance.
• Early treatment with standard multidrug therapy. Consider appropriate measures to maximise compliance.
• Most cases can be treated at home. There is no need to segregate cases from other household members, unless they are neonates or immunocompromised.

• Those treated in hospital who are smear positive (or pulmonary or laryngeal disease with results pending) should be segregated in a single room, preferably with measures to reduce airflow to other patient areas. Particular care is needed in units containing immunocompromised patients or if the case is suspected to have drug-resistant TB.
• Adults with smear-negative disease, nonpulmonary disease or those who have been on appropriate treatment for 2 weeks do not require isolation. Persons visiting children with TB in hospital (one of whom may be the source case) should be segregated from other hospital patients until they have been screened.
• Screen household contacts of cases of TB. For smear-positive cases, also assess other close contacts with household level exposure (e.g. boyfriend/girlfriend and frequent visitors).
• Inform and advise other contacts.
• Casual contacts need only be screened if the case is smear positive and either:
   (a) the contact is unusually susceptible to TB (e.g. young child or immunocompromised adult); or
   (b) the case appears to be highly infectious (e.g. more than 10% of contacts infected).
• Check that the index case and any secondary cases are not healthcare workers, teachers or others who work with susceptible people (Box 3.80.3).
• The recommendations of a systematic review of the evidence for investigation and management of contacts are shown in Figure 3.80.1.

Investigation of a cluster

• The aim is to discover whether there is an unrecognised infectious source.
• Check diagnosis of cases. Are they confirmed microbiologically? Beware the occasional 'pseudo-outbreak' (e.g. if all cases confirmed by same laboratory).
• Liaise with reference laboratory for genotyping of all isolates to look for potentially linked cases.

Box 3.80.3 How to manage specific TB scenarios

1 *If the case is a healthcare worker with patient contact* (or a patient found to have TB after admission onto an open ward):
- Decide how infectious the case is:
(a) respiratory or laryngeal TB?
(b) cough or cavities on chest X-ray?
(c) sputum smear and/or culture positive?
(d) results of screening of close contacts?
(e) duration of treatment + antibiotic sensitivity (e.g. multidrug resistant)?
(f) infection control procedures in place before isolation?
- Decide how long the case has been infectious, in particular duration of cough.
- If case is thought to be infectious, convene Incident Management Team including the following:
(a) hospital control of infection staff;
(b) senior hospital manager;
(c) local health protection consultant (CCDC);
(d) physician with expertise in TB;
(e) contact tracing services (TB health visitor);
(f) medical records manager;
(g) manager of affected ward/unit;
(h) occupational health;
(i) press officer,
- Draw up list of contacts. Consider:
(a) inpatients, outpatients, referrals from other consultants;
(b) other members of staff;
(c) classifying contacts by level of exposure (e.g. patients for which case was 'named nurse' could be classified higher exposure and other patients on ward as lower exposure. For patient index, higher exposure could be 8 hours in same bay or ward).
- Decide whether any of these contacts are particularly susceptible to TB (Box 3.80.2):
(a) ask medical and nursing staff who treat them;
(b) review case notes.
- Organise screening of highly susceptible contacts (remember incubation period of up to 3 months since last contact with case).
- Inform and advise other contacts and write to their GPs so that exposure is noted.
- Consider need for helpline and press release for worried patients.
- Reconsider actions when results of screening and culture results are known.
2 *If the case is a teacher or pupil at a school*
- If the teacher is potentially infectious, assess all children in relevant teaching groups during the last 3 months.
- Although children rarely infectious, if child case is sputum smear-positive, assess other children who share classes with the case.
- Consider other pupils and staff based on infectivity of index case, susceptibility of contact and proximity and duration of contact.
- Explain plan to staff and parents and prepare for press interest.
- Reassess in light of initial screening results.
- If potential source not found for child case in screening of household or in school and child not in a higher incidence group, consider screening of other staff.

Box 3.80.3 *(Continued)*

---

3. *If the case has recently travelled on an aircraft*
- Check if patient sputum smear (and preferably culture) positive.
- Was flight within last 3 months and over 8 hours in duration?
- Did the passenger have a frequent cough at time of flight or does patient have multidrug-resistant TB?
- If the criteria above are satisfied, ask the airline to identify passengers in the same part of the aircraft and contact them by letter.
- Letter to recommend passengers to contact their own doctor and give a central telephone number for advice.
- Inform health authorities for areas with affected passengers.

- Any clinical or epidemiological clues as to whether cases have recent or old infection:
  - **(a)** age and previous residence abroad;
  - **(b)** clinical and radiological signs;
  - **(c)** risk factors for new infection (e.g. contact with case or travel to high prevalence country); and
  - **(d)** risk factors for reactivation (e.g. diabetes, renal failure).
- Obtain microbiological samples on all non-confirmed cases.
- Undertake hypothesis-generating study. Include family links, social networks, leisure and hobbies, links to institutions, especially those containing highly susceptible individuals and/or overcrowding (hospitals, nursing homes, schools, jail, homeless hostels) and for travel to (or visitor from) a high prevalence country.
- Check drug sensitivities and compliance with treatment for known respiratory cases associated with cluster.

Control of an outbreak

- Undertake contact tracing for known cases to identify and treat undiscovered infectious cases (and others with infection or disease who would benefit from treatment).
- In outbreaks linked to hospitals:
  1 Look for an unsuspected infectious source, e.g.:
  (a) patient with multidrug-resistant TB remaining infectious despite prolonged therapy (check sensitivity results);

(b) smear-negative cases infecting highly susceptible contacts (check culture results);
(c) delayed diagnosis in AIDS cases (do not rely on classic clinical picture or Mantoux);
(d) healthcare worker, patient or visitor with undiagnosed TB (chronic cough unresponsive to antibiotics?).
2 Consider breakdown in infection control procedures, e.g.:
(a) procedures such as bronchoscopy, sputum induction and pentamidine inhalation may generate aerosols;
(b) inadequate isolation of sputum-positive patients;
(c) inadequate decontamination of multi-use equipment.

Suggested case-definition for an outbreak

Confirmed: clinically compatible illness with demonstration of infection with outbreak genotype.
Probable: culture or PCR positive or demonstration of AFB with clinically compatible illness and epidemiological link, but no genotype available.
Clinical: clinical diagnosis leading to initiation of antituberculous therapy in individual with epidemiological link to outbreak.

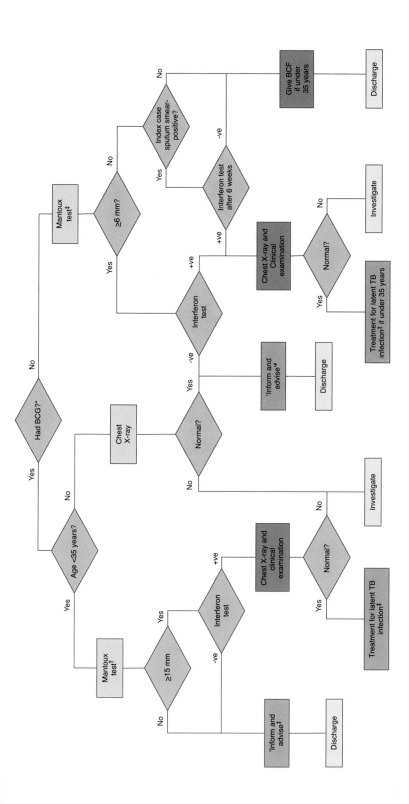

Fig. 3.80.1 Algorithm for examination of asymptomatic close contacts of patients with active tuberculosis. With permission from the National Collaborating Centre for Chronic Conditions, *Tuberculosis: clinical diagnosis and management of tuberculosis, and measures for its prevention and control*. London: Royal College of Physicians, 2006.

* Previous BCG vaccination cannot be accepted as evidence of immunity in HIV-infected patients
† A negative test in immunocompromised people does not exclude TB infection
‡ People advised to have treatment for latent TB infection, but who decline, should have 'inform and advise' information reinforced and chest X-ray follow-up at three and 22 months
For children aged between four weeks and two years old who are contacts of people with sputum smear-positive TB, use the algorithm in Figure 8

3.81 Tularaemia

Tularaemia (also known as rabbit fever, deer-fly fever, Ohara disease, Francis disease) is a zoonotic infection caused by the bacteria *Francisella tularensis* normally transmitted to humans from animal hosts. It is also a potential bioterrorism agent.

Suggested on-call action
None usually required.

Epidemiology

Tularaemia is endemic throughout the Northern Hemisphere. In Europe, outbreaks have been from Finland, Sweden, the Balkans and, most recently, Spain. The overall notification rate in the EU is 0.3 per 100,000; among males it is twice that of females. The highest rates are in the 45–64 years age group; most cases occur between July and September.

Clinical features

The clinical manifestations (ulceroglandular, oropharyngeal, oculoglandular, pneumonic, septicaemic and typhoidal) depend on the portal of entry. Symptoms include high fever, body aches, swollen lymph glands and difficulty swallowing. Fatalities occur mainly from typhoidal or pulmonary disease but are rare in Europe. With appropriate antibiotic treatment, the case fatality rate is negligible.

Laboratory confirmation

Diagnosis is usually clinical and confirmed by a rise in specific serum antibodies which are usually detectable after 2 weeks of the illness. Cross-reactions with *Brucella* species occur. Two biovars can cause human disease. Type A is more virulent than type B (case fatality rate 5–15% versus <1%). Type B strains occur across Northern Europe and Russia; the more severe type A is generally restricted to North America.

Transmission

Tularaemia is a zoonosis; reservoirs include wild rabbits, hares and muskrats as well as some domestic animals and ticks. The most prevalent modes of transmission includes arthropod bites, drinking water or food contaminated by rodents, handling of undercooked infected meat or inhalation of dust from contaminated hay. Tularaemia in Sweden and Finland is generally regarded as a mosquito-borne disease.

Acquisition

The incubation period is usually 3–5 days, but may be as long as 2 weeks. It depends upon strain virulence, type, inoculum size and portal of entry; as few as 10–50 type A organisms may cause infection by the inhalational route. Person-to-person transmission has not been reported.

Prevention

Health education to:
• avoid tick bites;
• avoid untreated potentially contaminated water; and
• ensure meat from rodents is cooked thoroughly.

Surveillance

• Tularaemia is notifiable in many countries (not the UK).
• Cases should be reported to the public health authorities so that assessments of risk can be made.
• Severe unexplained cases of sepsis or respiratory disease in otherwise healthy

individuals should be reported to local public health authorities.

Response to a case

No public health action is usually necessary.

Investigation of a cluster

- Search for a common source of infection related to arthropods, animal hosts, water or food.
- Consider deliberate release if two or more suspected cases are linked in time and place or a single confirmed case if not explained either by occupational risk or travel to an endemic area.

Control of an outbreak

- Investigate and control identified source.
- Emphasise prevention.

Response to a deliberate release

- Report to local and national public health authorities.
- Define exposed zone and identify individuals exposed within it (some may have left the scene).
- Cordon off exposed zone.
- Decontaminate those exposed: remove clothing and possessions, then shower with soap and water.
- Chemoprophylaxis (currently ciprofloxacin) as soon as possible for those exposed.
- Record contact details for all those exposed.
- Some health and emergency workers may also need prophylaxis.
- Police may take environmental samples.
- For more general information see Chapter 4.15 and specific advice on the Health Protection Agency website.

> **Suggested case-definition**
>
> Compatible clinical illness with laboratory confirmation of tularaemia.

3.82 Typhoid fever

Typhoid fever is a severe infection that is rare in developed countries, but is a risk for travellers abroad and can be spread by food handlers. Typhoid and paratyphoid (see Chapter 3.56) are both also known as enteric fever.

> **Suggested on-call action**
>
> - Exclude cases and contacts who are food handlers.
> - Exclude cases and symptomatic contacts in other risk groups (see below).

Epidemiology

The highest incidence is in south-central and South-East Asia (>100/100,000 cases pa); medium incidence areas are the rest of Asia, Africa, Latin America and the Caribbean and Oceania (except Australasia) (10–100 per 100,000); Europe, North America and the rest of the developed world are low incidence areas (<10 per 100,000). Incidence has been declining in Europe over the last decade. Cases are more common in late summer and in spring and are highest in young children. The majority of cases in Europe are imported (e.g. 90% of cases in UK are acquired abroad, most commonly in South Asia).

Clinical features

The onset may be insidious and non-specific. Fever is usually the earliest symptom, rising over a period of 2–3 days, and may be in a stepwise fashion. Headache and abdominal pain/tenderness may occur next, followed by anorexia, myalgia and fatigue. The most common symptoms reported in outbreaks are fever, headache and malaise. Other symptoms reported by a substantial minority of cases are diarrhoea, constipation, respiratory symptoms, abdominal pain, myalgia, vomiting and chills/rigors. Common signs include hepatomegaly, splenomegaly and rose spots. Fever commonly lasts for more than 1 week and may persist for 3 weeks.

Untreated typhoid has a case fatality rate of 10–15%; prompt treatment reduces this to under 1%. Relapses occur in 8–25% of cases, despite antibiotic treatment. Enteric fever should be considered when patients returning from an endemic or epidemic area develop a febrile illness.

Laboratory confirmation

Blood, stool, urine, rose spots, bone marrow and gastric or intestinal secretions can be cultured. Blood, urine and faeces culture are usually the first line: faeces are usually positive after the first week of illness and results should be available in 72 hours. The sensitivity of blood culture is about 60%.

Antibiotics may suppress *Salmonella* below detection levels for several weeks after completion of the course. However, bone marrow culture has 90% sensitivity, even after 5 days of antibiotic therapy. The Widal test on acute and convalescent sera may provide a retrospective diagnosis. Vi phage typing may be available for unexplained clusters; the most common in the UK are E1 and E9.

Transmission

Humans are the only reservoir for *S*. Typhi. Typhoid is spread from person to person via the faeco-oral route. Transmission can occur via contaminated food or water. In developed countries, transmission is predominantly from the consumption of foods contaminated by a human case or, occasionally,

an asymptomatic carrier. Fruit and vegetables washed in water contaminated by sewage may be a vehicle; the food vehicle may have been imported from abroad. Attack rates of about one-third have been reported from some food-borne outbreaks.

Secondary spread can occur in households. Direct person-to-person spread is rare, but is possible in poor hygienic conditions and spread can also occur via direct oro-anal contact.

Acquisition

The incubation period ranges from 3 to 40 days and varies with the size of the infecting dose. The average incubation period in outbreaks is about 14 days.

Cases are likely to be infectious for as long as faecal excretion continues, as the infectious dose is relatively low: the ID_{25} is probably about 10^5 organisms and the ID_{50} is about 10^7 organisms. Carriers often excrete $>10^5$ organisms/g stool. Half of cases are still excreting the organism after 2 weeks, despite treatment, 15% excrete for at least 4 weeks and 1–5% become chronic carriers. Prolonged asymptomatic carriage with intermittent detection in stool specimens may occur. Five consecutive negative faecal samples gives reasonable certainty of microbiological clearance, although about 95% of excretors are detected by three samples. Chronic urinary carriage of *S*. Typhi may occur, but is rare.

Repeated exposure (e.g. in endemic areas) leads to the development of natural immunity. However, immunity is not absolute.

Prevention

- Sanitation, clean water, handwashing and food hygiene.
- Two modern typhoid vaccines are available. Both are effective at preventing typhoid fever and side effects are rare. Vaccine is usually recommended for travellers from low-risk countries who are visiting higher incidence

countries, especially where hygiene and sanitation may be poor.

Surveillance

• Typhoid is notifiable in most countries, including the UK.
• Report on clinical suspicion to local public health authorities.

Response to a case

• Usually requires antibiotics: check antibiotic resistance of isolate.
• Advice on good personal and food hygiene to cases, carriers and contacts, especially handwashing.
• Enteric precautions for cases; consider isolation if hospitalised.
• Obtain food and travel history for the 3 weeks prior to onset of illness.
• Cases who have not visited an endemic country in the 3 weeks before onset should be investigated to determine the source of infection.
• Cases, excretors and carriers who are higher risk for spreading infection (see Box 2.2.1) should be excluded from work, school or nursery until no longer excreting the organism. Because of the higher risk of transmission from food handlers, microbiological clearance for this group is often defined (e.g. in UK guidance) as six consecutive negative specimens obtained 1 week apart and at least 3 weeks after the completion of treatment. For the other groups, only three such negatives are usually required.
• Contacts in high-risk groups are also excluded from work until microbiological clearance: this is often defined as two consecutive negative samples. Others thought to have the same exposure as the case (e.g. those in the same travel group) are usually treated as contacts.
• Exclude all other cases until clinically well for 48 hours with formed stools and hygiene advice has been given.

• Antibiotic clearance, under the care of an appropriate specialist, can be considered for chronic carriers.

Investigation of a cluster

• Investigate to ensure that secondary transmission has not occurred.
• Most clusters in developed countries will result from exposure to a common source abroad, or transmission within close family groups.
• Chains of transmission can be investigated through phage typing.

Control of an outbreak

• Outbreaks should be investigated as a matter of urgency.
• All cases and contacts should be investigated to identify the source of the outbreak.
• This could be due to contact with a chronic carrier, with faecal material or with contaminated food, milk, water or shellfish.
• Contacts should be observed and investigated if they develop symptoms suggestive of typhoid after appropriate specimens are taken.

Suggested case-definition for an outbreak
Probable: a clinically compatible case epidemiologically linked to a confirmed case in an outbreak.

3.83 Typhus, other Rickettsia, *Ehrlichia* and *Bartonella*

The order Rickettsiales includes the Rickettsiae and Ehrlichiae, small Gram-negative intracellular parasites; the classification is uncertain and genome analysis is likely to lead to a reconsideration. This chapter also covers the Bartonellae, Rickettsia-like organisms. Typhus refers to a number of illnesses caused by Rickettsiae (Table 3.83.1).

Clinical features

The clinical features depend upon the infecting organism. In typhus, following an infected arthropod bite, replication of the organism at the site may give rise to a characteristic skin lesion, a small painless ulcer with a black centre (an 'eschar'). The infection then becomes generalised with fever, which in severe infections is high and unremitting. If there is a rash, it appears around the fourth or fifth day of illness and may have either a dusky macular appearance or be petechial. In the most serious infections multiple organ damage may develop, usually towards the end of the second week.

Transmission

Transmission is by an arthropod vector, the natural host is typically a rodent. The epidemiology of disease depends upon the interaction of people with the vector; disease may result in conditions of poverty and poor hygiene, or with leisure and walking.

Prevention

Prevention is by reducing the incidence of vector bites through both personal and public health measures:
• Avoiding tick bite: wear long trousers, tucked into socks.
• Use repellents (permethrin can be sprayed on boots and clothing, DEET (*N,N*-diethyl-*meta*-toluamide) can be applied to the skin).
• Conduct body checks and remove ticks found using fine-tipped tweezers or fingers

shielded with a tissue, paper towel or rubber gloves. Grasp the tick close to the skin and pull upward steadily, twisting may break off the mouthparts (if this happens, remove with tweezers). The tick (saliva, hemolymph, gut) may contain infectious organisms so do not squeeze or handle with bare hands. Following removal, disinfect the bite site and wash hands with soap and water.
• In an epidemic of louse-borne disease, delousing measures with changing of clothes and impregnation with insecticide may be necessary.

Acquisition

There is no person-to-person spread.

Review the need for intervention if louse-borne disease is related to poor sanitation. Consider education campaigns for those exposed to vectors (e.g. walkers' exposure to ticks).

Response to a case

Rickettsial infection should be considered if there is fever with either the typical rash or an eschar and an appropriate travel history. Diagnosis is usually clinical. Treatment decisions must be based on epidemiological and clinical clues, and should not await laboratory confirmation. To confirm serologically use assays that detect antibodies to rickettsial antigens such as the indirect immunofluorescence antibody (IFA) test. Increased IgM titers are usually seen by the end of the first week of illness. Diagnostic levels of IgG antibody generally do not appear until 7–10 days after the onset of illness.

Ehrlichiosis can be confirmed using serology (IFA), polymerase chain reaction (PCR) may be available. Clusters of *Ehrlichia* (morulae) can be seen in infected cells.

Bartonellae may be cultured, Warthin–Starry staining of biopsy material may show bacilli, antibody tests and PCR may be available. Rickettsial infections are notifiable in most countries.

Table 3.83.1 Main diseases caused by Rickettsiae, Ehrlichia and Bartonellae

Disease and organism	Incubation period (days)	Mode of transmission and epidemiology	Clinical
Rickettsiae: typhus group			
Epidemic (louse-borne) typhus R. prowazekii	7–14	Vector: dog tick Host: rodents Human-to-human transmission: human body louse. Principally a disease of tropical highlands such as Ethiopia and the Andes. Infestation occurs where poverty and a cold climate coincide.	Relatively mild in children, mortality increases with age; untreated, about 50% of 50-year-olds will die. There is no eschar, usually a rash, often petechial. The high fever may be associated with severe headache, vomiting and epistaxis. Complications include diminished consciousness, pneumonia and renal failure.
Murine typhus R. typhi	7–14	Vector: flea Host: rat Found worldwide, particularly in tropical Asia	Resembles epidemic typhus, but milder
Rickettsiae: spotted fever group			
Rocky Mountain spotted fever R. rickettsii	3–14	Vector: dog tick Host: various, rodents most significant North American disease, occurs widely in the Eastern USA as well as in the Rocky Mountains	Severe illness. The rash is typically petechial and complications, including pneumonia and myocarditis, are common. Untreated, the mortality is around 20%.
Boutonneuse fever R. conorii, R. slovaca	5–8	Vector: tick Similar syndromes occur in the Mediterranean, Asia, Australia and Brazil	An eschar is usual, sometimes with regional lymphadenopathy, and a macular rash may occur; rarely fatal.
Rickettsialpox R. akari	7–14	Vector: mite Found in South and East Asia and in parts of Queensland, Australia. Also reported from Russia, Eastern USA and South Africa.	Disseminated vesicular rash, may be confused with chickenpox. Fatality is low.

Spotted fever rickettsiae have been found on all continents except Antarctica. Those causing human rickettsioses include *R. africae* (African tick bite fever), *R. japonica* (Japanese spotted fever), *R. sibirica* (North Asian tick typhus), *R. helvetica* (perimyocarditis), *R. australis* (Queensland tick typhus) and *R. honei* (Flinders Island spotted fever).

(Continued p. 244)

Table 3.83.1 (*Continued*)

Disease and organism	Incubation period (days)	Mode of transmission and epidemiology	Clinical
Rickettsiae: scrub typhus group			
Scrub typhus *Orientia tsutsugamushi*	6–21	Vector : mite Occurs in many parts of the world, including Japan, China, the Philippines, New Guinea, Indonesia, other South-West Pacific islands, South-East Asia, Northern Australia, India, Sri Lanka, Pakistan, Russia and Korea	Only fever, headache and swollen lymph nodes and in some cases myalgia, gastrointestinal complaints or cough. Mortality about 5% if untreated.
***Ehrlichia* and *Anaplasma*: intracytoplasmic bacteria that infect mononuclear cells and granulocytes. In contrast to spotted fevers, rash is rare and not petechial.**			
E. chaffeensis – E. canis group	3–16 days – may be longer	Vector: deer ticks Found in the USA	Human monocytic ehrlichiosis Illness similar to Rocky Mountain spotted fever
E. phagocytophila – E. equi group *Anaplasma phagocytophilum*		Vector: tick Host: small mammals, deer Found in North America, Europe. Renamed *Anaplasma*.	Human granulocytic anaplasmosis
***Bartonellae*: increasing importance as opportunistic parasites**			
Oroya fever and verruga peruana *B. bacilliformis*	21–84	Vector: sandfly Found in Peru, Ecuador and Colombia	Acute phase: (Carrion's disease, Oroya fever) fever, pallor, jaundice, hepato-splenomegaly, lymphadenopathy, severe haemolytic anaemia and transient immunosuppression. Chronic phase: (verruga peruana or Peruvian wart) cutaneus rash produced by a proliferation of endothelial cells.
Catscratch disease bacillary angiomatosis *B. henselae*	5–10	Vector: cat flea Host: domestic and feral cats Found worldwide	Usually causes self-limited regional adenopathy. Rare encephalopathy
Trench fever bacillary angiomatosis *B. quintana*	7–14	Vector: body louse Found worldwide. Associated with poor sanitation and poor personal hygiene; seen in homeless persons and those with AIDS.	Resembles epidemic typhus, but milder. Rash may be macular or maculopapular.

3.84 *Vibrio parahaemolyticus*

Vibrio parahaemolyticus causes a gastrointestinal infection that is particularly associated with consumption of contaminated seafood.

Suggested on-call action

If other cases are known to you or the reporting clinician/microbiologist then consult the local outbreak plan.

Epidemiology

V. parahaemolyticus food poisoning is rare in North and West Europe (e.g. 20–25 cases per year are reported in the UK), but may be more common in Southern Europe. It is responsible for over half of food-borne disease in Japan in summer months and is relatively common during the summer in coastal areas of the USA, the Caribbean, Bangladesh and South-East Asia. Most cases in the UK are in travellers returning from warmer countries, although serotype O3; K11 is reported from Spanish outbreaks. All ages are affected.

Clinical features

Characterised by explosive watery diarrhoea, usually accompanied by abdominal cramps. Nausea, vomiting and headache are common. Fever and chills occur in a minority of cases, as may bloody diarrhoea. The illness usually lasts 1–7 days (median of 3 days). Death is rare but may occur in very young children or elderly people with underlying disease. Occasionally, other *Vibrio* species, such as *Vibrio vunificans*, may cause illness, which is often non-gastrointestinal and particularly affects compromised hosts.

Skin infection has been reported following exposure of an open wound to contaminated warm seawater.

Laboratory confirmation

Diagnosis is dependent upon isolation of the organism from culture of a stool specimen or rectal swabs on selective media (warn the laboratory if organism suspected). Almost all pathogenic *V. parahaemolyticus* produce a haemolysin ('Kanagawa-positive') but most environmental isolates (and *Vibrio cholerae*) do not. DNA probes may also be used to demonstrate toxin capability.

The organism may also be cultured from food: at least 10^3 organisms/g would be expected. There are numerous serotypes but isolates from both food and faeces often contain a mixture of types.

Transmission

V. parahaemolyticus (and *V. vulnificans*) is ubiquitous in coastal waters of temperate and tropical countries. During the warm season (water at least 10°C, preferably over 22°C), the organism is found in salt water, fish and shellfish.

Transmission to humans is food-borne via consumption of raw or undercooked seafood; for example, oysters, clams, crab, scallops and shrimps (which may be imported), or food contaminated after cooking (e.g. by washing with seawater). The organism multiplies rapidly at room temperature (growth range 5–43°C, optimum 37°C): most outbreaks appear to involve food being held for several hours without refrigeration.

The organism is killed by temperatures of 80°C for 15 minutes and refrigeration is effective at controlling multiplication.

Acquisition

The incubation period is dependent upon the ingested dose: extremes of 4–96 hours have been reported, with the median for most outbreaks being 13–23 hours. The organism is non-communicable between humans. The minimum infectious dose is 10^6 organisms: despite this, there is usually a high attack rate in common source outbreaks. Immunity does not appear to develop in response to infection.

Prevention

• Care with seafood: maintain cold-chain, minimise time until consumption and cook thoroughly (or irradiate before eating raw).
• Avoid cross-contamination from raw seafood in kitchen. Do not use raw seawater to wash food.

Surveillance

Report to local public health departments and to national surveillance systems.

Response to a case

• Obtain details from case on foods consumed in 96 hours before onset (especially seafood) and any history of travel.
• Although person-to-person transmission is unusual, UK guidelines suggest cases in risk groups 1–4 (see Table 2.2.1) excluded from work/school for 48 hours after first normal stool.

Investigation of a cluster

• Plot epidemic curve: if all cases within 48 hours then a single exposure is likely. If more than 96 hours, assume continuing source as secondary spread is unlikely.
• Obtain food (especially seafood) and travel/recreation history for 96 hours before onset of each case.
• Organise laboratory testing of suspect foods.

Control of an outbreak

• Identify and rectify any of the following faults:
   (a) processes risking undercooking of seafood;
   (b) processes risking cross-contamination from seafood;
   (c) consumption of raw seafood without adequate temperature control; and
   (d) use of raw seawater.
• Reinforce food hygiene and handwashing.
• Report any suspected commercially produced food to relevant food safety authority.

Suggested case-definition for an outbreak

Confirmed: diarrhoea or abdominal cramps with *V. parahaemolyticus* identified in stool sample.
Clinical: watery diarrhoea and abdominal pain with onset 4–96 hours after exposure to suspect meal.

3.85 Viral haemorrhagic fevers

Viral haemorrhagic fevers (VHF) are severe, life-threatening viral infections caused by RNA viruses from several viral families. The disease syndromes are characterised by fever, malaise, vomiting, mucosal and gastrointestinal bleeding, oedema and hypotension. There is often multisystem involvement and the case fatality rate is high.

VHF are endemic in Africa, South America and some parts of Asia, the Middle East and Eastern Europe. About 20 cases of imported VHF were reported in England and Wales during the 10-year period to 2009. The environmental conditions in Western Europe do not support the natural reservoirs or vectors of these diseases. The risk of epidemic spread in the general population is negligible.

Suggested on-call action

• Undertake risk assessment.
• Contact Infectious Disease Unit and discuss with consultant.
• Ensure malaria excluded.
• Ensure clinical case is isolated, if appropriate arrange transfer to high security unit with special expertise.
• Ensure precautions in place for body fluids.
• Identify contacts and place under observation.
• Arrange press contact details.

Epidemiology

Each of the viruses grouped together has a different epidemiology (Table 3.85.1). The pattern of risk of infection depends upon the vector and host ranges; they are largely found in rural areas. The importance lies in their propensity to spread following exposure to body fluids. Large human outbreaks can result from person-to-person transmission; these may be associated with healthcare facilities.

Laboratory confirmation

The most common cause of VHF transmission in healthcare settings is in obtaining and handling laboratory specimens; blood and body fluids are likely to contain high concentrations of the virus. Therefore, most laboratory tests are discouraged in the initial assessment. Good laboratory practice guidelines must be in place and specimens must be taken and examined by experienced staff in appropriate facilities.

UK guidance is that specimens for virological investigations from moderate or high risk cases must be sent to a laboratory equipped to handle Hazard Group 4 biological agents (HPA, Colindale, and the Centre for Applied Microbiology and Research, Porton Down in

the UK). The appropriate specimen and investigation should be discussed first. Virus can be detected in body fluids. Newer techniques, such as reverse transcription polymerase chain reaction (RT-PCR) involve the detection of viral nucleic acid.

Post-mortem examination is a potential risk: if further tests are necessary to confirm the diagnosis, specialist advice should be sought.

Transmission

Person-to-person spread is through contact with infected body fluids of patients or cadavers. Zoonotic spread may occur from contact with other host species, such as bats or consumption of 'bushmeat' (Ebola, Marburg); consumption of raw milk or meat from infected animals (Congo–Crimean haemorrhagic fever, Rift Valley fever); contact with infected rodents or their excreta (arenaviruses, Hantaan, Omsk and Kyasnur Forest disease); insect vectors, mosquitoes (Rift Valley fever) or ticks (Congo–Crimean haemorrhagic fever, Omsk and Kyasnur Forest disease).

Surveillance

VHF are notifiable in most countries. Local and national public health authorities should be informed of cases immediately on clinical suspicion.

Response to a case

Many countries have specific guidelines for responding to a case or suspect case (in England and Wales the Guidelines of the Advisory Committee on Dangerous Pathogens: see Appendix 2).

Strict infection control precautions are required to protect those who may be exposed. In England and Wales the Control of Substances Hazardous to Health (COSHH) Regulations 1994 require employers to assess risks

Table 3.85.1 Viral haemorrhagic fevers

Virus family	Arenaviridae
Disease	Old World: Lassa fever New World: Junin (Argentine hemorrhagic fever), Machupo (Bolivian hemorrhagic fever), Guanarito (Venezuelan hemorrhagic fever), Sabia (Brazilian hemorrhagic fever) and other recently recognised viruses (Chapare, Flexal)
Natural distribution	Lassa: rural areas of West Africa Others: South America
Route of infection and transmission	Exposure to rodent urine, inhalation, ingestion or contact with broken skin Multimammate rat (Lassa) Nosocomial transmission through droplet and contact (Lassa)
Clinical features	Lassa: 80% cases asymptomatic. Otherwise gradual onset, malaise, fever, sore throat. Pharyngeal exudates common. Hypotension and shock. Albuminuria. Lassa responds to early treatment with ribavarin.
Incubation and infectious periods	Incubation: 6–21 days. Virus is present in body secretions, including the pharynx during the acute illness, and may be excreted in semen and urine for 2–3 months. Sexual intercourse must be avoided for 3 months.
Virus family	**Bunyaviridae**
Disease	RVF (Phlebovirus)
Natural distribution	Sub-Saharan Africa, Arabia. Recent epidemics occurred in Kenya, Somalia and Tanzania, Saudi Arabia and Yemen. Outbreaks in Egypt, Madagascar, Mauritania.
Route of infection and transmission	Mosquito, slaughter or consumption of infected animals. RVF is most commonly associated with mosquito-borne epidemics during years of unusually heavy rainfall.
Clinical features	May be mild illness associated with fever and liver abnormalities or progress to haemorrhage, encephalitis and retinitis. 1–10% patients – permanent vision loss. 1% case fatality
Incubation and infectious periods	Incubation: 2–6 days No person-to-person spread
Disease	Congo–Crimean haemorrhagic fever (Nairovirus)
Natural distribution	South Africa, the Balkans, the Middle East, Russia and Western China, and is highly endemic in Afghanistan, Iran, Pakistan and Turkey.
Route of infection and transmission	Ticks, slaughter or consumption of infected animals, usually domestic livestock. Nosocomial transmission often occurs.
Clinical features	Sudden onset of headache, high fever, back pain, joint pain, stomach pain, vomiting, red eyes, red throat and palatal petechiae, haemorrhagic features. Case fatality in hospitalised patients 10–50%.
Incubation and infectious periods	Incubation: 3–13 days
Disease	HFRS (see Chapter 3.29) HPS (see Chapter 3.29)
Virus family	**Filoviridae**
Disease	Marburg Ebola
Natural distribution	Ebola: Republic of Congo, Côte d'Ivoire, Democratic Republic of Congo, Gabon, Sudan and Uganda Marburg: Uganda, Kenya, Democratic Republic of Congo, Angola and possibly Zimbabwe
Route of infection and transmission	Animal host unknown, increasing evidence that the virus is present in bats. Pig to human transmission seen in a variant Ebola virus in the Philippines. Marburg has been transmitted from infected monkeys in laboratories.

Table 3.85.1 (*Continued*)

Virus family	Arenaviridae
Clinical features	Sudden onset, malaise, fever, myalgia, diarrhoea. Hypotension and shock. 50–90% case fatality rate for hospitalised cases.
Incubation and infectious periods	2–21 days
	Virus is present in body secretions, including the pharynx during the acute illness, may be excreted in semen for 2–3 months (Ebola).
Virus family	**Flaviviridaes**
Disease	Yellow fever (see Chapter 3.88)
	Dengue haemorrhagic fever (see Chapter 3.21)
Disease	OHF
	KFD
Natural distribution	OHF: Western Siberia
	KFD: Karnataka, India. 40–500 cases per year
Route of infection and transmission	KFD: tick. Host reservoir: rodents
	OHF: unknown: ?tick. Host reservoir: muskrat. Human infections occur by direct contact with their urine, faeces or blood.
Clinical features	Both conditions may follow a biphasic course. Fatality rate of 0.5–3%
Incubation and infectious periods	3–8 days
	No person-to-person spread

HFRS; hemorrhagic fever with renal syndrome; HPS, Hantavirus pulmonary syndrome; KFD, Kyasnur Forest disease; OHF, Omsk haemorrhagic fever; RVF, Rift Valley fever.

to employees and others in the workplace including, when appropriate, an assessment of the risk of VHF infection occurring at work.

Patient assessment and risk categorisation

VHF should be considered in the investigation of fever in a recent traveller and can usually be dismissed on epidemiological grounds. Patients should be assigned to risk groups (see checklist in the Guidelines) to ensure appropriate patient management and protection for the laboratory and clinical staff.

Minimum risk

This category includes febrile patients who have:
• not been in known endemic areas before the onset of illness; *or*
• been in endemic areas (or in contact with a known or suspected source of a VHF), but in whom the onset of illness was definitely more

than 21 days after their last contact with any potential source of infection.

Moderate risk

This category includes febrile patients who have:
• been in an endemic area during the 21 days before the onset of illness, but who have none of the additional risk factors that would place him or her in the high risk category; *or*
• not been in a known endemic area but who may have been in adjacent areas or countries during the 21 days before the onset of illness, and who have evidence of severe illness with organ failure and/or haemorrhage that could be due to a VHF and for which no alternative diagnosis is currently evident.

High risk

This category includes febrile patients who:
1 have been in an endemic area during the 3 weeks before illness; and
  • have lived in a house or stayed in a house for more than 4 hours where there were

ill, feverish persons known or strongly suspected to have a VHF; *or*

• took part in nursing or caring for ill, feverish patients known or strongly suspected to have a VHF, or had contact with the body fluids, tissue or the dead body of such a patient; *or*

• are a laboratory, health or other worker who has, or has been likely to have come into contact with the body fluids, tissues or the body of a human or animal known or strongly suspected to have a VHF; *or*

• were previously categorised as 'moderate' risk, but who have developed organ failure and/or haemorrhage;

2 have not been in an endemic area but during the 3 weeks before illness they:

• cared for a patient or animal known or strongly suspected to have a VHF or came into contact with the body fluids, tissues or dead body of such a patient or animal; *or*

• handled clinical specimens, tissues or laboratory cultures known or strongly suspected to contain the agent of a VHF.

The Public Health responsibility is to ensure the following:

• The patient is in the appropriate category of accommodation.

• Ambulance staff have been appropriately advised (liaise with ambulance control unit).

• Hospital staff have been appropriately advised (liaise with infection control doctor).

• Cases or contacts in other districts are followed up (liaise with appropriate staff).

• Specimens or contaminated material from before diagnosis suspected are dealt with appropriately.

• Contacts are identified and followed up appropriately.

• Any necessary disinfection of domestic and primary care premises is carried out.

• The body of any deceased case is appropriately dealt with.

• Appropriate agencies (Department of Health and Health Protection Agency in England and Wales) are informed.

• Arrangements are made for dealing with the media.

Initial management

Decisions on the management of a suspected case should be taken with an infectious disease specialist. An incident/outbreak control group should be convened to ensure that formal guidance is implemented correctly. Laboratory tests to exclude or confirm malaria should be undertaken as soon as possible for minimum and moderate risk patients:

• *Minimum risk*: admit (if requiring hospitalisation) under standard isolation and infection control procedures.

• *Moderate risk*: admit to high security infectious disease unit or intermediate isolation facilities and, apart from the malaria test, specimens should only be sent to a high security laboratory.

• *High risk*: admit to high security infectious disease unit, samples should only be sent to a high security laboratory and close contacts should be identified. Special precautions (ambulance category III) are required to transport moderate and high risk patients.

Management of contacts

Close contacts of a high risk or confirmed case should be kept under daily surveillance for a period of 21 days from the last possible date of exposure to infection. Close contacts are those who, after the onset of the patient's illness:

• had direct contact with the patient's blood, urine or secretions, or with clothing, bedding or other fomites soiled by the patient's blood, urine or secretions (not including saliva);

• cared for the patient or handled specimens from the patient – for example, household members, nurses, laboratory staff, ambulance crew, doctors or other staff;

• had direct contact with the body of a person who had died of VHF, either proven or in high or moderate risk categories, before the coffin was sealed;

• had direct contact with an animal infected with VHF, its blood, body fluids or corpse.

There need be no restriction on work or movement but the contact's temperature should be recorded daily and enquiry made about the presence of any suspicious symptoms. Those suffering any rise of temperature above 38°C should be kept under observation at home and, if fever persists for more than 24 hours, advice should be sought from a consultant in infectious or tropical diseases regarding the need for admission to an isolation unit.

When contact with a VHF patient has not been close, the risk of infection is minimal. Therefore there is no need to trace and/or follow up contacts that are not in the categories listed above.

3.86 Warts and verrucae

Warts are caused by infection of the epidermis with human papillomavirus (HPV). Various HPV genotypes affect different sites influenced by environmental and host factors.

Suggested on-call action
None usually required.

Epidemiology

Most people will have warts at some time in their life. The prevalence increases during childhood, peaks in adolescence and declines thereafter. The prevalence in children and adolescents in the UK is 4–5%. Warts are

more common in white ethnic groups. Warts clear spontaneously over time.

Clinical features

Various wart morphologies are recognised (Table 3.86.1).

Laboratory confirmation

The diagnosis can be confirmed histologically.

Transmission

Warts spread by direct contact or indirectly via contact with fomites or contaminated floors and surfaces. The attack rate is thought to be low. Auto-inoculation occurs as a result of scratching and shaving. Sexual transmission occurs.

Acquisition

The incubation period rages from 1 month to 2 years. A person with warts is infectious for as long as the warts persist. Warts are more common in immunocompromised people.

Prevention

• Health education, environmental hygiene in swimming pools and other communal

Table 3.86.1 Wart morphologies

Clinical type	Appearance	HPV type
Common warts (verrucae vulgaris)	Flesh-coloured or brown, keratotic papules	1, 2, 4, 57
Plane or flat warts (verrucae planae)	Smaller, flat topped, non-scaling, papules, cluster on hands, neck or face	3, 10
Plantar warts (verrucae plantaris)	Grow inwards and are painful, common in adolescents and children	1, 2, 4, 57
Condylomata acuminata (genital warts)	Occur in the genital tract, transmitted sexually (see Chapter 3.28)	6, 11

areas and avoiding direct contact with warts where practicable may reduce spread.

• Case reporting is not necessary.

• No single treatment is completely effective. Spontaneous regression is common and warts may be left untreated unless painful or unsightly.

• Children with warts do not have to stay away from school. Affected children can go swimming. Plantar warts should be covered if practicable in swimming pools, gymnasia and changing rooms.

Genital warts

Genital warts are caused by HPV infection and are the most frequently diagnosed viral sexually transmitted infection (STI) in the UK. Most genital warts are caused by low risk HPV types 6 and 11 and diagnosis is usually based on clinical appearance. However, asymptomatic HPV infections are also common.

Cervical cancer

HPV are implicated in the aetiology of cervical cancer, anogenital and head and neck cancers. In many areas of the world these diseases are a major cause of morbidity and mortality. For example, each year there are about 500,000 new cases of cervical cancer and 260,000 deaths worldwide. Most of these cases occur in developing countries where early detection by screening is not available. HPV types 16 and 18 cause about 70% of cervical cancers.

Two HPV vaccines have been available since 2006 and are being introduced in immunisation programmes in many high and some middle income countries. These vaccines may prevent 90% of pre-cancerous cervical lesions caused by the vaccine-related HPV types. The quadrivalent vaccine also prevents 90% of anogenital warts caused by HPV types 6 and 11. Both vaccines are safe and the World Health Organization (WHO) has recommended that they should be included in national immunisation programmes where it is feasible, affordable and cost-effective.

3.87 West Nile virus

An occasionally serious encephalitis caused by the West Nile virus (WNV).

Suggested on-call action
None unless unrecognised outbreak in which case inform Public Health Authorities.

Epidemiology

Acquired from a mosquito bite, the normal host is birds. Recognised in Africa, the Middle East, Southern and Eastern Europe (Czech Republic, France, Greece, Hungary, Italy, Portugal, Russia); there has been a recent increase in human cases in Southern Europe. Significant outbreaks have been reported in Greece, Romania, Russia and Israel. First reported in USA in 1999, the virus has now spread into Canada, Central America and the West Indies.

WNV, or other arboviral diseases, should be considered in adults >50 years with encephalitis or meningitis and who have visited endemic areas.

Clinical features

Usually asymptomatic or mild. Fewer than 1% have severe disease, typically aseptic meningitis or acute encephalitis associated with fever (characteristic if with acute flaccid paralysis). Severe illness is more common in the elderly. Symptoms and signs include fever, rash, pharyngitis and conjunctivitis, gastrointestinal symptoms, weakness, change in mental status, ataxia and extrapyramidal signs, optic neuritis, cranial nerve abnormalities, polyradiculitis, myelitis and seizures; myocarditis, pancreatitis and fulminant hepatitis have been described. Case fatality rates of 10–15% if hospitalized.

Laboratory confirmation

Virus-specific IgM can be detected in most cerebrospinal fluid (CSF) and serum specimens at the time of clinical presentation using IgM enzyme-linked immunosorbent assay (ELISA); polymerase chain reaction (PCR) is available. Paired serum samples should be tested. False positive results may be seen if recently exposed (vaccination or infection) to related flaviviruses (e.g. yellow fever, Japanese encephalitis, dengue).

Transmission

WNV is spread by the bite of a mosquito, infected by feeding on an infected bird. Transmission through blood transfusion, transplant, breast milk and transplacentally has been described. No person-to-person spread.

Acquisition

The incubation period is 5–60 days and depends on the species, route of transmission and infective dose, which may be as low 10–100 organisms. The duration of acquired immunity is uncertain.

Prevention

Avoidance of mosquito bites, especially for the elderly during periods of transmission.

Surveillance

Surveillance of virus in bird flocks and mosquitoes can inform risk. For case-definition see: http://ec.europa.eu/health/ph_threats/com/west_nile/wnv_case_def_en.pdf

Response to a case

If the first case, clinicians should be alerted to the presence of circulating WNV. Ensure public health advice about avoiding mosquito bites.

Response to a cluster and control of an outbreak

Mosquito control.

Additional information

• http://www.cdc.gov/ncidod/dvbid/westnile/index.htm
• http://www.hpa.org.uk/Topics/InfectiousDiseases/InfectionsAZ/WestNile Virus/

3.88 Whooping cough

Whooping cough (pertussis) is an acute bacterial respiratory infection caused by *Bordetella pertussis* (a related organism, *Bordetella parapertussis*, also causes a pertussis-like illness). Its public health importance lies in the severity of the disease, particularly in young infants, and its preventability by vaccination.

Suggested on-call action

• Start antibiotic treatment (erythromycin, azithromycin or clarithromycin).
• Exclude from nursery or school for 5 days from starting antibiotic treatment.

Epidemiology

Pertussis is well controlled in countries with good immunisation coverage. Where coverage is low, the disease has a cyclical pattern, with epidemics occurring at 3–4 yearly intervals. These epidemics affect young children;

infants under 6 months are particularly at risk.

The incidence of pertussis varies widely across Europe and has changed over time in many countries. In 2008, 18,807 cases of pertussis were reported by 28 EU countries. The overall notification rate was 5.28 per 100,000; highest rates were reported from Norway (82 per 100,000), the Netherlands (52 per 100,000) and Estonia (36 per 100,000). Variations in notification rates reflect different vaccine coverage and schedules but also differences in reporting and awareness of the disease. The World Health Organization (WHO) target was to reduce pertussis incidence to less than 1 per 100,000 in Europe by 2010.

The reported case fatality rate is 1 per 1000 overall, although it is higher in young infants, in whom pertussis is often not recognised. Enhanced surveillance using new laboratory methods such as polymerase chain reaction (PCR) diagnosis has significantly improved detection rates.

Clinical features

The initial illness starts with cough, cold and a fever. Over the next week, the cough gradually becomes paroxysmal; there are bouts of coughing which are terminated by the typical whoop, or by vomiting. The cough often lasts for 2–3 months. Young infants do not usually whoop, and coughing spasms may be followed by periods of apnoea. Adults and vaccinated children have a milder illness that lasts 2–3 weeks. Pertussis is being increasingly recognised as a cause of chronic cough in adults.

Laboratory confirmation

The classic method is culture from a pernasal swab, although the organism is difficult to grow, so sensitivity is low (although specificity is high). The sensitivity has been greatly improved by the advent of PCR diagnosis. Serology (EIA) is also available.

Transmission

Humans are the only reservoir. Transmission is by droplet spread from an infectious case, often an older sibling or parent. Carriers do not exist. Mild or subclinical cases among vaccinated individuals are also a source of infection.

Acquisition

The incubation period is 7–10 days, but may occasionally be up to 3 weeks. A case is highly infectious during the early stage of the illness, before the typical cough; infectiousness then decreases and the case is normally not infectious 3 weeks after the onset of paroxysmal cough, although in a proportion of cases (up to 20%) infectivity may persist for up to 6 weeks. The period of communicability may be shortened by antibiotic treatment. An attack of pertussis usually confers immunity, although second cases do sometimes occur.

Prevention

• Immunisation is highly effective at preventing illness, although its role in limiting transmission is less clear. Pertussis vaccine has also been shown to reduce the incidence of sudden infant death syndrome.
• There are two types of pertussis vaccine: killed whole-cell preparations and subunit acellular vaccines. Most countries in Europe now use acellular vaccines because of the lower incidence of side-effects. The vaccines are given in combination with diphtheria, tetanus, polio and Hib antigens, and sometimes also hepatitis B. Booster doses are recommended at various ages, usually in the second year of life. Some countries have started to introduce booster doses in older children, and booster vaccination of adolescents and adults is under consideration in many countries.
• It is important that pertussis vaccine is not delayed in infants, and that older siblings and

parents are fully vaccinated. The only true contraindication is a severe reaction to a previous dose.

Surveillance

• Pertussis is notifiable in most European countries.
• Laboratories should also report all clinically significant infections to the local and national surveillance centres.
• Serotyping should be performed in the national reference unit; surveillance of serotypes is important to monitor vaccine efficacy.

Response to a case

• Isolate, with respiratory precautions, in hospital.
• Start antibiotic treatment (erythromycin) and exclude from nursery or school for 5 days after treatment has started (course to continue for 14 days).
• Arrange for laboratory confirmation.
• Check vaccination status of case and household contacts, and arrange for vaccination if any are unvaccinated; report vaccines failures to the national surveillance unit.
• Erythromycin prophylaxis may be of value for unvaccinated household contacts of suspected or confirmed pertussis, particularly infants under 6 months of age, if given within 21 days of onset of case. The dose is 125 mg 6-hourly for children up to 2 years of age; 250 mg 6-hourly for children 2–8 years of age and 250–500 mg 6-hourly for children over 8 years of age and adults. Treatment should be continued for 7 days.

Investigation of a cluster

• Obtain laboratory confirmation, including serotyping.
• Check vaccination status of cases.
• Look for links to populations with low vaccine coverage. Consider potential sources of infection (e.g. unvaccinated adults).

Control of an outbreak

• Look for unvaccinated individuals and consider community-wide vaccination if coverage is low (NB three doses of vaccine are required for protection, so vaccination is a long-term outbreak control measure).
• Treatment of cases and erythromycin prophylaxis for unvaccinated contacts as above.
• Look for undiagnosed cases.
• Outbreaks in institutions can be controlled by a combination of case finding, antibiotic treatment and case exclusion.

Suggested case-definition for an outbreak

Clinical: 14 days or more of cough: *plus* one of:
• epidemiological link to a confirmed case, *or* one of
• paroxysms, whoop or post-coughing vomiting.
Confirmed: compatible symptoms with *B. pertussis* infection confirmed by culture, PCR or serology.

3.89 Yellow fever

An imported, acute flavivirus infection, which may be severe.

Epidemiology

Yellow fever is endemic in Central Africa and parts of South and Central America. Misidentification and inadequate surveillance systems means underreporting is common; the World Health Organization (WHO) estimates approximately 200,000 cases annually resulting in 30,000 deaths.

The insect vector is absent from Europe. Travellers to endemic areas are at risk. Imported cases are rare in Europe.

Clinical features

Cases are classified as inapparent, mild, moderately severe or malignant. Onset is sudden, with fever of 39–40°C. An initial tachycardia becomes a relative bradycardia given the fever. In mild cases, the illness ends after 1–3 days. In moderately severe and malignant cases, the fever falls suddenly 2–5 days after onset, a remission ensues of several hours or days; the fever recurs, albuminuria and epigastric tenderness with haematemesis appear, oliguria or anuria may occur and petechiae and mucosal haemorrhages are common. In malignant cases, delirium, convulsions and coma occur terminally.

Mortality of clinically diagnosed cases is up to 10% overall but as many infections are undiagnosed it is much lower.

Laboratory confirmation

Diagnosis is confirmed by virus isolation from blood, by a rising antibody titre (in absence of recent immunisation and after excluding cross-reactions to other flaviviruses) or at autopsy. Antigen or genome detection tests may be available.

Transmission

In sylvatic yellow fever, the virus is acquired from wild primates and transmitted by forest canopy mosquitoes. In urban yellow fever, the virus is acquired from a viraemic patient within the previous 2 weeks and transmitted by the *Aedes aegypti* mosquito.

Acquisition

Incubation lasts 3–6 days.

Prevention

• Active immunisation with the live attenuated vaccine effectively prevents cases.
• Vaccination requirements vary by country; information and vaccination centres addresses can be obtained from public health authorities.
• Eradication of urban yellow fever requires widespread mosquito control and mass immunisation.

Surveillance

Yellow fever is notifiable and should be reported to local public health authorities and to WHO.

Response to a case

• The case should be reported urgently to WHO (via national centre) and the country of origin.
• The case should be transferred to suitable isolation facilities and strict procedures such as those laid down by the Advisory Committee on Dangerous Pathogens (UK) followed.
• In an area where there is potential for further mosquito transmission, patients should be isolated in a screened room sprayed with residual insecticide.
• Hospital and laboratory personnel should be aware of the risk of transmission from inoculation.

Investigation of a cluster and control of an outbreak

Not usually relevant to Europe, but verify if cases have been to an infected area in the week before onset. Control of an outbreak is through mass immunisation and vector control.

3.90 Yersiniosis

Yersiniosis is an important cause of intestinal infection in many countries. *Yersinia enterocolitica* mainly causes enterocolitis, whereas *Yersinia pseudotuberculosis* mainly causes an appendicitis-like illness.

Suggested on-call action

• Exclude symptomatic cases in high-risk groups.
• If you or the reporting microbiologist/ clinician know of other cases, consult outbreak control plan.

Epidemiology

Although documented in temperate regions in all continents, *Y. enterocolitica* is more common in Northern Europe (particularly Scandinavia) and Canada, where it may be responsible for 2–4% of cases of diarrhoea. The incidence of reported infection is highest in those under 5 years old, followed by those aged 5–14 years. *Y. enterocolitica* occurs throughout the year, but may be higher from June to November.

Y. pseudotuberculosis is less common and has a worldwide distribution. Peak incidence is in winter.

Clinical features

Y. enterocolitica enteritis usually presents with diarrhoea, often with abdominal pain and fever. Less commonly reported symptoms include pharyngitis, vomiting; nausea; rash; bloody diarrhoea and headache. Illness duration ranges from 2 days to 6 weeks. Complications of *Y. enterocolitica* infection include reactive arthritis, erythema nodosum, septicaemia and unnecessary appendicectomy.

Y. pseudotuberculosis usually presents as mesenteric adenitis causing fever and right lower abdominal pain. Diarrhoea is less common than for *Y. enterocolitica*. Many cases result in appendicectomy. Illness lasts 1–37 days, with an average of about 18 days. Complications include reactive arthritis (relatively common), erythema nodosum and acute renal failure.

Laboratory confirmation

Diagnosis may be made by culture of faecal samples on selective media, with confirmatory biochemical testing. Serological diagnosis is available for both species. The laboratory should be informed if yersiniosis is suspected, as testing may not be undertaken routinely.

There are 11 species of *Yersinia*, although other species only rarely cause gastrointestinal infection. Not all strains are pathogenic and *Y. enterocolitica* and *Y. pseudotuberculosis* can be isolated from asymptomatic individuals. *Y. enterocolitica* is divided into six biotypes (1A, 1B, 2, 3, 4, 5), of which type 4 is the most common in Europe (and 1A is probably nonpathogenic), and over 50 serotypes, of which O3 and O9 are the most common in Europe. A phage typing scheme also exists.

Y. pseudotuberculosis may be confirmed by isolation from an excised mesenteric lymph node. All strains are biochemically homogenous and, although there are six serotypes, most human cases are serotype 1. Genotyping may be available in some countries.

Transmission

The most important reservoir of *Y. enterocolitica* in Europe is asymptomatic carriage in pigs. Other hosts are rodents, rabbits, sheep, goats, cattle, horses, dogs and cats.

Y. pseudotuberculosis is found in a number of mammals and birds, particularly rodents and poultry.

Humans usually acquire the infection orally via food, especially pork or pork products. Pork is easily contaminated in the abattoir and if eaten raw or undercooked may cause illness. Refrigeration offers little protection as the organism can multiply at 4°C. Milk, beef, dairy products, poultry products and water are potential sources of *Y. enterocolitica* outbreaks and vegetables such as tofu or bean sprouts have become contaminated from growing in contaminated water. Outbreaks of *Y. pseudotuberculosis* have been linked to raw carrots, lettuce and milk. The optimum temperature for growth is 22–29°C.

Other potential transmission routes are person to person (outbreaks have occurred in nurseries, schools and hospitals); direct contact with animals and contaminated blood products.

Acquisition

Excretion of both species in stool post-infection is common. The infectious dose (ID_{50}) of *Y. enterocolitica* is about 10^9 organisms. About 10^9/g *Y. enterocolitica* are excreted during the first 4 days of infection, about 10^4/g in the first 2–3 weeks and excretion can persist for months. Antibiotics may reduce the duration of excretion of both species in faeces.

The incubation period for *Y. enterocolitica* is usually 3–7 days, although extremes of 1–12 days are reported. *Y. pseudotuberculosis* has a reported range of 2–25 days, with a median of 5–8 days.

Natural infection confers immunity although the extent and duration is unclear. Maternal antibodies protect the newborn.

Prevention

• Good infection control during slaughtering of pigs.
• Good food handling practices and adequate cooking of meat, particularly pork.
• Avoidance of long-term refrigeration of meat.

• Pasteurisation of dairy products.
• Protection and treatment of drinking water.
• Washing of salad items to be eaten raw.
• Exclusion of blood donors with recent history of diarrhoea or fever.
• General measures to protect against gastrointestinal infection, including handwashing, safe disposal of human and animal/pet faeces, food hygiene and exclusion of cases with high risk of onward transmission.

Surveillance

• Cases of yersiniosis should be reported to local public health departments and to national surveillance systems.
• Clinicians should inform the local public health department of any increase in cases of mesenteric adenitis or appendicectomy.

Response to a case

• Give hygiene advice to case (enteric precautions).
• Report to public health authorities: compulsory notification in some European countries.
• Exclude case and symptomatic contacts if in risk group (see Box 2.2.1) until 48 hours after first normal stool. No microbiological clearance necessary.
• Obtain history of consumption of pork or pork products, raw or undercooked meat, milk, salad or water. Ask about sick pets, blood transfusions and exposure to animals/carcasses.

Investigation of a cluster

• Discuss case finding with local laboratory: need to change testing policy for routine specimens?
• Discuss further microbiological investigations of existing cases to discover if all one serotype or phage type.
• Conduct hypothesis-generating study. Questionnaire should include consumption of pork and pork products; consumption of raw or undercooked meats; salad items; source of milk; source of water; all other food consumed in last 12 days (25 days for

Y. pseudotuberculosis); contact with other cases; blood or blood product transfusions; hospital treatment; occupation; contact with animals (wild, agricultural or pet).

Control of an outbreak

• Exclude symptomatic cases in high risk groups and ensure enteric precautions followed.
• Reinforce food hygiene and handwashing.
• Look for ways in which food could have become contaminated (especially cross-contamination from raw pork), undercooked or stored too long in a refrigerator. Check that pasteurised milk could not become contaminated in dairy.
• Prevent use of unpasteurised milk. Prevent use of raw vegetables grown in untreated water, unless subsequently cleaned adequately.

Suggested case-definition for an outbreak

Clinical: diarrhoea or combination of fever and right lower abdominal pain with onset 4–7 days after exposure.
Confirmed: isolate of outbreak strain or serological positive with one of diarrhoea, fever, abdominal pain or vomiting beginning 1–12 days (2–25 days for *Y. pseudotuberculosis*) after exposure.

3.91 Other organisms

3.91.1 Helminths

For threadworms (pinworms) see Chapter 3.76 and for *Toxocara* see Chapter 3.78.

Intestinal roundworms

Most intestinal nematodes are not passed directly from person to person and so spread is rare in developed countries (Table 3.91.1a). Control is based on enteric precautions and early treatment of cases. The main exception is threadworm infection (see Chapter 3.76).

Filariae

Filariae produce larvae called microfilariae directly without an egg stage. Their life cycle involves an arthropod intermediate host, usually a biting insect which acts as a vector for the dissemination of the disease. At least 10 species infect humans. The incubation period is prolonged and may be more than a year. There is no person-to-person spread; individuals remain infectious for the insect vector if microfilariae are present. The endemic range of the diseases is determined by the insect vector (Table 3.91.1b).

Tapeworms

Humans are the only definitive host for the tapeworms *Taenia saginata* and *Taenia solium* and may also be accidental intermediate hosts for *T. solium*, giving rise to cysticercosis, and for *Echinococcus granulosus*, giving rise to hydatid disease.

Eggs, or whole detached segments (proglottids), are evacuated in the faeces of the definitive host and disseminate in the environment. Following ingestion by a suitable intermediate host they develop into invasive larvae in the gut, migrate through the tissues and settle as cysts at sites determined by the tropism of the parasite. When the intermediate host is eaten by a definitive host, allowing the cysts to develop into adults, the life cycle is completed (Table 3.91.1c).

Trematodes, flukes

Most flukes' life cycle involves molluscs, infection is acquired from an intermediate host, from cysts on water plants or direct penetration of skin. Human disease results either from the reaction to the eggs (schistosomes), obstruction (liver flukes) or inflammation at the site of attachment of intestinal flukes, which may lead to maladsorption. Chronic infection may result in malignancy. There is no person-to-person spread (Table 3.91.1d).

Table 3.91.1a Intestinal roundworms

Disease and organism	Mode of transmission	Clinical	Investigation	Epidemiology and public health action
Ascariasis *Ascaris lumbricoides*	Non-infective eggs excreted in faeces, become infectious after 2–3 weeks in soil and may survive many months. Infective eggs ingested from soil or foods contaminated by soil. Eggs hatch in duodenum. Larvae migrate in blood and lymphatics to lung and oropharynx where swallowed to develop into adult worms in small intestine. Adults live 6–12 months.	Migrating larvae may produce an eosinophilic pneumonia. Asymptomatic patient may pass an adult worm by vomiting or per rectum. Heavy infection may produce abdominal cramps and may cause intestinal obstruction. Even moderate infections can lead to malnutrition in children.	Identification of the eggs in faeces. Occasionally, adult worms are passed in the stool or vomited.	Worldwide but concentrated in tropical and subtropical areas with poor sanitation. Estimated that more than 1 billion persons are infected making ascariasis the world's most prevalent intestinal helminth infection. Uncooked and unwashed vegetables should be avoided in areas where human faeces (night soil) is used as fertiliser. There is no risk of transmission from a case in Europe if basic hygienic precautions are taken.
Whipworm infection *Trichuris trichiura*	Non-infective eggs excreted in faeces to develop in soil over 10–14 days. Ingested from soil or via contaminated food or water. No migration to other tissues. Adult worms may live 7–10 years.	Infection is often asymptomatic. Heavy infection causes abdominal pain, anorexia and diarrhoea and may retard growth. Rarely, weight loss, anaemia and rectal prolapse may occur.	Identification of the eggs in faeces.	The parasite is found principally in the tropics and subtropics. Prevention rests upon adequate sanitation and good personal hygiene.

| Hookworm infection Ancylostoma duodenale or Necator americanus | Eggs passed in human stool hatch in 1–2 days and release larvae, which mature over 5–8 days and may then penetrate human skin (often foot), migrate to the lungs via blood vessels, ascend to epiglottis and are swallowed. Adult worms may live 2–10 years. Occasionally, cat or dog hookworms may infect humans. | Most cases are asymptomatic. Migration of larvae may cause an eosinophilic pneumonia. Adult worms in the intestine may cause colicky pain and non-specific symptoms. Chronic infection may lead to iron deficiency anaemia and hypoproteinaemia. | Identification of the eggs in faeces. | A. duodenale is widely distributed in the Mediterranean, India, China, Japan and South America. N. americanus is the predominant hookworm of Central and South Africa, Southern Asia, Melanesia, the Caribbean and Polynesia. About 25% of the world's population is infected with hookworms. Preventing defecation where others may come into contact with the stool. Avoiding direct skin contact with the soil. Wearing shoes. Periodic mass deworming may be effective in high risk populations. |

(Continued p. 262)

Table 3.91.1a *(Continued)*

Disease and organism	Mode of transmission	Clinical	Investigation	Epidemiology and public health action
Strongyloidiasis *Strongyloides stercoralis*	Adult worms live in the duodenum and jejunum. Released eggs hatch immediately and larvae are then passed in faeces. After a few days the larvae can penetrate the skin of humans, migrate through the lungs, and reach the intestine, where they complete maturation in about 2 weeks. Filariform larvae can bypass the soil phase and directly penetrate the colon or the skin. Transmission is often due to exposure of bare skin to larvae in contaminated soil in unsanitary conditions. Faeco-oral transmission may occur in mental institutions and daycare centres. Self-reinfection may occur and can result in extremely high worm burdens (hyperinfection syndrome).	Most cases are asymptomatic. There may be non-specific abdominal symptoms. An enteritis, protein losing enteropathy, urticaria and pulmonary symptoms are seen less frequently. Larva currens, a serpiginous, migratory, urticarial lesion, is pathognomonic. The hyperinfection syndrome and disseminated strongyloidiasis are usually seen in persons with impaired immunity. Immunosuppression may lead to overwhelming hyperinfection in persons with previously asymptomatic infection. Hyperinfection produces serious gastrointestinal symptoms including haemorrhage, pulmonary infiltration, hepatitis and may involve the CNS. Even with treatment the mortality is over 50%.	Larvae can be identified in stool 25% of the time. Repeat examination of concentrated stool is necessary.	Endemic throughout the tropics and subtropics. Prevention of primary infections is as for hookworms. To prevent hyperinfection syndrome, patients with possible exposure to *Strongyloides* (even in the distant past), should undergo several stool examinations and, if necessary, a string test or duodenal aspiration before receiving immunosuppressive therapy including steroids.

| Trichinosis
Trichinella sp,
especially
T. spiralis | Infectious cysts are acquired from eating undercooked meat from infected carnivores or omnivores (pigs). Larvae develop in the small intestine, penetrate the mucosa and become adults in 6–8 days. Mature females release larvae for 4–6 weeks, before dying or being expelled. Larvae pass though the intestinal wall and travel to striated muscle cells, where they encyst over 1–3 months. The cycle continues when encysted larvae are ingested by another carnivore. | Gastrointestinal symptoms are absent or mild; nausea, abdominal cramps and diarrhoea may occur during the first week. The characteristic syndrome of periorbital oedema, myalgia, fever and subconjunctival haemorrhages and petechiae appears in weeks 2–3. Soreness may affect the muscles of respiration, speech, mastication and swallowing. Heavy infection may cause severe dyspnoea, multisystem disease or fatal myocarditis. Most symptoms and signs resolve by the third month. | There are no specific tests for the intestinal stage. Eosinophilia peaks 2–4 weeks after infection. Muscle enzymes are elevated in 50% of patients. A muscle biopsy may disclose larvae, inflammation and cysts. Serology can give false negative results, especially if performed early. They are of most value if initially negative and turn positive. | Trichinosis occurs worldwide. The life cycle is maintained by animals that are fed on (e.g. pigs) or that hunt (e.g. bears) other animals whose striated muscles contain encysted infective larvae (e.g. rodents). There have been outbreaks in Europe associated with imported horsemeat.
Trichinosis is prevented by cooking meat thoroughly (55°C (140°F) throughout). Larvae can also be killed by freezing at −15°C (5°F) for 3 weeks or −18°C (0°F) for 1 day.
Meat should be inspected before being sold.
There is no person-to-person spread.
Investigate clusters for a common contaminated food source. |

(*Continued p. 264*)

Table 3.91.1a (*Continued*)

Disease and organism	Mode of transmission	Clinical	Investigation	Epidemiology and public health action
Capillariasis *Capillaria philippinensis* Intestinal capillariasis	Larvae acquired from gut of undercooked fish. Mature and multiply in human gut.	Gastrointestinal symptoms: weight loss, diarrhoea, abdominal pain; may be fatal.	Faeces microscopy.	Philippines. Avoid raw whole fish.
C. hepatica Hepatic capillariasis	Eggs are present in soil or food contaminated with faeces of infected rodents. Larvae migrate to and mature in liver.	Fever, eosinophilia, hepatomegaly.	Liver imaging and biopsy.	Found on all continents in rodents, rare in humans.
C. aerophila Lung worm pulmonary capillariasis	Similar to *C. hepatica except* host is often dog or cat and final maturation is in lung.	Cough, wheeze.	Eggs in nasal or tracheal lavage.	Found on all continents, rare in humans.

Table 3.91.1b Filariae

Disease and organism	Mode of transmission	Clinical	Investigation	Epidemiology and public health action
Lymphatic filariasis (elephantiasis), *Wuchereria bancrofti*, *Brugia malayi*	Adult worms inhabit the lymphatics; the microfilariae, which have a strong diurnal periodicity, appear briefly in the peripheral blood around midnight when they can be ingested by mosquitos, which are the vectors.	Cause of elephantiasis. Fever and lymphangitis may occur early in the disease, the most serious consequences are the chronic sequelae of lymphatic damage caused by dying worms. Gross lymphoedema, most often of the legs or genitals, and chyluria are typical features.	Definitive diagnosis is by recognition of the microfilariae (in a midnight sample of blood for *W. bancrofti*). Serology provides supportive evidence but there may be cross-reactions with other nematode infections.	*W. bancrofti* has a widespread distribution in South Asia, the Pacific islands, tropical Africa and some parts of South America. Two species of *Brugia*, restricted to South-East Asia, give rise to a similar syndrome. Eliminating vector breeding sites.
Onchocerciasis (river blindness), *Onchocerca volvulus*	Microfilariae in the skin are ingested by a black fly of the genus *Simulium*.	The adult *Onchocerca* lives in the subcutaneous tissues. Clinical consequences are caused by the inflammation resulting from death of the microfilariae. In the skin this causes a chronic dermatitis. Most significant is damage to the eye. The inflammatory process may involve all the structures between the cornea and the optic nerve. Blindness occurs after 20 years or more of heavy infection.	Diagnosis depends on detecting microfilariae in superficial snips of skin.	Primarily an African disease although there are some foci in Central America. Eliminate vector breeding sites.

(*Continued p. 266*)

265

Table 3.91.1b Filariae

Disease and organism	Mode of transmission	Clinical	Investigation	Epidemiology and public health action
Loiasis: *Loa loa* (African eye worm)	Adult *Loa loa* are migratory and roam widely in the subcutaneous tissues and may become visible on passing under the conjunctiva of the eye. The microfilariae appear with a diurnal periodicity in the blood around midday.	Many cases asymptomatic, symptoms include 'Calabar swellings', diffuse areas of subcutaneous oedema, usually distally on the limbs, which last a few days.	Diagnosis is by recognising the microfilariae in midday blood.	Rainforests of West and Central Africa Eliminate vector breeding sites.
Dracontiasis Dracunculiasis *Dracunculus medinensis* (Guinea worm)	The disease is acquired by drinking water containing Cyclops ('water fleas') which harbour larvae. The larvae invade into the body cavity mature and mate. The gravid female, about 60 cm long, then makes her way to the lower extremities where she penetrates to the surface, giving rise to an irritating ulcer. Contact with water causes her to release larvae through this defect where they may be able to infect new Cyclops.	The chronic ulceration, and associated secondary infection, may be a severe problem in conditions of poor hygiene. Death of the worm causes intense inflammation.	Recognition of larvae or adult worm.	Now only Sudan, Ghana, Mali and Ethiopia. Eradication planned. Provision of clean drinking water. Filtering drinking water. Treat water with larvicides.

Table 3.91.1c Tapeworms (cestodes)

Disease and organism	Mode of transmission	Clinical	Investigation	Epidemiology and public health action
Taeniasis *Taenia saginata, T. solium*	Infection is acquired by eating undercooked infected pork or beef.	Adult *T. saginata* (beef tapeworm) may grow to 10 m and *T. solium* (pork tapeworm) to 4 m. However, infection is usually asymptomatic. Abdominal pains are sometimes reported. Detached motile segments (proglottids) of *T. saginata* may be noticed as they emerge from the anus.	Taeniasis infections are usually diagnosed because of eggs or proglottids in the faeces	Occurs in most countries where beef or pork is eaten undercooked. Rare in North-West Europe. Basic hygienic precautions. Exclusion of cases of pork tapeworm in risk groups 1–4 (see Box 2.2.1) until treated. Regular deworming of pets.
Dwarf tapeworm *Hymenolepis nana*	Eggs excreted in human faeces are infectious. May spread faeco-orally or via contaminated food. May be auto-infection.	Asymptomatic or mild abdominal discomfort. May be anorexia, dizziness, diarrhoea.	Identification of characteristic eggs in faeces.	Occurs in Asia, South-East Europe, Africa, Latin America. Occasionally found in institutions or the immunocompromised. Basic hygiene precautions. Exclusion of risk groups 1–4 until treated.
Fish tapeworm *Diphyllobothrium latum*	Acquired by eating undercooked fish.	Causes B$_{12}$ deficiency.	Identification of eggs in faeces.	Consider screening household. Worldwide, rare in North-West Europe. Avoid raw, smoked or undercooked fish.

(*Continued p. 268*)

Table 3.91.1c Tapeworms (cestodes)

Disease and organism	Mode of transmission	Clinical	Investigation	Epidemiology and public health action
Cysticercosis Due to the pork tapeworm (*Taenia solium*)	If eggs excreted by a human carrier of the pork tapeworm are ingested, the cysticerci preferentially settle in skeletal muscle and central nervous system, where they act as space-occupying lesions.	Clinical features may include epilepsy, raised intracranial pressure and chronic basal meningitis.	Diagnosis has been much advanced by modern imaging techniques, which may be supported by serology or by evidence of cysticerci in other tissues. Definitive identification of parasite segments and eggs, and serology is available from reference laboratory	Cysticercosis occurs in most countries where beef or pork is eaten undercooked and person-to-person transmission occurs. Rare in North-West Europe. Hydatid is found in most sheep and cattle raising parts of the world. Treatment of Hydatid disease and Cysticercosis should be undertaken by specialists. Poor hygiene and close contact with infected animals and ingestion of undercooked infected meat are all risk factors.
Hydatid disease Due to the dog tapeworm *Echinococcus granulosus*, or *E. multilocularis*	Humans acquire hydatid cysts, the metacestodes of *Echinococcus sp.* by ingesting eggs excreted in the faeces of an infected dog.	The most common sites for hydatid cysts are liver, lung and bone. The cysts expand slowly over several years. Occasional leaks may cause hypersensitivity phenomena such as generalised urticaria and can seed further cysts at distant sites. Symptoms are most often due to the mass effect of the lesion.	An appropriate imaging technique, such as ultrasound of the abdomen, will reveal the diagnosis, and may be supported by serology.	
Sparganosis Infection by larvae of *Spirometra* tapeworm *Spirometra*	Exposure to contaminated water or to flesh of an infected frog used as poultice (South-East Asia).	Larvae develop into cysts in subcutaneous tissue.	Microscopy of lesion.	Avoid frog poultices. Water sanitation.

Table 3.91.1d Flukes (trematodes)

Disease and organism	Mode of transmission	Clinical	Investigation	Epidemiology and public health action
Schistosomiasis, Bilharzia, Swimmers' itch Blood flukes, *Schistosoma haematobium*, *S. mansoni*, *S. japonicum*	Contact with water (swimming, wading) containing infected snails and hence cercariae which penetrate the skin and enter the bloodstream. Maturation takes place in mesenteric or portal veins. Eggs are laid into the blood vessels and erode through the wall to be excreted,	Acute systemic illness (Katayama fever) may manifest 2–6 weeks after exposure. Pruritic rash. May present as an 'outbreak'. *S. mansoni* and *S. japonicum* mature in mesenteric veins, causing intestinal disease and eggs in the faeces; *S. haematobium* in veins draining the bladder and causes cystitis and eggs in the urine. Chronic infection can produce malignancy.	Stool/urine examination. Rectal snip. ELISA.	Africa, Middle East South America, Asia. Remove snail breeding sites. Reduce exposure to contaminated water. Proper disposal of faeces, urine. Identify exposure to contaminated bathing site.
Lung fluke *Paragonimus westermani*	Eating uncook crustacea (prawns), crabs.	Cough, wheeze.	Sputum examination.	Asia, South America.
Liver fluke *Fasciola hepatica*	Eating contaminated water plants.	Fluke may obstruct biliary ducts.	Stool examination.	
Oriental liver fluke Chlonorchiasis *Chlonorchis senensis*	Eating undercooked or raw fish.	Chronic liver disease. Cholangiocarcinoma.	Stool/duodenal aspirate examination for eggs.	South-East Asia, China. Cook fish, educate public.
Intestinal flukes *Fasciolopsis buski* There are large numbers of intestinal flukes fasciolipsis is shown as an exemplar.	Eggs in human faeces contaminate fresh water. These hatch into miracidia which infect snails. A maturation cycle produces cercariae which encyst on plants which are consumed by humans.	Most infected people are asymptomatic. Large numbers of worms provoke mucous discharge and may cause obstruction. Mucosal damage causes complications.	Eggs in faeces.	Endemic in Far East, South-East Asia.

3.91.2 Other protozoal diseases

For *Entamoeba* (amoebiasis) see Chapter 3.1; for *Cryptosporidium* see Chapter 3.18; for *Cyclospora* see Chapter 3.19; for *Giardia* see Chapter 3.27; for *Plasmodium* (malaria) see Chapter 3.48; for *Toxoplasma* see Chapter 3.79; and for *Trichomonas* see Chapter 2.7.

Leishmaniasis

Leishmania are flagellate protozoan parasites transmitted by the bite of sand flies. Cutaneous leishmaniasis is the most common form of disease, visceral leishmaniasis occurs when parasites have migrated to vital organs.

There are a number of species of *Leishmania*, these include the *Leishmania donovani* complex; the *L. mexicana* complex; *L. tropica*; *L. major*; *L. aethiopica*; and the subgenus *Viannia*. The different species are not distinguishable morphologically and can be differentiated by DNA sequence or monoclonal antibodies (Table 3.91.2a).

Trypanosomiasis

There are three trypanosomes pathogenic to humans: the causes of African trypanosomiasis, *T. brucei gambiense* and *T. brucei rhodesiense*, and *T. cruzi*, the cause of South American trypanosomiasis (Table 3.91.2b).

Babesiosis

Infection with bovine or rodent *Babesia* spp., which cause a malaria-like illness (Table 3.91.2c).

Table 3.91.2a Leishmaniasis

Incubation period	Cutaneous : a few days to more than 6 months. Visceral: usually 2–4 months, may be prolonged.
Infectious period	As long as there are parasites present, this may be many years. Person-to-person spread is reported.
Epidemiology	Tropical and subtropical areas of the Mediterranean, Middle East, Indian subcontinent. Mucocutaneous disease is found in South America.
Clinical	Cutaneous: the lesions begin as a small itching papule with increasing infiltration of the dermis. The lesion becomes crusted which, when scratched, produces a shallow discharging ulcer. Mucocutaneous (espundia): progressive involvement of destructive cutaneous lesions. Visceral (kala azar): a primary lesion resembling cutaneous leishmaniasis may occur. The onset is usually insidious. Patients present with anorexia, malaise and weight loss, and may complain of abdominal discomfort due to splenic enlargement. Anaemia and cachexia are present and the liver and spleen are enlarged. Fever is intermittent and undulant with often two spikes in 1 day. Untreated patients undergo a slow decline and die usually from secondary infections after about 2 years.
Investigation	Amastigotes of *Leishmaniasis donovani* may be found by direct microscopy of slit skin smears (cutaneous disease), bone marrow or splenic aspirate. Occasionally, amastigotes may be demonstrated in the buffy coat cells.
Mode of transmission and public health action	Transmitted to humans by the bite of a sand fly. Infective blood meals may come from another human or an animal reservoir host. This may be a dog or rodent, depending on the species of *Leishmania*. Measures to break transmission cycle. Cover the cutaneous lesion. No isolation required. Rare direct person-to-person spread.

Table 3.91.2b Trypanosomiasis

Disease and organism	African trypanosomiasis. *Trypanosoma brucei gambiense.* *Trypanosoma brucei rhodesiense.*	South American trypanosomiasis Chagas' disease *Trypanosoma cruzi*
Incubation period	*T.b. gambiense*: few days to months *T.b. rhodesiense:* few days to 2–3 weeks	1–2 weeks for acute disease. Many years for chronic
Epidemiology	Estimated 40,000 deaths a year. *T.b. gambiense*: West and Central Africa, river and lakeside areas. Humans are the main reservoir. *T.b. rhodesiense:* Southern and Eastern Africa, wild antelope (particularly the bushbuck) is reservoir.	Estimates of 16 million people infected and 50,000 deaths a year in South America.
Clinical	*T.b. gambiense*: chronic course and can last several years. *T.b. rhodesiense:* acute, untreated infection can cause death in a few months and usually before 1 year. Initial sign is a papule that develops into an indurated nodule (chancre) at the bite site. The diagnosis should be suspected in a patient with fever and lymphadenopathy who has recently resided in an endemic area. Death occurs as a result of encephalitis, which may be insidious.	In many instances acute infection is asymptomatic or unrecognised. A local inflammatory reaction at the site of the bite with regional lymphadenopathy, generalized adenopathy and hepatomegaly may also be found. Acute infection is complicated by myocarditis in about 15% of cases, and most deaths are due to this complication. The latent stage follows and this asymptomatic period may last for up to 25 years. The final stage, Chagas' disease, is characterised by cardiomyopathy and intractable congestive cardiac failure.
Investigation	Parasites may be demonstrated by Giemsa-stained films of the peripheral blood during the early stages of infection, in the CSF, and sometimes in a lymph node aspirate. Serological tests are largely useful for screening, the wb-CATT may be useful in diagnosis.	Examination of peripheral blood for parasites. Parasites may be concentrated by centrifugation and lysis of the red cells. *T. cruzi* may be cultured *in vitro* or in mice. In xenobiotic culture laboratory-reared triatomid bugs are fed on the patient with suspected disease. After 30 days trypomastigotes are sought in the insect's gut. An antibody ELISA is available, this is most useful in excluding Chagas' disease in those from endemic areas and in sero-epidemiological surveys. PCR may be available.
Mode of transmission and public health action	Bite of the tsetse fly Elimination of the tsetse flies. There are no control implications outside endemic areas. No person-to-person spread.	Infective organisms, excreted in the faeces of biting triatomid bugs, living in cracks in poorly constructed houses, are inoculated into the bite when the victim scratches. Transfusion of blood and blood products may cause transmission. Improve the quality of housing construction. Spraying houses with residual insecticide. No control implications outside endemic areas. No person-to-person spread.

Table 3.91.2c Babesiosis

Incubation period	1–4 weeks, may be up to 9 weeks
Epidemiology	USA (Long Island, Massachusetts), Ireland, UK, France, Japan, Korea, China, Mexico, South Africa and Egypt.
Clinical	Most cases are asymptomatic or mild fever. May be similar to malaria, with fever, chills and severe haemolytic anemia with organ failure. Splenectomised patients are at increased risk.
Investigation	Blood film, PCR.
Mode of transmission and public health action	Tick-bite. Similar transmission and epidemiology to Lyme disease and ehrlichiosis. Transfusion associated. Avoid tick bites.

3.91.3 Fungi and actinomycetes

For ringworm (tinea) see Chapter 3.65.

Fungal infection can be broadly classified according to the site of infection.
• Superficial mycoses: confined to the hair, nails and outer layers of skin.
• Subcutaneous mycoses: confined to the subcutaneous tissue and rarely spread systemically; usually caused by soil organisms which gain entry through trauma.
• Systemic mycoses: involve organs and may be disseminated.

Life-threatening fungal infection has increased due to the rising prevalence of immunocompromise, resulting from disease (HIV, cancers) or immunosuppressive treatments (particularly due to opportunistic mycoses, fungi of low inherent virulence) (Table 3.91.3a). In addition, changing patterns of behaviour are bringing larger populations in contact with potentially pathogenic fungi such as in the South West USA.

Investigation and treatment of serious fungal disease is complex and should be undertaken in collaboration with an infectious disease specialist/microbiologist. Further information is available from http://www.idsociety.org/content.aspx?id=9200 and www.doctorfungus.org.

3.91.4 Rare viruses

Person-to-person spread is rare with these viruses; however, it may occur in some of them (e.g. monkeypox). Public health action comprises identifying the mode of transmission and reducing exposure (Table 3.91.4a). Expert advice should be sought.

3.91.5 Bites, stings and venoms

Epidemiology

Although Western Europe has few indigenous venomous species, the pet trade has increased the likelihood of exposure to exotic animals that may bite or sting.

Bites

Human, dog and cat

These bites frequently become infected. The bite should be cleaned and dead tissue removed. Infecting organisms are usually derived from the oral flora; these may include streptococci, *Pasteurella* and anaerobes. Antibiotics covering the likely organisms should be given if there is evidence of infection. Consider rabies if any possibility of bat bite or exposure to imported animal.

Table 3.91.3a Fungal infections

Disease, organism, epidemiology, investigation and public health relevance	Clinical
Actinomycosis *Actinomyces israelii* Actinomycetes are bacteria formerly classified with fungi as they can be grown on fungal media and form long branching chains. Species of *Actinomyces* are amongst the causes of mycetoma (see below) Occurrence: worldwide Investigation: microscopy. Identify sulphur granules. Transmission: endogenous organism. Public health relevence: none.	A chronic suppurative, granulomatous disease. May present with jaw, tooth abscess, abscesses may also be found in the thorax and abdomen. Lesion often drains pus.
Aspergillosis *Aspergillus fumigatus, A. flavus* Occurrence: worldwide Incubation period: days to weeks. Investigation: serum precipitins, microscopy of sputum. Culture confirmation. Galactomannan antigen positivity. Transmission: inhalation of organism found in damp hay, decaying vegetation, soil, household dust, building materials, ornamental plants, food and water. Public health relevance: clusters may occur where the immunocompromised are gathered together. Environmental investigation should be carried out to determine the source. Nosocomial infection may be associated with dust exposure during building renovation. Occasional outbreaks of cutaneous infection traced to contaminated biomedical devices.	Chronic pulmonary disease. Invasive disease in the immunocompromised, most frequently involves the lungs and sinuses. May disseminate and involve brain, bones and other organs. Also causes allergic sinusitis and allergic bronchopulmonary disease. If severe granulocytopenia persists, mortality rate can be very high (up to 100% in patients with cerebral abscesses). Patient outcome depends on resolution of granulocytopaenia and early institution of effective antifungal drug therapy.
Blastomycosis *Blastomyces dermatitidis* Occurrence: Central and South-East USA, Central and South Africa, India, Near and Middle East. Incubation: weeks to many months. Investigation: microscopy, culture, serology. Transmission: inhalation, exposures to wooded sites and moist soil enriched with decomposing organic debris (farmers, forestry workers, hunters and campers at risk). Public health relevance: identify likely exposure – often not determined.	Picture similar to TB. Symptomatic infection (50% of cases) usually presents as a flu-like illness with fever, chills, productive cough, myalgia, arthralgia and pleuritic chest pain. Some patients fail to recover and develop chronic pulmonary infection or widespread disseminated infection (affecting the skin, bones and genitourinary tract). Occasionally affects the meninges. Mortality rate is about 5%.

(Continued p. 274)

Table 3.91.3a (*Continued*)

Disease, organism, epidemiology, investigation and public health relevance	Clinical
Candidiasis *Candida albicans* is the most common cause of candidiasis. Occurrence: worldwide. Investigation: microscopy and culture. Transmission: endogenous organisms. Public health relevance: none unless contaminated devices considered.	Candidiasis may be classified as superficial or deep. Deep: the alimentary tract and intravascular catheters are the main routes of entry for visceral candidiasis. The main predisposing factors are prolonged courses of broad-spectrum antibiotics, vascular catheters, cytotoxic chemotherapy and corticosteroids. Superficial: candidiasis of the mouth and throat, also known as a 'thrush' or oropharyngeal candidiasi or vulvovaginal candidiasis (VVC). Women with VVC usually experience genital itching or burning, with or without a 'cottage cheese-like' vaginal discharge. Males may have an itchy rash on the penis. Risk factors: pregnancy, diabetes mellitus, broad-spectrum antibiotics, corticosteroids and immunosuppression.
Chromoblastomycosis *Chromomycosis* Occurence: rural areas in tropical or subtropical climates. Investigation: microscopy. Transmission: implantation. Public health relevence: none.	A chronic localised infection of the skin and subcutaneous tissue following the implantation of the aetiological agent. The mycosis usually remains localised with keloid formation. Many different fungi may cause this disease.
Coccidioidomycosis *Coccidioides immitis* Occurrence: North and South America arid and desert areas. Incubation: weeks to years. Investigation: microscopy, culture, serology. Transmission: inhalation after disturbance of contaminated soil. Occupational exposure in farmers, etc. Present in pigeon, chicken droppings. Public health relevance: anti-dust measures in endemic areas. Risk groups: persons in areas with endemic disease who are exposed to dust (construction or agricultural workers and archeologists). High risk: African-Americans and Asians, pregnant women during third trimester and immunocompromised persons.	Symptomatic infection usually presents as flu-like illness. Some patients develop chronic pulmonary infection or widespread disseminated infection (affecting meninges, soft tissues, joints and bone). Severe pulmonary disease may develop in HIV-infected persons. Meningitis may lead to permanent damage. Mortality high in HIV-infected persons with diffuse lung disease.

Table 3.91.3a (*Continued*)

Disease, organism, epidemiology, investigation and public health relevance	Clinical
Cryptococcosis *Cryptococcus neoformans* Occurrence: worldwide. Investigation: direct microscopy with Indian ink staining; antigen detection is more sensitive. Transmission: inhalation of air-borne yeast cells, isolated from the soil, usually in association with bird droppings. Less common *C. neoformans var. gattii* isolated from eucalyptus trees in tropical and subtropical regions. Public health relevance: none.	Principally a disease of the immunosuppressed and occurs most commonly in AIDS. Initial pulmonary infection is often asymptomatic. Most patients present with disseminated infection, especially meningoencephalitis. Resembles tuberculous meningitis with subacute onset and similar CSF findings. Meningitis may lead to permanent neurologic damage. Mortality rate is about 12%.
Histoplasmosis *Histoplasma capsulatum* Incubation: weeks to years. Occurrence: North and South America (Ohio and Mississipi river valleys), Africa, India and South-East Asia. Investigation: culture, skin testing, serology. Transmission: found in soil and in bird and bat droppings. Infection is acquired by the inhalation of spores; spreading chicken manure and bat caves have been identified. Public health relevaence: identify likely exposure – often not determined.	Symptomatic infection usually presents as a flu-like illness with fever, cough, headaches and myalgias. Illness may resemble acute pneumonia, chronic, apical, chest infection mimicking tuberculosis or (in the immunocompromised) a fulminant disseminated infection. Asymptomatic infection is very common in endemic areas. Resolution may leave multiple miliary calcifications on the chest X-ray. Some patients develop chronic pulmonary infection or widespread disseminated infection.
Mycetoma, Madura foot, Actinomycosis *Madurella mycetoma* Investigation: microscopy, culture, biopsy. Public health relevance: none.	Localised chronic granulomatous infections with multiple discharging sinuses and slowly progressive destruction of underlying structures including bone occur in many tropical countries and are known collectively as mycetomas. They may be caused by true fungi such as *Madurella mycetoma*, or by actinomycetes such as *Streptomyces somaliensis* or *Nocardia brasiliensis*. Organisms typically inoculated through the skin by thorns. After some delay, a painless swelling appears which subsequently breaks down and discharges pus. A network of sinuses and chronic inflammatory tissue extends over a period of months, destroying surrounding structures. Bacterial secondary infection commonly exacerbates the problem. The most common site is the foot. *Actinomyces israelii* typically causes multiple abscesses around the mouth, in the chest, or at the terminal ileum. Drug treatment depends upon the organism so microbiological diagnosis is essential.

(*Continued p. 276*)

Table 3.91.3a (*Continued*)

Disease, organism, epidemiology, investigation and public health relevance	Clinical
Mycotic keratitis Occurrence: worldwide. Investigation: slit lamp, microscopy. Transmission: may be iatrogenic. Public health relevance: investigate for contaminated contact cleaning fluid and iatrogenic transmission.	Corneal infection caused by fungi or yeast. The risk factors include trauma, contact lens usage, chronic ocular surface diseases, surgery and corneal anesthetic abuse. Fungal keratitis is a serious condition that requires prolonged treatment and close follow-up.
Nocardiosis *Nocardia asteroides, N. brasiliensis* Occurence: worldwide. Investigation: microscopy. Transmission: soil organisms. Endogenous in sputum. Public health relevance: none.	Causes severe systemic opportunistic infections, brain abscess and occasionally chronic chest infections in the immunocompetent.
Onychomycosis *Trichophyton rubrum* Tinea unguium, 'ringworm of the nail' The dermatophytes are the most common cause Public health relevance: none.	Onychomycosis refers to the invasion of the nail plate by a fungus. Infection may be due to a dermatophyte, yeast or non-dermatophyte mould. The disease is twice as frequent among men than women, and increases with age. Diabetics are about three times more likely to be affected. Immunosuppressed individuals are at increased risk.
Opportunistic mycoses Public health relevance: ensure there are no clusters associated with contaminated preparations, building works, etc.	Fungal infection is associated with immunosupression. Immunosupression may be due to underlying disease (e.g. malignancy, diabetes mellitus, HIV) or pharmacological. Fungi account for about 10% of all nosocomial infections in the USA. The most common reported were *Candida* spp. (85.6%), followed by *Aspergillus* spp. (1.3%). *C. albicans* accounted for 76% of all *Candida* spp. infections. Other fungal pathogens (e.g. *Malassezia, Trichosporon, Fusarium* and *Acremonium*) represented 11% of the nosocomial fungal pathogens. Fungal infection should be considered in all immunosuppressed patients with an unexplained fever. Diagnostic tests for fungi are improving; mycological advice should be sought early so that appropriate specimens are sent. *Candida* septicaemia in a transplant recipient or periorbital mucormycosis in a diabetic patient require prompt treatment if the patient is to survive.

Table 3.91.3a (*Continued*)

Disease, organism, epidemiology, investigation and public health relevance	Clinical
Paracoccidioidomycosis *Paracoccidioides brasiliensis* South American blastomycosis Occurrence: Central and South America. Incubation: up to 20 years. Investigation: microscopy, serology. Transmission: from soil. Public health relevance: none.	Chronic granulomatous disease of mucous membranes, skin and pulmonary system. Classic triad of symptoms: pulmonary lesions, edentulous mouth, cervical lymphadenopathy. Organism invades mucous membranes of the mouth causing the teeth to fall out. White plaques are found on the buccal mucosa.
Pityriasis versicolor *Malassezia furfur* Investigation: view scrapings under Wood's lamp. Public health relevance: avoid sharing of towels, etc.	*M. furfur* colonises oily areas of the skin, especially the scalp, back and chest causing characteristic discolored or depigmented lesions of the skin. Young people around puberty are most commonly affected.
Sporotrichosis *Sporothrix schenckii* Occurrence: found in sphagnum moss, in hay, in other plant materials and in the soil. Incubation: 1–12 weeks. Investigation: microscopy of swab, biopsy. Transmission: enters the skin through small cuts or punctures from thorns, barbs, pine needles or wires. Public health relevance: outbreaks have occurred among nursery workers handling sphagnum moss, rose gardeners, children playing on baled hay and greenhouse workers. Wearing gloves and long sleeves when handling materials that may cause minor skin breaks. Avoid skin contact with sphagnum moss.	Skin infection; people handling thorny plants, sphagnum moss or hay are at increased risk. Usually starts with a small, painless, red, pink or purple nodule resembling an insect bite. This appears where the fungus entered through a break on the skin. Additional nodules follow; these ulcerate and are slow to heal. Joint, lung and CNS infection have occurred but are rare. Usually, they occur in the immunocompromised.
Zygomycosis/Mucormycosis *Rhizopus, Rhizomucor, Absidia, Mucor* Investigation: microscopy, biopsy. Transmission: inhalation of spores. Public health relevance: none.	Invasive sinopulmonary infections such as the rhinocerebral syndrome, which occurs in diabetics with ketoacidosis, present with pain, fever, orbital cellulitis and proptosis. The palate, the facial bones and nasal septum may be destroyed. Mucormycosis (phycomycosis) is an infection caused by a fungus of the group Mucorales. The other common site of infection is the lung. Rarely, the skin and digestive system are involved.

Table 3.91.4a Rare potentially imported viral infections

Viral species	Infection	Clinical	Incubation period	Vector/transmission	Geographical spread
Arenaviridae	Venezuelan (Guanarito virus), Argentine (Junin virus), Bolivian (Machupo virus) haemorrhagic fevers	Fever, prostration and haemorrhagic features	7–16 days	Wild rodents	South America
	Lujo virus	Fever, prostration and haemorrhagic features		Unknown	South Africa
	Lymphocytic choriomeningitis	Meningoencephalitis	8–13 days	Common house mouse, hamster, cell lines	USA, South America, Europe
Bunyaviridae	Bunyamwera virus	Fever, headache, non-specific	3–12 days	Midge	All continents except Australia and Antarctica
	Oropouche	Fever, headache, non-specific	3–12 days	Midge	Central and South America
	Phleboviruses: Sandfly fever	Fever, headache, non-specific	3–12 days	*Phlebotomus* flies and mosquitoes	Africa and some parts of Asia and Mediterranean
	Rift Valley fever	Fever, haemorrhagic features	3–12 days	Handling animal tissues	Central Asia, Africa
	California encephalitis	Meningo-encephalitis	5–15 days	Mosquito	Midwest USA
	LaCrosse virus				
Flaviviridae	Powassan encephalitis	Fever, encephalitis	7–14 days	Tick-borne (*Ixodes*)	USA, Canada, Russia
	Russian spring–summer encephalitis	Fever, encephalitis	7–14 days	Tick-borne (*Ixodes*)	Russia
	Louping ill	Fever, encephalitis	7–14 days	Tick-borne (*Ixodes*)	UK
	St. Louis encephalitis	Encephalitis, hepatitis	5–15 days	Mosquito	Americas
	Omsk haemorrhagic fever (OHF)	Fever, diarrhoea, vomiting, haemorrhage	3–8 days	Tick bite	OHF: Far East
	Kyasanur Forest disease (KFD)				KFD: Far East, particularly India
	Alkhurma haemorrhagic fever (AHD)				AHD: Saudi Arabia
	West Nile fever	Fever, meningism	3–12 days	Mosquito	USA, Eastern Europe, Eastern Mediterranean
	Zika virus	Fever, conjunctivitis, arthralgia	2–4 days	Mosquito	Africa, South-East Asia, Micronesia

Family	Virus	Disease/symptoms	Incubation	Host	Geographic location
Paramyxoviridae	Hendra virus	High fever, myalgia, respiratory disease, encephalitis	4–18 days	Horses	Australia
	Nipah virus			Pigs, Fruitbats	Malaysia
Poxviridae	Monkeypox	Fever, rash, similar to smallpox	c. 12 days	Monkeys, squirrels, prairie dogs	Central Africa
	Cowpox	Cutaneous pustules		Cats, rodents	Unclear
	Parapoxvirus orf (sheep and goats)	Cutaneous pustules	3–7 days	Sheep, goats, cattle	Worldwide
	Bovine papular stomatitis (cattle)	Milker's nodule			
	Pseudocowpox virus (paravaccinia virus)				
	American equine encephalitides (EE)	Fever, chills, encephalitis	5–15 days	Mosquito	USA and Canada (Florida only for EEE)
	Eastern EE				South and Central Americas (VEE)
	Western EE				
	Everglades EE (EEE)				
	Venezuelan EE (VEE)				
Togaviridae	Barmah Forest	Fever arthritis rash	3–11 days	Mosquito	Australia
	Ross River				Australia, South Pacific
	Chickungunya				Africa, South-East Asia
	Sindbis				Africa, Asia, Europe, Philippines, Australia
	O'nyong-nyong				East Africa

Venomous snakes

There are few venomous snakes in Europe; however, bites may arise from imported snakes. Venomous snakebites are medical emergencies; a poisons centre should be contacted. The symptoms and signs depend upon the species and size of snake, the volume of venom injected, the location of the bite (central bites tend to be more severe than peripheral) and the age, size and health of the victim.

The victim should avoid exertion and be urgently moved to the nearest medical facility. Rings, watches and constrictive clothing should be removed and the injured part immobilised in a functional position just below heart level. Tourniquets, incision and suction are contraindicated.

Attempts should be made to identify the snake so that the appropriate antivenom can be provided.

Spiders

Venomous spiders may be introduced as novelty pets. In the event of a bite every attempt should be made to identify the spider and a poisons centre should be contacted.

Other arthropods

There are a large number of other biting arthropods, mosquitoes, fleas, lice, bedbugs sand flies, horseflies; none of these are venomous. The lesions produced vary from small papules to large ulcers. Dermatitis may also occur. Bites can be complicated by sensitivity reactions or infection; in hypersensitive persons, they can be fatal.

Ticks

Ticks may transmit infection such as Lyme disease or relapsing fever. Ascending flaccid paralysis may occur when toxin-secreting ticks remain attached for several days. Symptoms and signs include anorexia, lethargy, weakness, incoordination and ascending flaccid paralysis. Tick paralysis may be confused with Guillain–Barré syndrome, botulism, myasthenia gravis or spinal cord tumour. Bulbar or respiratory paralysis may develop. Tick paralysis is rapidly reversible on removal of the tick (or ticks) and may require only symptomatic treatment.

Mites

Mite bites are common. Chiggers are mite larvae that feed in the skin, causing a pruritic dermatitis. There may be sensitisation.

Centipedes and millipedes

Some centipedes can inflict a painful bite, with some localised swelling and erythema. Lymphangitis and lymphadenitis are common. Millipedes can secrete a toxin that can cause local skin irritation and, in severe cases, marked erythema, vesiculation and necrosis. Some species can spray a secretion that causes conjunctival reactions.

Stings

Bees and wasps

The average person can tolerate approximately 20 stings/kg body weight. One sting can cause a fatal anaphylactic reaction in a hypersensitive person.

Stings may remain in the skin and should be removed. An ice cube will reduce pain. Persons known to be hypersensitive should carry epinephrine with them.

Scorpions

Stings from pet scorpions should be treated as potentially dangerous as the species may be difficult to determine. The victim should be observed. Information on antivenoms should be obtained from a poisons centre.

3.91.6 Chemical food-borne illness

Scombrotoxin fish poisoning

Caused by excess histamine, a consequence of inadequate refrigeration of tuna, mackerel and other fish, leading to diarrhoea, flushing, headache and sweating, sometimes accompanied by nausea, abdominal pain, burning in the mouth, tingling and palpitations. Onset is 10 minutes to 2 hours after consumption and symptoms usually resolve over 12 hours. Antihistamines may reduce severity. Histamine level of fish can be tested.

Ciguatera

Poisoning caused by eating fish contaminated with toxins produced by dinoflagellates and associated with fish caught in tropical reef waters. Ciguatoxin is very heat-resistant and not detoxified by conventional cooking. May occur in imported fish.

Gastrointestinal and neurological symptoms occur. Symptoms can last years with long-term disability or relapses.

Shellfish poisoning

Associated with consumption of filter-feeding bivalve shellfish or crustacea (e.g. mussels, clams, oysters, scallops and crabs) that have consumed toxin-producing algae, sometimes after 'red tides'. The various toxins can be measured in a specialist laboratory.

Paralytic

Caused by saxitoxins produced by certain algae. Causes neurological symptoms: dizziness, tingling, drowsiness and muscular paralysis. Severe cases may suffer respiratory failure and death. There may occasionally be gastrointestinal symptoms. Onset is 30 minutes to 2 hours after consumption.

Diarrhetic

Caused by okadaic acid and other toxins in algae. Causes diarrhoea, nausea, vomiting and abdominal pain, with onset 30 minutes to 12 hours after consumption. Illness lasts 3–4 days. Toxin may be detected in shellfish.

Amnesic

Caused by domoic acid, in addition to gastrointestinal symptoms can cause short-term memory loss and brain damage.

Neurotoxic

Caused by brevetoxins, causes neurological (slurred speech) as well as gastrointestinal symptoms.

Phytohaemagglutinin poisoning

Caused by inadequate preparation of pulses such as red kidney beans, butter beans and lentils. Causes nausea and vomiting, followed by abdominal pain and diarrhoea, with onset 30 minutes to 12 hours after consumption.

Mushroom poisoning

Due to cyclopeptides and amatoxins consumed in *Amanita phalloides* (death cap), *Amanita verna*, *Amanita virosa* and some *Galerina* and *Lepiota* species. Causes colic, nausea, vomiting and diarrhoea, which – after apparent recovery – may be followed by liver or kidney failure with appreciable mortality. The advice of a regional poisons centre is vital for both investigation and treatment.

Others

- Gastrointestinal illness caused by heavy metal poisoning (e.g. from food containers).
- Intoxication (alcohol-like) caused by mushrooms.
- Gastrointestinal, liver and renal illness caused by aflatoxins (e.g. fungal contamination of cereals).
- Neurological illness caused by pesticides.
- Puffer fish poisoning (Japan, Thailand).

Section 4
Services and organisations

4.1 Surveillance of communicable disease

The effective management of infectious disease depends on good surveillance, which has been defined as the continuing scrutiny of all aspects of the occurrence and spread of a disease through the systematic collection, collation and analysis of data and the prompt dissemination of the resulting information to those who need to know so that action can result. The account of surveillance in this section is based on the UK model but similar arrangements can be found in most other European countries.

Purpose of surveillance

• Surveillance allows individual cases of infection to be identified so that action can be taken to prevent spread.
• Surveillance measures the incidence of infectious disease. Changes in incidence may signal an outbreak, which may need further investigation and the introduction of special control measures.
• Surveillance tracks changes in the occurrence and risk factors of infectious disease and can indicate if sections of the population are at increased risk of infection as a result of environmental or behavioural factors. This allows specific interventions to be targeted at those groups.
• Surveillance allows existing control measures to be evaluated, and if new control measures are introduced, continuing surveillance will allow their effectiveness to be measured. A fall in the incidence of an infection may allow existing control measures to be relaxed.
• Syndromic surveillance or surveillance based on clinical case-definitions may lead to the identification of new emerging infections

of public health importance. Further formal surveillance of these new infections will allow the epidemiology of these infections to be described and will produce hypotheses about aetiology and risk factors.

Principles of surveillance

A good surveillance system consists of the following key steps:
• There should be a case-definition, which includes clinical and/or microbiological criteria.
• Cases of infection are identified from a variety of sources including reports from clinicians and laboratories. The case or an informant, who may be a relative, friend or medical or nursing attendant, is contacted by telephone, visit or letter, depending on the degree of urgency. A data set is collected for each case. The data that are collected depend on the nature of the infection. For all infections, the following minimum data set is usually collected: name; date of birth; sex; address; ethnic group; place of work; occupation; name of GP; recent travel; immunisation history; date of illness; clinical description of illness. For food-borne infections, food histories and food preferences may be recorded. For infections that are spread from person-to-person, the names and addresses of contacts may be requested, and for infections with an environmental source such as Legionnaires' disease, places visited and routes taken may be recorded. For some infections where intervention is required, additional data are collected. For example, in the case of meningococcal infection the names of close household contacts may be recorded so that chemoprophylaxis and immunisation may be offered. For rare or novel infections, or where there is a need to find out more about the epidemiology, an enhanced data set may be collected or there may be a request for laboratory data to confirm the diagnosis. An example of this is the serological confirmation of clinical

Communicable Disease Control and Health Protection Handbook, Third Edition. Jeremy Hawker, Norman Begg, Iain Blair, Ralf Reintjes, Julius Weinberg and Karl Ekdahl.
© 2012 Jeremy Hawker, Norman Begg, Iain Blair, Ralf Reintjes, Julius Weinberg and Karl Ekdahl.
Published 2012 by Blackwell Publishing Ltd.

reports of measles, mumps and rubella using salivary antibody testing.

- Data are recorded on specially designed data collection forms and collated in a computerised database. Increasingly, data may be entered directly into a database that may be accessed via an Internet website. Data may be downloaded from databases used for patient management.
- One of the first uses of the data is to ensure that the cases satisfy the case-definition. The database then allows analysis of the data and the production of summary statistics including frequency counts and rates, if suitable denominators are available. This permits the epidemiology of the infection to be described in terms of person, place and time and the detection of clusters of outbreaks. Local data can be shared and merged to produce data sets at national or even international level.
- Interpretation of the data and summary statistics leads to information on trends and risk factors, which are disseminated so that action can be taken. Dissemination can take place in a variety of ways. Increasingly, data are available online but may also be found in local and national newsletters and journals (see Section 5 for country-specific details).
- Feedback to local data providers is important. It demonstrates the usefulness of the data and creates reliance on it. This in turn will lead to improvement in case ascertainment and data quality. Local data may be sent to GPs, hospital clinicians, microbiologists, environmental health professionals and health service managers.
- There should be continuing surveillance to evaluate the effect of interventions.

Sources of surveillance data

A number of data sources are available for the surveillance of infectious diseases. Many cases of infection are subclinical. These cases can only be detected by serological surveys. Clinical infection that does not lead to a medical consultation can be measured by population surveys or reported to a telephone helpline. Cases that are seen by a doctor may be reported via a primary care reporting scheme or statutory notification system. Cases that are investigated by laboratory tests may be detected by a laboratory reporting system, and those that are admitted to hospital will be counted by a hospital information system. Finally, the small proportion of infections that result in death will be detected by the death notification system. When designing a surveillance system it is important to ensure that the most appropriate data source is utilised. For example, it is not sensible to rely on laboratory reports for the surveillance of pertussis, which is only rarely diagnosed by the laboratory. In England and Wales, the main routine data collecting systems are as follows.

Statutory notifications of infectious disease

All EU countries have statutory reporting of certain notifiable diseases: the system for each European country is described in the relevant chapter of Section 5 but since 2008 all EU Member States and EEA countries have reported data on communicable diseases to the European Surveillance System (TESSy), which is a flexible system for the collection, validation, cleaning, analysis and dissemination of data (http://www.ecdc.europa.eu/en/activities/surveillance/tessy/pages/tessy.aspx). Statutory notifications are an important way of monitoring trends in infectious disease, such as whooping cough, where the diagnosis is rarely confirmed by laboratory test. The list of notifiable diseases varies by country: the current list of notifiable infectious diseases in England and Wales is shown in Table 4.1.1. Any clinician suspecting these diagnoses is required to notify the proper officer of the local authority, who is usually the Consultant in Communicable Disease Control (CCDC) and the proper officer sends a weekly return to the Health Protection Agency (HPA) by e-mail and the data are collated and published on their website. New regulations in UK also require the notification of other infections (such as those caused by new or emerging diseases)

Table 4.1.1 Notifiable diseases example: diseases notifiable in England under the Health Protection (Notification) Regulations 2010

Rare infections	Common infections
Acute encephalitis	Acute infectious hepatitis
Acute poliomyelitis	Acute meningitis
Anthrax	Food poisoning
Botulism	Enteric fever (typhoid or paratyphoid fever)
Brucellosis	Haemolytic uraemic syndrome (HUS)
Cholera	Infectious bloody diarrhoea
Diphtheria	Invasive group A streptococcal disease and scarlet fever
Plague	Legionnaires' disease
Rabies	Malaria
SARS	Meningococcal septicaemia
Smallpox	Measles
Tetanus	Mumps
Leprosy	Rubella
Typhus	Tuberculosis
Viral haemorrhagic fever (VHF)	Whooping cough
Yellow fever	

or contamination, such as with chemicals or radiation, that may pose a significant risk to public health.

Laboratory reporting system

The other main source of surveillance data is from laboratory diagnoses and each country has a system to obtain the key diagnoses of interest. Although the data are usually of high quality, they are limited to infections for which there is a suitable laboratory test and infections that are easy to diagnose clinically tend to be poorly covered. Trends are difficult to interpret, because the data are sensitive to changes in testing or reporting by laboratories. In addition, because data are based on place of treatment rather than place of residence, denominators are not usually available and because negatives are not usually reported, neither the number of specimens tested nor the population at risk is known with certainty. In England, HPA laboratories, NHS hospital laboratories and private laboratories should be able to offer a full diagnostic service for all common pathogenic microorganisms. If the laboratory is unable to carry out the work, then specimens are forwarded to a suitable reference laboratory. Medical

microbiologists ensure that results of clinical significance are notified to the requesting clinician. In the UK, the 2010 Health Protection (Notification) Regulations also require diagnostic laboratories to notify the HPA within 7 days when certain causative agents are detected in human samples. Reports of micro-organisms of public health significance should also be reported to the local Health Protection Unit (HPU) so that public health action can be taken. This should be in accordance with previously agreed arrangements covered by a written policy. Typical arrangements for reporting to the CCDC are shown in Table 4.1.2. Ideally, results should be sent electronically within 24 hours but infections requiring immediate public health action should be reported urgently by telephone. The data set that the laboratory forwards to the CCDC and HPA will depend on the data that is included on the request form by the requesting clinician and is often limited. If additional clinical and epidemiological data are available (Table 4.1.3) then the inclusion of these data in reports from laboratories is welcomed. Data that is received by the HPA is collated, analysed and published regularly in the *Health Protection Report* which is available weekly on the HPA website.

Table 4.1.2 Laboratory reporting of infectious diseases to the CCDC: statutory list in England

Infection	Likely to be urgent?
Viral infections	
Viral haemorrhagic fever (CCHF, Ebola, Lassa, Marburg)	Yes
Chikungunya virus, dengue, Hanta	No, unless thought to be UK acquired
Viral hepatitis (all forms)	All acute cases and any chronic cases who might represent a high risk to others, such as healthcare workers who perform exposure-prone procedures
Influenza virus	No, unless known to be a new subtype of the virus or associated with known cluster or closed communities such as care homes
Measles	Yes
Mumps	No
Polio virus	Yes
Rabies virus	Yes
Rubella virus	No
SARS coronavirus	Yes
Varicella zoster virus	No
Variola virus	Yes
West Nile virus	No, unless thought to be UK acquired
Yellow fever virus	No, unless thought to be UK acquired
Bacterial infections	
Bacillus anthracis	Yes
Bacillus cereus	No, unless part of a known cluster
Bordetella pertussis	Yes, if diagnosed during acute phase
Brucella spp	No, unless thought to be UK acquired
Burkholderia mallei/pseudomallei	Yes
Campylobacter spp	No, unless part of a known cluster
Chlamydophila psittaci	Yes, if diagnosed during acute phase or part of a known cluster
Clostridium botulinum	Yes
Clostridium perfringens	No, unless known to be part of a cluster
Clostridium tetani	No, unless associated with injecting drug use
Corynebacterium spp	Yes
Coxiella burnetii	Yes, if diagnosed during acute phase or part of a known cluster
Francisella tularenis	Yes
Haemophilus influenzae	Yes
Legionella spp	Yes
Listeria monocytogenes	Yes
Mycobacterium tuberculosis	No, unless healthcare worker or suspected cluster or multidrug-resistance
Neisseria meningitidis	Yes
Salmonella spp	Yes, if *S. typhi* or *S. paratyphi* or suspected outbreak or food handler or closed communities such as care homes. No, if sporadic case of other *Salmonella* species
Shigella spp	Yes, except *Sh. sonnei* unless suspected outbreak or food handler or closed communities such as care homes
Streptococcus pneumoniae	No, unless part of a known cluster
Streptococcus pyogenes	Yes
Verocytotoxigenic *Escherichia coli*	Yes
Vibrio cholerae	Yes
Yersinia pestis	Yes

Table 4.1.2 (*Continued*)

Infection	Likely to be urgent?
Protozoan infections	
Cryptosporidium	No, unless part of a known cluster, known food handler or evidence of increase above expected numbers
Entamoeba histolytica	No, unless known to be part of a cluster or known food handler
Giardia lamblia	No, unless part of a known cluster, known food handler or evidence of increase above expected numbers
Plasmodium falciparum, P. vivax, P. ovale, P. malariae and *P. knowlesi*	No, unless thought to be UK acquired

CCHF, Congo–Crimean haemorrhagic fever; SARS, severe acute respiratory syndrome.

Reporting from primary care

Forty percent of the population consult their GP at least once each year and 30% of consultations will be for an infection. A number of European countries have surveillance systems that capture data from a sample of general practices. The data can be related to a defined population so that rates can be calculated for a selection of common diseases that are not notifiable, for which laboratory confirmation is not usually obtained and that do not usually result in admission to hospital. Primary care based systems are particularly useful in the surveillance of influenza and influenza-like illness. In England, the Royal College of General Practitioners (RCGP) Weekly Returns Service is a network of 100 general practices covering a combined population of 900,000 that collect data on consultations and episodes of illness diagnosed in general practice. This has recently been supplemented by a larger system based on routine computerised GP data (QSurveillance). Data from both these systems can be accessed via the HPA website.

Syndromic surveillance

The purpose of syndromic surveillance is to identify promptly an increase in symptoms

Table 4.1.3 Data to be included in laboratory reports when available (to CCDC/HPA in England)

Epidemiological features/risk factors	Clinical/syndrome features
Recent travel abroad, dates, places	Died
Country of birth, dates of arrival	Bacteraemia
Outbreak	Conjunctivitis
Hospital acquired	Bronchiolitis
Sexual orientation	Arthritis
Animal contact	Meningitis
Transplant recipient	Invasive
Blood recipient	Pneumonia
Vaccine status	Croup
Immunocompromised	Enteric fever
Pregnancy	Haemolytic uraemic syndrome (HUS)
Injecting drug use	Asymptomatic
Congenital infection	
Food source, vehicle	
Transmission (person to person, water-borne, animal, food-borne)	

in a population due to the early stages of disease that may be due to exposure to an environmental or biological agent. One such national system is based on NHS Direct, which is a nurse-led telephone helpline with 22 call centres in England and Wales. Data on 10 syndromes are collated daily. These include cough, cold and influenza, fever, diarrhoea, vomiting, eye problems, double vision, difficulty in breathing, rash and lumps. Significant increases in call rates may be due to the deliberate release of a biological or chemical agent but are more likely to represent seasonal patterns in common infections.

Hospital data

Data are available from hospital information systems on infectious diseases that result in admission to hospital. This is a useful source of data on more severe diseases likely to result in admission to hospital, although data are often not sufficiently timely for some routine surveillance functions.

Sexually transmitted diseases

See Chapter 2.7 and Table 3.39.2.

Death certification and registration

Mortality data on communicable disease are of limited use because communicable diseases rarely cause death directly. Exceptions are deaths due to influenza, AIDS and TB. However, not all deaths due to infection are coded as such, and data may not be sufficiently timely for all surveillance functions.

International surveillance

International surveillance data can be found on the website of the World Health Organization (http://www.who.int/en/). Surveillance is undertaken by individual European countries and summary data are available through Eurosurveillance, a multiformat journal (www.eurosurveillance.org). See also Chapter 5.2.

Enhanced surveillance

Many European countries have established enhanced surveillance systems for infections and hazards of particular public health importance. These systems may collect a more detailed data set from informants, they may combine epidemiological and microbiological data including genotyping or they may use multiple sources of data. In the UK, such systems have been established for meningococcal disease, tuberculosis, listeriosis, enteric fevers, invasive streptococcal infection, antimicrobial resistance, travel-associated *Legionella* infection, zoonoses, influenza, infections in prisons, outbreaks of infectious intestinal disease and water-borne infections and water quality. Often, the systems are discontinued once the recent epidemiology of the infection has been clarified.

Other sources of data

Data may be collected by organisations that do not have specific communicable disease control duties which is useful for surveillance of certain conditions. For example, the British Paediatric Surveillance Unit of the Royal College of Paediatrics and Child Health co-ordinates active surveillance of uncommon paediatric conditions. A reporting card is sent each month to consultant paediatricians in the UK. They indicate if they have seen a case that month and return the card. An investigator then contacts the paediatrician for further information. Conditions of infective origin that are under surveillance include HIV/AIDS, congenital neonatal infections, toxic shock syndrome and acute flaccid paralysis.

Other local reporting arrangements may include histopathology laboratories (for TB), haematology laboratories (for malaria), pharmacies, genitourinary medicine (GUM) clinics, chest clinics and drug teams. The CCDC should agree a local surveillance protocol, publicise case definitions and remind clinicians annually of their responsibility to report infections.

4.2 Managing infectious disease incidents and outbreaks

An infectious disease incident may be defined in one of the following ways:

• Two or more persons with the same disease or symptoms or the same organism isolated from a diagnostic sample, who are linked through common exposure, personal characteristics, time or location.

• A greater than expected rate of infection compared with the usual background rate for a particular place and time.

• A single case of a rare or serious disease such as diphtheria, rabies, viral haemorrhagic fever or polio.

• A suspected or actual event involving exposure to an infectious agent (e.g. HIV infected healthcare worker, white powder incident, failure of decontamination procedures).

• Actual or potential microbial or chemical contamination of food or water.

The first two of these categories may also be described as an outbreak. The control of an outbreak of infectious disease depends on early detection followed by a rapid structured investigation to uncover the source of infection and the route of transmission. This is followed by the application of appropriate control measures to prevent further cases. Outbreaks of infectious disease are usually investigated and managed by an informal team comprising epidemiologists (e.g. the local health protection team), microbiologists (e.g. a medical microbiologist from the local hospital or health protection laboratory) and environmental health (e.g. an environmental health officer (EHO) from the local authority). Consideration should be given to convening an outbreak control team to oversee management if:

• the outbreak affects a large number of people;

• it involves a serious infection;

• it affects a wide geographical area; or

• there is significant public or political interest.

A written outbreak control plan detailing the steps that should be taken is an essential requirement. Incident management may be more effective if an incident control room is established. Accommodation that can be used as an incident room within local authority or health premises should be identified in the outbreak control plan. In circumstances where there are likely to be significant numbers of enquiries from members of the public, for example during a look-back exercise following identification of a healthcare worker infected with hepatitis B, a dedicated telephone helpline may be established. Telephone helplines can deal with large numbers of people needing information, counselling or reassurance and they can be used for case finding. Setting up an incident room and telephone helpline are useful parts of an outbreak exercise or simulation (Box 4.2.1).

Detection

An outbreak will be recognised by case reports, complaints or as a result of routine surveillance.

An outbreak of haemorrhagic colitis due to consumption of cold turkey roll contaminated with Escherichia coli O157 was discovered when several people who had attended the same christening party were admitted to the infectious disease ward at a local hospital.

An outbreak of gastroenteritis due to Salmonella Panama infection due to the sale of contaminated cold meats from a market stall was detected when the local public health laboratory isolated this unusual organism from several faecal samples sent in by GPs from patients with diarrhoea.

An outbreak of food-borne viral gastroenteritis affecting people who had attended a wedding reception at a hotel came to light when affected guests complained to the local environmental health department.

An outbreak due to the common strain of Salmonella enteritidis PT4 was uncovered when environmental health officers questioned several people, initially reported as sporadic cases by clinicians and laboratories, with this infection in a

---

Box 4.2.1 Setting up an incident room and telephone helpline

The incident room
- Dedicated use.
- 24-hour access and security.
- Large enough for the incident team their equipment and files.
- Sufficient telephone lines.
- A dedicated fax machine.
- Computer with access to the Internet and e-mail.
- Access to photocopying facilities.
- Filing systems for storing all communications, minutes of meetings, notes of decisions, etc.

Helpline
- Decision taken by the outbreak control team.
- Part of the local emergency plan.
- A subgroup should take responsibility for planning and establishing the helplines.
- The group should include a public health physician; a person with the authority to make financial decisions; a telecommunications expert; administrative support.
- The purpose of the helpline must be clear.
- List of staff needed to staff the line.
- Needs of minority ethnic groups and the hearing impaired should be considered.
- Early liaison with clinical specialists to ensure that staff are properly briefed.
- Question and answer and frequently asked question sheets should be developed.
- Mechanisms to deal with unexpected calls or complex queries.
- Training to deal with obscene, silent or threatening calls.
- Staff may have to deal with anxious and distressed callers and should be properly supported.
- Facilities to call back may be required.
- Briefing materials and procedures should be reviewed regularly to identify any inadequacies.
- All calls should be logged.
- A minimum data set would include date and time of call; sex, age and postcode of caller; and the appropriateness of the call.
- Further data collection would depend upon the nature of the helpline.
- Headsets rather than handsets should be provided so that helpline workers can keep their hands free to make notes or use computer terminals.
- Media can be used to publicise the helpline.
- It can be difficult to estimate the number of telephone lines required; the limiting factor may be the number of people available to staff the lines. Most calls arrive in the first few days, so the maximum number of lines should be available at the start of an incident; excess lines can then be closed down.
- Calls can first be screened by an experienced person who then allocates them appropriately, or calls can be taken by a first-line person, who passes on difficult calls.
- Four-hour shifts are generally used, some may be able to do two shifts.
- A supervisor is needed for each shift to deal with briefings and administration and cover staff breaks.
- The hours that the helpline is open will depend on circumstances.
- It should include the evening so that those working shifts or with children can call (e.g. 08.00 to 21.00 hours).
- Hours may need to be adjusted to cope with anxieties raised by media coverage (e.g. keeping the helpline open until midnight if the issue is covered in the evening).
- An answering machine message giving the opening hours should be available when closed.
- After the incident the helpline should be reviewed; lessons learned can be recorded and a formal report prepared for the health authority.

Midlands town. They all reported buying and eating bakery products from a mobile shop. Further investigations revealed that custard mix used in the preparation of trifle had become contaminated with raw egg.

Systematic investigation

The reasons for investigating an outbreak are to identify and control the source of infection and route of transmission to prevent further cases, to identify others at risk, to prevent similar outbreaks in the future, to describe new diseases and learn more about known diseases, to teach and learn epidemiology, to address public concern and to gather evidence for legal action.

A systematic approach to the investigation of an outbreak consists of nine stages.

Establishing that a problem exists

A report of an outbreak of infection may be mistaken. It may result from increased clinical or laboratory detection of cases, changes in reporting patterns, changes in the size of the at-risk population or false positive laboratory tests.

Recent increases in the number of cases of tuberculosis after many years of decline may be due to increases in the size of certain population subgroups that are at increased risk of tuberculosis. These would include the elderly, the homeless and those who have migrated from areas of the world where the incidence of tuberculosis remains high.

An outbreak of cryptosporidiosis was due to false positive laboratory tests. The microbiology technician mistook fat globules for oocysts of the protozoon Cryptosporidium parvum in faecal smears.

Other pseudo-outbreaks due to laboratory contamination were recognised because cases, despite having identical microbiological results, had no detectable epidemiological links, inconclusive clinical diagnoses and were only reported by one laboratory.

Confirming the diagnosis

Cases can be diagnosed either clinically or by laboratory investigations. At an early stage it is important to produce and adhere to a clear case-definition. This is particularly important with previously unrecognised diseases in which proper definitions are needed before epidemiological studies can proceed.

In 1989, an investigation was started into an outbreak of atypical pneumonia affecting men of working age in the Birmingham area. Four weeks elapsed before the laboratory confirmed the diagnosis as Q fever and progress could be made with the epidemiological investigation. Cases of Q fever were defined as patients with onset of an acute febrile illness between 27 March and 3 July and a fourfold rise in titre of complement fixing antibodies to phase II antigen of C. burnetii, a sustained phase II titre of ≥ 256, or the presence of specific IgM on an indirect immunofluoresence test.

Immediate control measures

Control measures involve controlling the source of infection, interrupting transmission or protecting those at risk.

Case finding

In an episode of infection, the cases that are first noticed may only be a small proportion of the total population affected and may not be representative of that population. Efforts must be made to search for additional cases. This allows the extent of the incident to be quantified, it allows a more accurate picture of the range of illness that people have experienced, it allows individual cases to be treated and control measures to be taken, and it provides subjects for further descriptive and analytical epidemiology. There are several ways of searching for additional cases:

• Notifications of infectious disease.
• Requests for laboratory tests and reports of positive results.
• People attending their GP, the local accident and emergency department, hospital inpatients and outpatients.

- Reports from the occupational health departments of large local businesses.
- Telephone helplines, including NHS Direct.
- Reports from schools of absenteeism and illness.
- Household enquiries.
- Appeals through TV, radio and local newspapers.
- Screening tests applied to communities and population subgroups.

In a local outbreak of Salmonella Panama infection a fax message was sent to all microbiologists in the region asking them to report isolates of Salmonella Panama to the investigating team.

In the 1989 outbreak of Q fever local GPs were telephoned and local occupational health departments were contacted to enquire about cases of atypical pneumonia or unexplained respiratory disease.

Local public health teams and microbiologists can be alerted by fax or e-mail. In the past they have been asked to report cases of Legionnaires' disease associated with a Midlands industrial site, cases of meningitis associated with a university hall of residence and food-borne infection associated with hotels and social gatherings.

Collection of data

A set of data is collected from each of the cases. This includes name, age, sex, address, occupation, name of GP, recent travel, immunisation history, date of illness and clinical description of illness. Data should also be collected about exposure to possible sources of the infection. In the case of a food-borne infection this would include a recent food history. In the case of infection spread by person-to-person contact, the case would be questioned about contact with other affected persons. In the case of an infection spread by the air-borne route, cases would be questioned about places they had visited. It is preferable to collect these data by administering a detailed semi-structured questionnaire in a face-to-face interview. This allows the interviewer to ask probing questions which may sometimes uncover previously unsuspected associations between cases. Telephone interviews or

self-completion questionnaires are less helpful at this stage of an investigation.

In an investigation of a possible national outbreak of Salmonella Newport infection that was thought to be food-borne, very detailed questioning was undertaken about the food that had been consumed in the 7 days prior to illness. This included asking specifically what food items had been eaten at each meal. In addition, respondents were asked if they had eaten particular food items and if so where these had been purchased and the brand that had been purchased.

In the investigation of an outbreak of Legionnaires' disease thought to have an environmental source, cases were asked to indicate on a map the exact places they had visited in the 10 days prior to illness. In addition, they were asked specifically if they had visited particular locations that had been mentioned by other respondents.

It may be necessary to re-interview early cases to ask about possible exposures that are reported by later cases.

In the investigation of the Salmonella Panama outbreak, it was not until the seventh case was interviewed that the market stall was mentioned for a second time. The early cases were questioned again and all but one reported buying or receiving items that could be traced to this stall.

Descriptive epidemiology

Important data items on each case are summarised in a table often called a *line listing* in which each column represents an important variable and each row represents a different case. This format ensures key information on each case is available and allows updating and the addition of new cases. Cases are described by the three epidemiological parameters of time, place and person. Describing cases by person includes clinical features, age, sex, occupation, social class, ethnic group, food history, travel, leisure activity. Describing cases by place includes home address, work address and often travel. Describing cases by time involves plotting the epidemic curve, a frequency distribution of date or time of onset. This may allow the incubation period to be estimated which, with the clinical features, may give some clues as to the causative

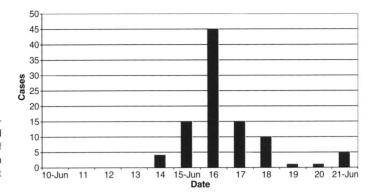

Fig. 4.2.1 Outbreak of *Campylobacter* gastroenteritis associated with consumption of unpastuerised milk at a boarding school (point source).

organism (see Table 2.2.1). The incubation period should be related to events that may have occurred in the environment of the cases and which may indicate possible sources of infection.

In a national outbreak of Salmonella Ealing infection, those affected were mainly infants. This suggested a connection with a widely distributed infant food. Dried baby milk was subsequently found to be the source of infection. A national outbreak of Salmonella Napoli infection affecting mainly children was found to be due to contaminated chocolate bars.

Figure 4.2.1 shows the epidemic curve that would occur in a milk-borne *Campylobacter* outbreak due to delivery and consumption of contaminated milk on one particular day (point source outbreak). Figure 4.2.2 shows the epidemic curve in a similar out-

break in which contaminated milk was consumed at the school over several days (continuing source outbreak). Figure 4.2.3 shows the epidemic curve in a community outbreak of measles where the infection is spread from person to person (propagated outbreak). There is a smooth epidemic curve with distinct peaks at intervals of the incubation period.

Generating a hypothesis

A detailed epidemiological description of typical cases may well provide the investigators with a hypothesis regarding the source of infection or the route of transmission. A description of atypical cases may also be helpful.

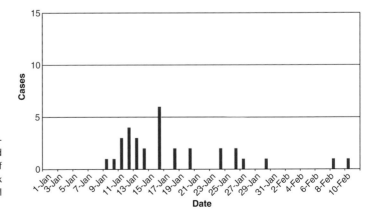

Fig. 4.2.2 Outbreak of *Campylobacter* gastroenteritis associated with consumption of unpastuerised milk at a boarding school (continuing source).

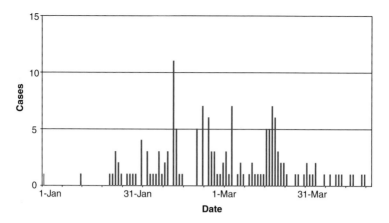

Fig. 4.2.3 Outbreak of measles in a community (propagated outbreak).

Testing the hypothesis

Finding that consumption of a particular food, visiting a particular place or being involved in a certain activity is occurring frequently among cases is only a first step. These risk factors may also be common among those who have not been ill. To confirm an association between a risk factor and disease, further microbiological or environmental investigations may be required, or an analytical epidemiological study may be necessary. This can be either a cohort study or a case–control study.

• *Case–control study*: a case–control study compares exposures in people who are ill (the cases) with exposure in people who are not ill (the controls). Case–control studies are most useful when the at-risk population cannot be accurately defined (e.g. when cases are laboratory reports of infection in the general population). Controls can be selected from a GP's practice list, from the primary care trust's patient register, from the laboratory that reported the case, from people nominated by the case or from neighbours selected at random from nearby houses.

• *Cohort study*: a cohort study is a type of natural experiment in which a proportion of a population is exposed to a factor, while the remainder is not. The incidence or attack rate of infection amongst exposed persons is compared with the rate amongst unexposed per-

sons. For example, following a food poisoning outbreak at a social gathering, thought to be due to consumption of contaminated chocolate mousse, the cohort (all those who attended) is divided into those who ate the mousse (the exposed) and those who did not (the unexposed).

• *Collecting the data*: a set of data are collected from both cases and control or from the exposed and unexposed persons within the cohort. A case-definition should be agreed and sample size calculation should be performed to ensure that the study has adequate statistical power. To avoid any bias the data must be collected from each subject in exactly the same way. Usually this is done by questionnaire. Unlike the hypothesis-generating questionnaire, the questionnaire for an analytical study is often shorter, more structured and uses mostly closed questions. It may be administered at interview, by telephone or it may be a self-completion postal questionnaire. Questionnaires should be piloted before use. If several interviewers are to be used they should be adequately briefed and provided with instructions to ensure the questionnaire is administered in a consistent way.

• *Analysis*: In both cohort and case–control studies initial analysis is by a 2×2 table. In cohort studies the ratio of incidence in exposed to incidence in unexposed is calculated. This is the relative risk. In case–control studies the odds of exposure in the cases is compared with the odds of exposure in the controls. This is the odds ratio, which usually approximates the relative risk. Confidence intervals for these estimates can be calculated and tests of statistical significance applied. Computer programs that will perform these calculations are freely available (e.g. Epi-Info). Where more than one exposure is associated with illness, multiple regression analyses can help eliminate confounding variables.

In an outbreak of cryptosporidiosis in Kent at the end of 1990, the hypothesis was that infection was associated with the consumption of cold drinking water supplied by the local water company. This was tested using a case–control study. Cases were defined as people living locally who had had a diarrhoeal illness between 1 December 1990 and 31 January 1991, with oocysts present in a faecal sample. Cases were excluded if they had travelled abroad or if an-

other household member had diarrhoea in the 4 weeks before the onset of their illness. The names and addresses of controls were obtained from the patient list held by the health authority. They were matched with the cases for sex, age group and GP or health centre. They were excluded if they had been abroad within 4 weeks of the onset of illness in their matched cases or if they themselves had diarrhoea since 1 December 1990. Five names and addresses of controls were obtained for each case. For each case and control a questionnaire was completed by a member of the investigating team during a telephone interview. The questionnaire asked about illness and consumption of various food items, including milk, salad, meat and cheese. Participants were also asked about the consumption of cold tap water both at home and outside the home, consumption of untreated, filtered or bottle water and exposure to recreational water. The results are shown in Table 4.2.1. There was a dose–response relationship with the quantity of tap water consumed.

Table 4.2.1 Cryptosporidiosis in Kent, December 1990. Odds ratios for exposure to select factors

	Case		Control			95% CI on
	Y	N	Y	N	Odds ratio*	odds ratio
Unpasteurised milk	0	29	0	80	N/A	N/A
Lettuce	16	11	51	29	0.83	0.31–2.22
Fresh raw vegetables	2	6	56	23	1.51	0.5–5.12
Unpasteurised cheese	0	29	10	69	0	0–1.15
Contact with farm animals	0	27	0	80	N/A	N/A
Tap water	19	7	33	47	3.87[†]	1.35–12.03[‡]
Y = >1 cup/day						
N = <1 cup/day						
Water consumed	15	10	23	51	3.33	1.18–9.49
outside the home						
Water filtered	0	29	8	72	0	0–1.57
Bottled water	0	29	16	64	0	0–0.63[§]
Swimming pool	5	23	16	64	0.87	0.22–2.87
Rivers	2	26	1	79	6.08	0.3–363

*The odds ratio is the odds of exposure in the cases divided by the odds of exposure in the controls. An odds ratio of 1 indicates no association.
[†]Consumption of tap water is nearly four times as likely in cases as in controls.
[‡]The 95% confidence interval (CI) does not include 1, indicating that this is a significant association that is unlikely to be due to chance.
[§]Controls are significantly more likely than cases to have been exposed to bottle water (i.e. there is a protective effect).

Table 4.2.2 *Salmonella* infection in a south coast hotel, Christmas 1988. Relative risk of infection for consumption of selected foods (significant items only)

Food	Ill		Not ill		Relative risk*	95% CI on relative risk
	Ate	Did not eat	Ate	Did not eat		
Chocolate mousse	66	2	21	14	6.07[†]	1.65–2.31[‡]
Lemon mousse	60	4	25	12	2.82	1.2–6.67[§]
Crème caramel	55	9	24	13	1.7	1.01–2.57[§]

*The relative risk (RR) is the risk of illness in the exposed divided by the risk of illness in the unexposed. A RR of 1 indicates no difference and therefore no association between illness and exposure. The relative risk can only be calculated for cohort or cross-sectional studies.
[†]Illness is six times more likely in those who ate chocolate mousse.
[‡]The 95% confidence interval (CI) does not include 1, so the results are unlikely to have occurred by chance.
[§]There are weaker but none the less significant associations between illness and lemon mousse and crème caramel.

An outbreak of Salmonella Enteritidis PT 4 infection affected a party of 136 elderly people staying at a hotel on the south coast of England over Christmas and New Year 1988/89. The hypothesis was that illness was associated with consumption of contaminated food items served in the hotel restaurant. This was tested with a cohort study. The cohort was guests and staff at the hotel. Cases were defined as members of staff or guests who had gastrointestinal symptoms between 23 and 29 December. All members of the cohort were asked to complete a questionnaire during an interview with an EHO, which enquired about symptoms and food eaten in the hotel. Attack rates for those who did and did not eat certain food items were compared and relative risks were calculated. Consumption of three food items (Table 4.2.2) were significantly associated with illness. All these items contained fresh egg, the presumed source of infection in this outbreak.

Further control measures and declaring the outbreak over

Once the source and route of transmission are known further control measures may be required. Surveillance to detect new cases and updating of the epidemic curve will allow the outbreak control team to set criteria for declaring the end of the outbreak.

4.3 Infection prevention and control in the community

Introduction

The community is defined as all settings that are outside major hospitals. Care settings in the community are those that provide health and social care and include community hospitals, care homes, home-care services, schools, nurseries and prisons. Other community settings are workplaces, leisure centres, hotels, restaurants, communal areas and individual homes. Many infectious diseases have the capacity to spread within community settings where people, some of whom may be particularly susceptible, share eating and living accommodation. In recent years the control of infection in community settings has become important because of an increase in the number of services providing health and social care in the community and an increase in the scope and complexity of the interventions that they provide. Community infection control services have developed in response to this. These comprise surveillance, investigation and risk assessment, advice, support and leadership on standard precautions, development and implementation of policies and guidelines, training, audit, advice on immunisation and decontamination, management of outbreaks and use of antimicrobials.

Administrative arrangements for the prevention and control of infection in the community

Prevention and control of infection in the community depends on joint working between many different agencies and individuals including the commissioners of health and social care services, the specialist health protection service, local health protection teams, care homes, GPs, hospitals and other independent providers of health and social care for adults and children.

Control measures for community infection

Control measures for community infection can be directed at the source of infection, the route of transmission, or susceptible people can be offered protection with antibiotics or immunisation. The measures may involve the person or case, his or her contacts, the environment and the wider community. Ideally, control measures should be evidence-based or at least based on consensus and best practice.

Person

The case is contacted by visit, telephone or letter and details are recorded on a specific case report form. Diagnostic samples may be requested (e.g. faecal samples in the case of suspected gastrointestinal infections). Control measures are based on an assessment of the risk that the case may spread infection. Guidelines are available to assist with this risk assessment. For example, with gastrointestinal infections the case may be assigned to one of four risk groups: food handler, health or social care worker, child aged less than 5 years, or older child or adult with low standards of personal hygiene. Factors such as type of employment, availability of sanitary facilities and standards of personal hygiene should also be considered. The case may be isolated until no longer infectious. The extent of this isolation will vary. Usually, isolation at home will be sufficient. However, strict isolation for highly infectious or virulent infections that spread by both the air-borne route as well as direct contact may necessitate admission to an infectious diseases unit. It may be necessary to exclude infectious cases from school or work. The case may be kept under surveillance, examined clinically or undergo laboratory investigations. He or she may be treated to reduce the communicable period or family and household contacts and medical and nursing attendants may be advised to adopt certain precautions to reduce the risk of transmission. Precautions that are advised to prevent transmission of blood-borne pathogens include advice not to share personal items, careful use and disposal of needles and other sharp instruments, careful disposal of clinical waste, safe sex and careful attention to blood spillages. Enteric precautions for gastrointestinal infections comprise use of gloves and gowns, sanitary disposal of faeces and nappies, attention to personal hygiene including handwashing, regular cleaning and use of appropriate disinfectants. The case may be advised to restrict contact with young children and others who may be particularly susceptible to infection. He or she may be advised not to prepare food for other household members. Advice should be reinforced with written material such as leaflets, or a video may be available. Legal powers are available (see Box 4.3.1 for national example).

Contacts

Contacts of a case of infectious disease may be at risk of acquiring infection themselves, they may risk spreading infection to others, or they may be the source of infection. It is important to have a definition of a contact and conduct a risk assessment. For example, a contact of a case of gastrointestinal infection is someone who has been exposed to the excreta of a case. With typhoid this

---

Box 4.3.1 Public health law: English example

In the UK the Public Health (Control of Disease) Act 1984 has recently been amended by the Health and Social Care Act 2008 to produce three new sets of Health Protection Regulations 2010 dealing with notification of infectious diseases and local authority and justices of the peace (JPs) powers and duties to take action to protect public health from infection or contamination, if this cannot be done by voluntary cooperation. Examples of local authority powers are keeping a child away from school, requiring a headteacher to provide a list of contact details of pupils attending their school and disinfecting or decontaminating premises or articles. JPs can make orders to control things, premises and people. For example, a JP can require that a person is medically examined, detained in hospital or is disinfected or decontaminated.

---

definition would be extended to those exposed to the same source as the case, such as those who were on the same visit abroad. A contact of a case of meningococcal infection is someone who has spent a night under the same roof as the case in the 7 days before onset, or has had mouth-kissing contact. Contacts may be subjected to clinical or laboratory examination. For example, in the case of diphtheria and typhoid, they may be offered advice, placed under surveillance, asked for laboratory specimens or offered prophylaxis with antibiotics or immunisation. In some circumstances contacts may be excluded from school or work.

Environment

In some circumstances it may be appropriate to investigate the environment of a case of infection. This may involve inspection and laboratory investigation of home or work. Examples are food-borne infections, gastrointestinal infections and Legionnaires' disease. Legal powers may be used to control the environment, including powers to seize, destroy and prohibit the use of certain objects. This may be necessary in the event of infection caused by a contaminated foodstuff. It may be appropriate to advise on cleaning and disinfection.

Community

The occurrence of cases of infection will have an effect on the wider community. For example, a case of Legionnaires' disease or tu-

berculosis may generate considerable anxiety in the workforce. Meningitis and hepatitis B will have a similar effect in schools on staff, pupils and parents. Scabies in daycare centres and head lice in schools are other examples. It is helpful to keep all sections of the community informed about certain cases of infection. This can be done by letter or public meeting. In some circumstances it may be appropriate to set up a telephone advice line or website. In addition, it can be helpful to inform local newspapers, radio, television and politicians. All sections of the community have information needs with respect to the prevention and control of infectious disease. Advice is available from a range of health professionals. This can be reinforced by leaflets, videos and through the media. In community settings such as schools, nursing homes, residential homes and primary care it is helpful to make available written guidelines on infection control in the form of a manual or handbook. These materials can subsequently form the basis for training and audit in infection control.

Prevention of infectious disease

Activity to prevent infection can be directed at the host or the environment.

Host

Risk behaviour may be changed by health education campaigns. These may be national or local, and may be aimed at the general population or targeted at those who are particularly at risk. Infections that have been the subject of national health education campaigns include HIV infection, sexually transmitted infections (STIs), *Salmonella*, *Listeria*, and *E. coli* verocytotoxin producing *E. coli* (VTEC) infection. Health services offer diagnosis, screening, treatment, prophylaxis and immunisation. Examples are routine and selective immunisation, services for tuberculosis screening, treatment for newly arrived immigrants and services for STI diagnosis and treatment.

Environment

Specified public agencies in most countries have legal powers to control aspects of the environment that could be a source of infection including supplies of food and water, disposal of sewage, waste management and pest control. In the UK, most of these powers rest with Local Authority environmental health departments. There are usually specific powers in relation to food safety; for example, in the UK, the Food Safety Act 1990 provides a framework for a range of regulations that govern the activity of food businesses, the composition and labelling of foods, chemical safety, food hygiene and the control of specific foodstuffs. The day-to-day work of enforcement is mainly the responsibility of Local Authority staff, but the Food Standards Agency enforces some regulations. Regulations and codes of practice place obligations on food businesses to ensure their activities are carried out in a hygienic way including arrangements governing food handlers' fitness to work. Staff handling food or working in a food handling area must report diarrhoea and vomiting symptoms to management immediately and managers must exclude staff with these symptoms from working with or around open food.

Measures for the prevention and control of infection in specific community settings

Specific national guidelines are available in many countries for control of infection in community settings. Foe example, the UK Department of Health has developed a Code of Practice for health and adult social care on the prevention and control of infections and related guidance. Under the Health and Social Care Act (2008) this is legally binding on NHS hospitals and care providers and will be extended to all providers of health and social care in 2010.

Box 4.3.2 comprises a checklist for the community infection prevention and control (CIPC) measures that should be in place in community settings. These settings include community hospitals, care homes, GP and primary care clinics, dental clinics, home care services, schools, nurseries and prisons. Other settings include tattooists and body-piercing premises, swimming pools and gymnasia. Not all these measures will be relevant for every setting.

Infection Control Guidelines for specific community settings and specific infections of community relevance

A range of manuals, handbooks and guidelines have been developed covering selected community settings. In addition, specific infections are of particular importance in the community. In some cases, international consensus guidelines are available from the European Centre for Disease Prevention and Control (ECDC), WHO and others and some of these can be found at http://www.ecdc.europa.eu/en/publications/guidance/Pages/index.aspx and http://www.who.int/rpc/guidelines/en/index.html.

Many useful community guidelines are available in the UK and these can offer guidance to professionals in other countries where local guidelines are not available. The key community infection control guidelines are as follow:

• Best practice guidance on the control of infection in care homes and clarification of roles and responsibilities is detailed in this recent publication from the Department

Box 4.3.2 Checklist for community infection prevention and control (CIPC) measures

- Clear management accountability for CIPC.
- CIPC is part of clinical governance and quality framework.
- Named person with operational responsibility for CIPC.
- Programme of policy review and updating, training and audit.
- Arrangements for seeking advice on risk assessment and application of appropriate control measures.
- Arrangements for surveillance, recording and reporting of cases of infection and outbreaks and incidents. Outbreaks and incidents should be reported to the Health Protection Unit (HPU). The HPU will advise what action is required. An outbreak may be defined as symptoms in two or more residents which may indicate a possible outbreak are cough and/or fever (e.g. influenza), diarrhoea and/or vomiting (e.g. *Clostridium difficile*/norovirus/food poisoning) and itchy skin lesion or rash (e.g. scabies).
- Handbook or procedure manual detailing.
    (a) Standard precautions: hand hygiene; and use of personal protective equipment (gloves, aprons, masks, eye protection).
    (b) Aseptic technique for clinical procedures to prevent contamination of wounds and other susceptible body sites (including minimising exposure of susceptible site, using a 'no-touch' approach if appropriate, hand decontamination, using sterile or non-sterile gloves as appropriate, use of disposable plastic apron, ensuring all equipment and materials are sterile, not re-using single-use items).
    (c) Safe handling and disposal of sharps.
    (d) Management of waste.
    (e) Managing spillages of blood, vomit, diarrhoea.
    (f) Collection and transport of specimens.
    (g) Decontaminating equipment and the environment including cleaning, disinfection and sterilisation.
    (h) Maintaining a clean and safe clinical environment including vaccine storage.
    (i) Laundry and linen management.
    (j) Placing patients with infections in appropriate accommodation including isolation.
    (k) Circumstances where droplet, air-borne or contact precautions are required.
- Arrangements for meeting the occupational health needs of staff.
    (a) Prevention of occupational exposure to blood-borne viruses (BBV) including prevention of sharps injuries.
    (b) Management of occupational exposure to BBVs and post-exposure prophylaxis.
    (c) Management of exposure to rash illnesses.
    (d) Health of pregnant staff.
    (e) Pre-employment assessment (TB, HIV).
    (f) Immunisation of staff (influenza, varicella, MMR, hepatitis B).
- Antibiotic formulary or equivalent to ensure appropriate use of antimicrobials.
- Information for patients, relatives, visitors and staff.
- Access to reference book or poster detailing the epidemiology and control measures for common infections of public health significance.

Box 4.3.3 *(Continued)*
• Guidance on specific procedures and practices such as that published by the Health Protection Agency, the Department of Health, the National Institute for Health and Clinical Excellence and professional bodies such as the Royal College of Nursing. This guidance covers management of urinary catheters, enteral feeding, peripheral and central vascular devices and respiratory support equipment. • Arrangements for responding to outbreaks of infection including reporting, closure of wards, departments and premises to new admissions, restrictions on visitors, staff absenteeism and business continuity planning.

of Health. Available at http://www.dh.gov.uk/en/Publicationsandstatistics/Publications/PublicationsPolicyAndGuidance/DH_4136381 (accessed March 2011).

• 'Essential steps to safe, clean care' provides a framework for community organisations to apply best practice to prevent and manage infections. Available at http://www.dh.gov.uk/prod_consum_dh/groups/dh_digitalassets/documents/digitalasset/dh_081719.pdf (accessed March 2011).

• GP and primary care clinics: guidance is available from the Infection Control Nurses Association (Rayfield, 2003). Dental clinics: guidance is available from the British Dental Association: http://www.udp.org.uk/resources/bda-cross-infection.pdf#search=%22infection%20control%20in%20dentistry%22 (accessed March 2011).

• Schools, nurseries: guidance is available from the Health Protection Agency http://www.hpa.org.uk/webw/HPAweb&HPAwebStandard/HPAweb_C/1203496946639?p=1158945066455 (accessed March 2011).

• Prisons should have a comprehensive written policy on communicable disease control, including an outbreak control plan. Guidance is available from Offender Health (a partnership between the Ministry of Justice and the Department of Health) http://www.dh.gov.uk/en/Healthcare/Offenderhealth/index.htm (accessed March 2011).

• Guidance is also available on the HPA Prison Infection Prevention Team website: http://www.hpa.org.uk/Topics/Infectious Diseases/InfectionsAZ/PrisonInfection PreventionTeam/ (accessed March 2011).

• Tattooists and body-piercing premises: under the Local Government (Miscellaneous Provisions) Act 1982 no person may carry out procedures that involve skin penetration (electrolysis, acupuncture, tattooing, ear-piercing) unless they are registered with their local environmental health department. Medical practitioners are exempt. Many local authorities publish guidelines. An example is at http://www.salford.gov.uk/piercinginfectioncontroladvice.pdf#search=%22infection%20control%20guidelines%20for%20tattooists%22 (accessed March 2011).

• The Health and Safety Executive has produced guidance related to body piercing, tattooing and scarification http//www.hse.gov.uk/LAU/LACS/76-2app.htm (accessed March 2011).

• In addition, trade organisations publish guidelines for their members. An example is Habia which serves the hair, beauty, nails and spa industries http://www.habia.org (accessed March 2011).

• Swimming pools: the risks of *Legionella* infection in spa pools are covered in http://www.hpa.org.uk/web/HPAweb&HPAwebStandard/HPAweb_C/1200471665170 (accessed March 2011).

• The Pool Water Treatment Advisory Group is an independent, industry group that publishes standards for swimming pool water treatment and quality http://www.pwtag.org/index.php (accessed March 2011).

• The Federation of Tour Operators has published guidelines for hotel swimming pool operators at http://www.fto.co.uk/assets/documents/fto_cryptosporidum%20Global%20V2.pdf (accessed October 2010).

• Undertakers and funeral homes: guidance on infection control for funeral workers (Bakhshi, 2001) and the infection risk from human cadavers can be found at http://www.hpa.org.uk/cdph/issues/CDPHVol4/no4/funeral%20workers.pdf#search=%22deceased%22 (accessed March 2011) and http://hse.gov.uk/pubns/web01.pdf#search=%22funeral%22 (accessed March 2011).

• Guidelines on the management of Panton–Valentine leukocidin (PVL) producing *S. aureus* at http://www.hpa.org.uk/webw/HPAweb&HPAwebStandard/HPAweb_C/1195733827175 (accessed March 2011).

• Guidance on methicillin-resistant *Staphylococcus aureus* (MRSA) for nursing staff is available at http://www.lesionicutaneecroniche.it/PDF/BIBLIOTECA/INFEZIONI/Wipe_it_out-MRSA-guidance_for_nursing_staff.pdf (accessed March 2011).

• MRSA Information leaflets are avalable for hospital patients at http://www.hpa.org.uk/webw/HPAweb&HPAwebStandard/HPAweb_C/1203496949853?p=1153846674382 (accessed March 2011).

• MRSA information leaflets are avalable for hospital patients at http://www.hillingdon.nhs.uk/uploads/MRSA_Advice.pdf (accessed March 2011).

• *Clostridium difficile* associated infection (CDI): http://www.hpa.org.uk/webw/HPAweb&Page&HPAwebAutoListName/Page/1179745281238?p=1179745281238 (accessed March 2011).

• CDI patient information leaflets: http://www.nnuh.nhs.uk/viewdoc.asp?ID=653&t=Leaflet(accessed March 2011).

• Head lice: updated evidence-based guidelines on head lice available at www.phmeg.org.uk (accessed March 2011).

Further disease-specific and non-community-specific guidelines are given in Appendix 2.

4.4 Healthcare-associated infection

Healthcare-associated infections (HCAI) are those that occur in patients or healthcare workers as a result of healthcare interventions. Hospital-acquired infections are those acquired during a stay in hospital. Most HCAI relates to hospitals although as more vulnerable patients are cared for outside hospital more HCAI may be seen in community settings. HCAI includes bacteraemias, urinary infections, chest infections, skin infections and surgical wound infections. The microorganisms that typically cause HCAI include MRSA, *Clostridium difficile*, Gram-negative organisms such as Acinetobacter, Enterobacter, Escherichia coli, Klebsiella, Proteus and Pseudomonas and Gram-positive organisms such as Enterococcus, Staphylococci, pyogenic streptococci and S. pneumoniae. Infections that are more commonly community acquired such as TB, norovirus and influenza can also spread in healthcare settings and may present management challenges. Most cases of HCAI are sporadic but outbreaks and clusters can occur.

Impact of HCAI

The emergence of HCAI as a problem is explained by the classic balance between host, agent and environment. Patients are more susceptible because of age and underlying conditions, organisms may be resistant to antibiotics, treatment is more invasive and more intensive and hospitals are busier. HCAI have an impact because they complicate other medical and surgical conditions, add to length of stay and treatment costs, cause anxiety and discomfort and may lead to disability and even death. HCAIs are a worldwide problem. In industrialised countries, since the mid-1980s, HCAI prevalence in hospitals has been stable at 5–10%. A 2006 survey found an overall prevalence of HCAIs in English hospitals of 8.2%. Patients with an MRSA bacteraemia spend on average an additional 10 days in hospital and for *C. difficile*, the additional length of stay is 21 days. The estimated additional cost of HCAI infection is £4000–10,000 per inpatient episode.

Risk factors for HCAI

Hospital patients with underlying disease, particularly the old and young and those with weakened immune systems are at greatest risk of HCAI. Invasive devices and procedures including surgery, pressure sores, intensive care, previous exposure to antimicrobial agents and previous hospital admission add to the risk.

Surveillance of HCAI

Most European countries have HCAI surveillance programmes. For example EARS-Net is the European Antimicrobial Resistance Surveillance Network, a Europe-wide network of national surveillance systems providing reference data on antimicrobial resistance for public health purposes. Voluntary surveillance schemes have been in place in England for some years based on laboratory reporting of alert organisms. Recently, mandatory schemes have been introduced for MRSA bacteraemia, *C. difficile* diarrhoea, glycopeptide-resistant enterococcal bacteraemia and surgical site infections.

Control of HCAI

HCAI is an indicator of the quality of patient care and HCAI incidents result in morbidity, cost and adverse publicity. Control of HCAI is an important aspect of patient safety and should be subject to strict oversight by health service managers. Control measures for HCAI comprise a range of activities which aim to prevent HCAI and limit the spread of community-acquired infection in healthcare settings. In a large US study, programmes of HCAI surveillance and control were associated with a 32% reduction in infection rates. In the UK, there is agreement that a 10–15% reduction in HCAI is achievable. Such a reduction would result in the release of considerable resources for use in other aspects of patient care. Control of HCAI comprises surveillance (Table 4.4.1.) and infection control practice (Table 4.4.2.). Evidence-based guidelines have been published on handwashing, use of personal protective equipment, handling sharps, care of urinary catheters, enteral feeding and care of central venous catheters. Guidelines, recommendations and summaries of best practice from a wide range of authoritative sources are available on nearly all aspects of the control of HCAI.

Management arrangements for the control of HCAI

Effective management arrangements are vital for effective control of HCAI. In the UK The UK Department of Health has developed a Code of Practice for health and adult social care on the prevention and control of infections and related guidance. Under the Health and Social Care Act (2008) this is legally binding on NHS hospitals and will be extended to all providers of healthcare in 2010. Overall responsibility rests with the hospital chief executive and hospital board and the Director of Infection Prevention and Control (DIPC). There should be an infection control team (ICT) comprising an infection control doctor (ICD), one or more infection control nurses (ICN) and clerical support. There should also be a multidisciplinary infection control committee (ICC). In acute hospitals the ICD is usually a medical microbiologist. Current roles and responsibilities for HCAI in England are summarised in Table 4.4.3. (see also Table 4.4.2.).

Table 4.4.1. Surveillance of HCAI

Surveillance	Examples
Laboratory-based surveillance of alert organisms detected in clinical specimens. Data should be collated using a computerised database to allow data retrieval and analysis. Weekly, monthly and annual totals and antibiotic resistance patterns should be reported. Infection rates may be calculated using appropriate denominators (admissions, discharges, occupied bed-days, days of device usage). Surveillance data should be widely circulated and discussed. An annual report should be compiled.	MRSA and other resistant *S aureus* *Clostridium difficile* TB *Streptococcus pyogenes* (Streptococcus Group A) *Streptococcus agalactiae* (Streptococcus Group B) Penicillin-resistant *S pneumoniae* Multi-resistant Gram negative bacilli (including ESBL *E. coli*) *Legionella spp.* Glycopeptide-resistant enterococci *Neisseria* spp. *Salmonella, Shigella or Campylobacter* *Escherichia coli* O157 Any unusual bacteria Rotavirus Norovirus Respiratory syncytial virus Varicella zoster Influenza virus Rubella Parvovirus Measles Pseudomonas aeruginosa Strenotrophomonas maltophilia (Xanthomonas maltophilia) Fungi: In special units, Candida species, Aspergillus
Other laboratory-based surveillance.	Blood cultures, CSF, vascular catheters, postoperative wound swabs, urine samples, etc
Surveillance by ward staff of alert conditions	Patient admitted with any infection Post surgical sepsis Diarrhoea or vomiting Diarrhoea with blood Cellulitis Tuberculosis (chronic productive cough) Exanthemata (acute rash illness) Chicken pox or shingles Mumps, measles, rubella, parvovirus Whooping cough Diphtheria Scabies Meningitis Viral hepatitis Pyrexia of unknown origin Typhoid and paratyphoid fevers
Targeted surveillance	Liaison with special units and wards (intensive care, oncology, etc.) or particular subgroups of patients to enquire about infections, incidents and outbreaks

Table 4.4.2. Control of HCAI

Infection control measures	
Developing and implementing policies and procedures Written policies should be collated in an infection control manual. Policies should be audited, reviewed and updated regularly Outbreak and incident control plans should be exercised if not in regular use	• hand washing • PPE • handling sharps • antibiotic usage • clinical procedures • disposal of waste • outbreaks and incidents • decontamination, sterilization and disinfection; • management of patients at risk of acquiring or transmitting infection • use of isolation facilities • management of specific communicable diseases • laundry • catering (including food hygiene) • domestic cleaning • mortuary procedures • engineering and building services (including Legionella infection) • equipment purchasing; • new building; • staff immunisation (hepatitis B, influenza, BCG) • other aspects of occupational health (sharps injuries) • operating theatres • transfer and discharge of patients; • pest control.
Staff training and education Carrying out audits	Induction Annual update • hand hygiene • clinical practices (isolation, protective clothing, catheter care) • environmental cleaning and hygiene • ward kitchen areas • waste disposal • sharps management • care of linen • decontamination of equipment.
Advice	• proposed building constructions • purchase of equipment and consumables • tenders for other services

Relationships between hospitals and community health services

HCAI may present after a patient has been discharged from hospital. Hospitals are responsible for passing relevant information to the GP and to community nursing staff who in turn should provide feedback to the hospital, both to the ICT and the consultant who has treated the patient, both for surveillance purposes and to alert the ICT when a potentially infected patient is to be admitted to hospital. Collaboration between community staff, the ICT and the CCDC is encouraged by the appointment of community infection control nurses.

Table 4.4.3. Example of roles and responsibilities for HCAI (England, 2010)

Department of Health	• Sets overall policy • Publish guidance • Provide expertise • Provide public information
Strategic Heath Authorities* Monitor *(independent regulator of NHS foundation trusts)	• Manages performance of NHS hospitals
Hospital Trust Chief Executive	• Ensure effective arrangements for HCAI • Core part of governance and patient safety • Promote low levels of HCAI • Appoint DIPC
Director of Infection Prevention and Control	• Oversee policies and work of ICT • Report directly to CE and board • Challenge poor practice • Assess impact of policies • Produce annual report
Infection Control Committee	• Endorse policies • Advises and supports implementation • Oversees work of ICT • Agrees annual programme and monitors progress
Infection Control Team	• 24-hour advice on control of HCAI • Annual programme of activity • Surveillance of HCAI • Audit of compliance with policies • Education and training
Modern Matron	• Champion importance of HCAI • Promote hand washing and hospital hygiene
Primary Care Trusts*	• Same responsibilities as acute trusts • Advice on infection control in community premises • Appoint DIPC, community ICN, set up ICC • As commissioners of health services ensure that hospitals have arrangements for HCAI
Health Protection Agency*	• Deliver national surveillance programmes • Monitor and assist in management of HCAI outbreaks
Consultants for Communicable Disease Control and team* (employed by HPA)	• Surveillance, prevention and control of infection • Management of outbreaks • Advice to PCTs • Liaison with ICTs • Epidemiological advice
Care Quality Commission	• Reviews infection control arrangements in Trusts

*Some of these bodies may be reformed as part of proposed changes to UK health services in 2010

Outbreaks of infection in hospital

Infectious diseases can spread readily within hospitals amongst staff and patients who may be more susceptible to infection as a result of illness or treatment. Despite high standards of infection control practice, outbreaks of infection or infectious disease incidents may occur.

Recognition of an outbreak

An outbreak is an incident in which two or more people who are thought to have had a common exposure, experience a similar illness or proven infection. Outbreaks in hospital are either detected by the laboratory or by nursing or medical staff. Cases of infection and outbreaks are reported to the ICT.

Action

Hospitals should have written plans for responding to infectious disease incidents. These should cover the following:
• Recognition of an outbreak.
• Circumstances in which the ICD or CCDC would take the lead.
• Initial investigation by ICD and ICN which determines whether or not an outbreak exists.
• If the outbreak is confined to hospital, whether it can be dealt with by the ICT or if an outbreak control group is needed. A major outbreak is one in which large numbers of people are affected, where the organism involved is particularly pathogenic or where there is potential for spread within the hospital and the community.
• The outbreak to be reported to appropriate authorities (e.g. Health Protection Agency (HPA) and Strategic Health Authority).
• If the outbreak is not confined to hospital the CCDC would be involved and the district outbreak plan would be implemented as appropriate
• Outbreaks of limited extent will be dealt with by the ICT along with the relevant clinicians and nurses.

• It would be usual for the CCDC to be informed, although he or she may already know of the outbreak through regular contact with the ICD.
• If the disease involved is statutorily notifiable, the medical staff responsible for the patient(s) must notify the CCDC.
• In any infectious disease incident where food or water is implicated, a local authority environmental health officer should be informed.

Initial investigation of a hospital outbreak

This should consist of the following:
• Collect information on all cases occurring on all wards and units.
• Establish a case definition; request laboratory tests.
• Ensure provision of medical and nursing care for affected patients, including appropriate precautions to prevent secondary spread.
• Consider antibiotic prophylaxis or immunisation if appropriate (not usually applicable for gastrointestinal infections)
• Consider catering arrangements, disinfection, hand washing, laundry, food samples, environmental samples and microbiological or serological screening of those at risk.
• If a food borne or water borne infection is suspected, the EHO will conduct an environmental investigation, including inspection of kitchen, food handling and storage practices, review of illness amongst staff, requesting faecal samples from members of staff if necessary, review of menus, waste handling and pest-control.
• Implement control measures, for example:
  (a) patient isolation/cohort nursing;
  (b) restriction of transfers and/or discharges;
  (c) staff education in infection control procedures;
  (d) clear instructions and information for ward staff, cleaners, etc.;
  (e) information to patients' relatives and visitors.

- Decide when the outbreak is over.
- Communicate with SHA, HPA and media as appropriate.

Community outbreak affecting the hospital

Hospitals should have plans for responding to a major community outbreak affecting the hospital. Major outbreaks of infectious disease in the community may place heavy demands on hospital services. Acute outbreaks developing over a few hours are generally toxin-mediated. Non-acute outbreaks, due for example to influenza, develop over days or weeks. The ICT role would include advising on the collection of microbiological samples and advising on any control of infection measures. The hospital may activate its Major Incident Plan and convene a an outbreak control group. The hospital response will involve clinical and managerial staff. Consideration should be given to: admissions policy; appropriate management of patients; opening up additional beds; consequences of staff illness; communications with media, community staff and GPs.

4.5 Antimicrobial resistance

Resistance to an antimicrobial is defined as the ability to multiply in the presence of concentrations of the antimicrobial higher than those found in humans receiving therapeutic doses. Resistance may be a characteristic of a particular species of micro-organism or may appear in strains of previously susceptible species. Micro-organisms naturally develop resistance to antimicrobials and all antimicrobials have the potential to induce resistance. The development of resistance is a consequence of mutation or gene transfer and there are various mechanisms that may result in resistance to other, even unrelated, antimicrobials.

Impact of antimicrobial resistance

Antimicrobial resistance leads to valuable treatments becoming ineffective, increases morbidity and mortality, complicates decision making and adds to healthcare costs. Outbreaks caused by resistant organisms may lead to closure of facilities. Bacteria, viruses, protozoa, yeasts and parasites can all exhibit resistance. The epidemiology varies by organism and antimicrobial. Problems may be confined to particular healthcare environments (e.g. *Acinetobacter sp* in intensive care units), widespread within healthcare environments (MRSA), geographically widespread but circumscribed (chloroquine resistance in *Plasmodium falciparum*) or worldwide (penicillin resistance in *Staphylococcus aureus*).

Risk factors for antimicrobial resistance

The prevalence of resistance varies in place and time, by organism and antimicrobial. The total consumption (not just inappropriate use) is the main factor in the development of resistance. Use that leads to inappropriate low level exposure such as inadequate dosage or length of treatment, poor adherence and/or substandard preparations may particularly promote the development of resistance. Inappropriate use of antibiotics adds to the burden of antimicrobial use without benefit to the patient and may expose the individual to adverse effects. As the major factor is antimicrobial consumption, the facilities most at risk are those with high rates of antimicrobial use and the individuals most likely to harbour resistant organisms are those with the most exposure to antimicrobials, particularly if inadequately prescribed.

Surveillance for antimicrobial resistance

Surveillance for antimicrobial resistance monitors changes in microbial populations.

Box 4.5.1 Surveillance methods for antimicrobial resistance

- Alert organism identification and tracking.
- Enhanced routine surveillance.
- Specific targeted surveys.

This aims to identify trends in resistance, the emergence of new resistance patterns and identifies outbreaks. The outputs of surveillance should aid clinical decision making, the formulation of prescribing and containment policy and the monitoring of interventions. In addition, surveillance data should alert practitioners to the presence of an acute problem. Tests for antimicrobial sensitivity are usually performed for patients who may have failed empirical therapy or have other complications. Therefore it is often difficult to draw robust inferences about the prevalence of resistance from microbiological data. A number of surveillance methods are commonly used in understanding antimicrobial resistance (Box 4.5.1).

Surveillance of antimicrobial resistance should be directed towards the organisms that are most problematic. For example, in hospitals, Gram-negative coliforms and MRSA; in genitourinary medicine (GUM) clinics, resistant gonococci; in chest clinics, resistant *Mycobacterium tuberculosis*; and in AIDS clinics, antiviral-resistant HIV subtypes (see also Table 4.4.1.).

Surveillance data for various organisms is available from national centres and from the European Antimicrobial Resistance Surveillance Network (EARS-Net), at http://www.ecdc.europa.eu/en/activities/surveillance/EARS-Net/Pages/index.aspx.

Control of antimicrobial resistance

The key tools for combating antimicrobial resistance are those of public health: surveillance to understand the extent of the problem and policy development and implementation for hygiene, patient management and antimicrobial use. Antimicrobial resistance programmes should reduce the burden of disease and the spread of infection through hygiene and infection control measures, ensuring access to and better use of appropriate antimicrobials, strengthening surveillance and putting in place appropriate policies and legislation. A key step for reducing the spread of antimicrobial resistance is preventing unnecessary and inappropriate use of antimicrobials (Box 4.5.2). Unnecessary use would be when there is no clinical indication (viral upper respiratory tract infection) and inappropriate use would be prophylaxis when there is no evidence of benefit. Effective infection control measures will reduce the need for antibiotics to be prescribed by preventing the acquisition of both sensitive and resistant organisms (see Table 4.4.2.).

The European Centre for Disease Prevention and Control (ECDC) has since 2008 organised a European Antibiotic Awareness Day (EAAD), which takes place in the week of 18 November every year (http://ecdc.europa.eu/en/EAAD/). EAAD is a platform for national awareness-raising campaign activities, which are now carried out in more than 35 countries.

Action in an outbreak caused by a resistant organism (see also Chapter 4.4).

- Collect information on all cases occurring throughout facility.
- Establish a case-definition; request laboratory tests.
- Ensure provision of medical and nursing care for affected patients, including appropriate precautions to prevent secondary spread.
- Consider sensitivity patterns and treatment options for those who require antimicrobials.
- Implement control measures, for example:
  (a) patient isolation/cohort nursing;
  (b) restriction of transfers and/or discharges;

Box 4.5.2 Key steps in an antimicrobial resistance control programme

Reduce antimicrobial use and ensure optimal use of antimicrobials:
• Develop and maintain guidelines for antimicrobial treatment and prophylaxis.
• Use alternative interventions, such as antiseptics, where possible.
• Reduce need for antimicrobials through vaccination, minimizing the time during which a patient is immunocompromised and minimise use of interventions that may introduce infection, such as catheterisation.
• Education of health professionals and patients.
Reducing the transmission of antibiotic resistance:
• Hand hygiene.
• Effective infection control measures.
• Consider isolation of colonized or infected cases.
• Consider screening of those coming from high risk areas.
• Develop early recognition of resistance through surveillance and rapid diagnostic techniques.
Information and leadership:
• Ensure senior level responsibility for effective oversight of antimicrobial resistance and antimicrobial prescribing.
• Establish surveillance of resistance and antimicrobial prescribing and ensure feedback of surveillance data.
• Become involved with public campaigns such as EAAD, an annual event usually held in November which aims to raise awareness on how to use antibiotics in a responsible way that will help keep them effective for the future.

(c) staff education in infection control procedures;
(d) clear instructions and information for ward staff, cleaners, etc.; and
(e) information to patients' relatives and visitors.
• Consider catering arrangements, disinfection, handwashing, laundry, food samples, environmental samples, and microbiological or serological screening of those at risk.
• Decide when the outbreak is over.
• Communicate with Public Health Authorities and media as appropriate.

4.6 Risks to and from healthcare workers

Healthcare workers (HCWs) are at risk of acquiring infection because of exposure at work.

They are also a potential source of infection for those they are caring for, particularly those with impaired resistance to infections.

HCWs are an important sentinel group. Unexplained illness amongst HCWs may be an early sign of an unusual or novel outbreak, as occurred with SARS.

HCWs can be considered according to the level of probable exposure to infectious disease risks. Target groups for preventative interventions can then be identified following a risk assessment based upon the likelihood of transmission (Table 4.6.1) and disease-specific risks identified and controlled (Table 4.6.2).

Lookback studies

Purpose

The purpose of lookback studies is to:
• determine those at risk of acquiring a communicable disease following an exposure, usually related to healthcare;

Table 4.6.1 Exposure categories for healthcare workers (HCWs)

Category I	Clinical and other staff, including those in primary care, who have regular, clinical contact with patients
Category II	Laboratory and mortuary staff who have direct contact with potentially infectious clinical specimens
Category III	Non-clinical ancillary staff who have social contact with patients, but not usually of a prolonged or close nature
Category IV	Maintenance staff (e.g. engineers, gardeners)

Table 4.6.2 Specific disease risks

Infection	Target group	Rationale	Comments
Diarrhoea	Category I	Personal and patient protection	Staff with diarrhoea should report to occupational health.
Diphtheria	Category I staff caring for patients with diphtheria Category II staff	Personal protection	National immunisation programme should ensure immunity. Category II staff should have immunity checked.
Hepatitis A	Category I staff working in institutions for patients with learning disabilities Category II laboratory staff who may handle the virus Category IV maintenance staff exposed to sewage	Personal protection	Immunisation may be offered following a risk assessment.
Hepatitis B	Category I and II staff with exposure to blood, blood-stained body fluids and tissues	Personal and patient protection	Immunisation may be offered to other groups of staff following a risk assessment.
Hepatitis C	Category I and II staff with exposure to blood, blood-stained body fluids and tissues	Personal and patient protection	See section on lookback exercises.
HIV	Category I and II staff	Personal and patient protection	See section on lookback exercises. Risk assessment to be undertaken, particularly if exposure to TB.
Influenza	Category I staff	Personal and possibly patient protection	Annual immunisation should be offered by occupational health service.
Poliomyelitis	All HCWs	Personal protection	National immunisation programme should ensure immunity.
Rabies	Those directly caring for rabid patients	Personal protection	Immunisation

(*Continued on p. 314*)

Table 4.6.2 (*Continued*)

Infection	Target group	Rationale	Comments
Rubella	Category I HCWs working in maternity departments	For patient protection	National immunisation programme should ensure immunity. HCWs in high-risk areas should have documented immunity.
SARS	Important for all Category I and II staff	Personal and patient protection	Ensure surveillance of HCW in contact with SARS patients is in place.
TB	Important for all Category I and II staff	Personal and patient protection	Staff without a BCG scar or documented BCG immunisation should be tuberculin tested and offered BCG. Staff should report possible TB symptoms promptly.
Tetanus	Category III staff at higher risk of tetanus-prone wounds (e.g. gardeners)	Personal protection	National immunisation programme should ensure immunity.
Varicella	Category I–III HCWs with patient contact, especial attention to those working in high risk clinical areas such as maternity and oncology	Patient protection Varicella-zoster vaccine recommended for all non-immune HCWs with patient contact (i.e. categories I–III)	Varicella-zoster vaccine now licensed in many European countries (incl UK). Varicella-zoster antibodies to be checked. Non-immune staff to be excluded from high-risk areas 7–21 days following exposure.

BCG, bacille Calmette–Guérin; SARS, severe acute respiratory syndrome.

- inform exposed individuals about the risk to which they have been exposed;
- determine whom, amongst those exposed, has been infected;
- prevent further transmissions and/or clinical disease;
- provide appropriate interventions (treatment, counselling, etc.) for those exposed, both infected and uninfected; and
- advance understanding about reducing and quantifying exposure risks.

Context

Lookback exercises are usually carried out following exposure or suspected exposure to blood-borne viruses (hepatitis B, hepatitis C virus or HIV) within a healthcare setting (e.g. exposure to a surgeon with hepatitis B, or to contaminated instruments). Similar exercises may be recommended for potential exposures to other infections, such as TB and Creutzfeldt–Jakob disease (CJD). When lookback studies are being undertaken there may well be heightened media interest. Procedures for managing this should be established early to ensure confidence in the service is maintained, mechanisms for providing reassurance may need to be established, including for the 'worried well'. The importance of preserving the confidentiality of the HCW and contacts should be emphasised.

HIV

Guidance on lookback exercises is given by the UK Expert Advisory Group on AIDS

Table 4.6.3 Lookback exercises for HIV exposure from HCW

When to carry out a lookback	EAGA recommends 'that all patients who have undergone an exposure prone procedure (EPP) where the infected HCW was the sole or main operator should, as far as practicable be notified of this'.
What is an EPP?	A procedure in which there is a risk that injury to the HCW may result in exposure of the patient's open tissues to the blood of the HCW. This usually involves operations in which the HCWs fingers are not visible whilst exposed to sharp objects.

	Risk of exposure*	Definition	Examples
	High	Major operations	Vaginal or abdominal hysterectomy, caesarean section, prolapse repair, salpingectomy
Low	Other procedures, suturing or sharp instruments	Laparoscopy, forceps delivery, episiotomy repair, incision of Bartholin's abscess	
	None	Procedures that do not involve suturing or sharp instruments	Manual removal of placenta, dilatation and curettage, cystoscopy, spontaneous vaginal delivery

Methods	Establish incident management team.
	Ensure overall co-ordination is clear.
	Establish helplines.
	Ensure that GPs are kept informed.
	Define EPP. It may be necessary to define high and low risk procedures in order to concentrate resources on those most at risk.
	Identify those exposed. This may involve extensive searches through hospital records, operating theatre registers, etc.
	Contact exposed patients. This may be personally by GPs or their staff, or by letter. The method will need to be sensitive to the risk, and to the need of those contacted for support and counselling. It is important to ensure that helplines/counselling is in place, and that there are clear algorithms for the care of those identified.
	Ensure close liaison with press office throughout.
Transmission risk	A number of lookback studies have been carried out following exposure to HIV infected HCWs. Studies of over 30,000 patients (about half of whom have undergone testing) have shown no evidence of transmission of HIV to patients. Two incidents, a Florida dentist who transmitted infection to six patients and a French orthopaedic surgeon who infected one patient have been reported. The risk of transmission from an HIV infected HCW to a patient following an EPP is likely to be low.
Sources of further advice	EAGA; national specialist CDC/HPA; ECDC; Department of Health.

CDC, Communicable Disease Control; EAGA, UK Expert Advisory Group on AIDS; ECDC, European Centre for Disease Prevention and Control; EPP, exposure-prone procedure; HP, Health Protection Agency.
*From Commun Dis Public Health, 1999, **2**: 127.

Table 4.6.4 Lookback exercises for hepatitis B virus (HBV) exposure from HCW

When to carry out a lookback	There is no formal guidance. However, the recommendations given by EAGA for HIV lookback exercises are helpful. Notification exercises should not extend beyond 12 months unless high rates of transmission have been documented.
What is an EPP?	A procedure in which gloved hands may be in contact with sharp instruments, needle tips and sharp tissues (spicules of bone or teeth) inside a patient's open body cavity, wound or confined anatomical space where the hands or fingertips may not be completely visible at all times.
Methods	As above
	The incubation period for HBV (2–6 months) is such that exposed patients may be identified during the period before seroconversion.
	Serum should be taken from patients on identification and they should be retested 6 months after exposure to identify seroconversions.
	DNA sequencing of fragments of HBV DNA may be useful to establish transmission.
Interventions	Hepatitis B immunoglobulin is effective up to 1 week after exposure and should be offered to individuals at risk.
	The value of hepatitis B vaccination is unclear and there is probably little merit in using hepatitis B vaccine more than 2 weeks after exposure.
	Systems will need to be put in place for ensuring that those who do not clear the virus are followed up and if appropriate offered treatment for chronic HBV.
Transmission risk	Transmission rates identified in incidents involving surgical staff in the UK have ranged from 0.9 to 20% depending on the procedures and other factors.
Sources of further advice	Expert Advisory Group on Hepatitis; national CDC/HPA: ECDC; Department of Health.

CDC, Communicable Disease Control; ECDC, European Centre for Disease Prevention and Control; EPP, exposure-prone procedure; HP, Health Protection Agency.

(EAGA) (see Appendix 2). These are summarised in Table 4.6.3.

Hepatitis B

HCWs who carry hepatitis B virus (HBV) may infect patients who become exposed to their serum. The UK Health Departments require all HCWs who undertake exposure prone procedures (EPPs) to be vaccinated against HBV, and their subsequent immunity to be documented. Non-responders to vaccination should be investigated for evidence of chronic HBV infection. HCWs who are hepatitis e antigen positive may not undertake EPPs be-

cause of the significant risk they pose to patients.

In spite of the recommendations for immunisation and restriction placed upon practice, a number of events have still occurred where patients have been exposed to an infected HCW, or to the risk of transmission in a healthcare setting (Table 4.6.4).

Hepatitis C

HCWs who carry hepatitis C virus may infect patients who become exposed to their serum; however, the risk of transmission is much lower than the risk of transmission for HBV

Table 4.6.5 Lookback exercises for hepatitis C virus (HCV) exposure from HCW

When to carry out a lookback	As for hepatitis B
What is an EPP?	As for hepatitis B
Methods	Serum should be taken from those exposed on identification. Advice should be sought on the when repeat testing should be performed. It is recommended that serum is obtained from HCWs exposed to a known positive source at baseline, 6, 12 and 24 weeks and tested for HCV RNA at 6 and 12 weeks and anti-HCV at 12 and 24 weeks. Genotyping may be useful to establish transmission.
Interventions	Although there is some disagreement over the effectiveness of early treatment in preventing progression of disease most experts favour treatment of patients with acute hepatitis C.
Sources of further advice	Expert Advisory Group on Hepatitis; national CDC/HPA: ECDC; Department of Health. See Appendix 2 for guidance on the risks and management of occupational exposure to hepatitis C.

CDC, Communicable Disease Control; ECDC, European Centre for Disease Prevention and Control; EPP, exposure-prone procedure; HPA, Health Protection Agency.

from an e antigen positive surgeon. HCWs are not restricted in carrying out EPPs unless they have been shown to transmit hepatitis C. They should be advised on adherence to precautions for the control of blood-borne infection by the occupational health department (Table 4.6.5).

4.7 Co-ordination of immunisation services

Role of the immunisation co-ordinator

Effective immunisation services require the co-ordination of the inputs of many different professionals and agencies. Each local health organisation should delegate a particular person (or persons) to take on special responsibility for implementing improvements to immunisation programmes at local level. The main functions of this immunisation co-ordinator are as follows:
• To ensure that an appropriate strategy, with the aim of ensuring that every child (in the absence of genuine contraindications) receives immunisation, is devised and implemented.
• To ensure that appropriate resources are in place to support the strategy.
• To ensure that appropriate local policies and procedures, based on models of good practice, are in place to support the strategy.
• To act as a local source of advice and information on immunisation issues for both the public and professionals.
• To co-ordinate the role of all those involved with immunisation in primary care, child health services, hospitals, educational establishments and elsewhere, and to gain their commitment to the strategy and its aims.
• To chair the District Immunisation Committee (DIC) and ensure delivery of its identified responsibilities (see below).
• To ensure that training and updating of all staff involved in immunisation is available.
• To ensure that up-to-date and reliable figures on immunisation uptake rates are available.
• To ensure that non-immunised children are identified and followed up.
• To investigate the reasons for poor uptake figures and to promote appropriate methods to overcome identified problems.

• To ensure that appropriate audit is carried out on the availability effectiveness and efficiency of local immunisation services.

The separation of functions in some national health services means that some of the above list may be delegated to other individuals. The functions may be split as:

• *Health services commissioning organisation*: assume overall responsibility for delivery of service and national targets, including provision of services, training, public information and collection of vaccine uptake data.

• *Public health specialist service*: provide strategic leadership, co-ordination, expert advice and support to health services in areas in discharging their responsibilities.

• *Paediatric and community health services*: provision of expert clinical advice, supporting clinical services for complex cases and, where appropriate, maintenance of the child health (immunisation) database.

District Immunisation Committee

The immunisation co-ordinator should be supported by a DIC. An appropriate membership might be:

• public health service local immunisation lead/co-ordinator (Chair);
• health service commissioning organisation immunisation leads/co-ordinators;
• community paediatrician;
• information manager (child health/immunisation database);
• community services manager;
• community services commissioner;
• GP;
• community nurses, including practice nurse;
• pharmacist; and
• health promotion officer.

The terms of reference of the DIC could be as follows:

• To review and advise on immunisation policies within the district and to develop an integrated district-wide strategy in order to achieve the maximum immunisation up-

take within the district, in line with national guidelines.

• To implement and monitor the local immunisation programme.

• To ensure accurate information is maintained to support the immunisation programme and shared appropriately.

• To ensure the organisation of an efficient and effective recall system.

• To ensure an accurate record of all immunisations given to any child in the district is provided to any professional caring for that child and the parent/carer.

• To ensure appropriate training and updating is available on an ongoing basis for all staff involved in the immunisation programme.

• To ensure that advice is given on the appropriate systems for the storage of vaccines.

• To co-ordinate health promotion activities within the district on immunisation issues.

• To ensure organisation of an efficient patient recall system.

• To ensure that a source of clinical management advice concerning the immunisation programme is available within the district.

• To ensure that a rapid response is possible should a particular immunisation need arise.

Immunisation uptake rates

The theoretical aim of immunisation services is to achieve herd immunity against those diseases transmitted from person to person (e.g. measles) and to protect everyone against those with other sources (e.g. tetanus). Many countries have set general targets for immunisation uptake based on WHO recommendations for (Table 4.7.1):

• 95% of children to receive three primary doses of diphtheria, tetanus, polio and pertussis in the first year of life and one dose of MMR by their second birthday;

• 75% uptake of annual influenza immunisation in recommended groups.

Many districts fail to achieve these targets. These districts are often those with the highest population density and therefore where a higher than average uptake is needed to achieve herd immunity (Box 4.7.1). Many

Table 4.7.1 Routine immunisation schedule: UK example. (Currently no EU-wide consensus schedule. http://www.euvac.net/graphics/euvac/vaccination/vaccination.html)

Age	Vaccine
Neonates	BCG (high risk groups only)
	Hepatitis B (high risk groups only)
2, 3 + 4 months	3 dose primary course of:
	Diphtheria/tetanus/pertussis/polio/Hib (DTaP/IPV/Hib)
	2 doses of meningococcus C (MenC) and pneumococcal
	(PCV) vaccines
12–14 months	Booster dose of Hib/MenC
	1 dose primary course of measles/mumps/rubella (MMR)
	Booster dose of PCV
3–5 years	4th dose of diphtheria/tetanus/pertussis/polio (dTaP/IPV or DTaP/IPV)
	Booster dose of MMR
12–13 years (girls only)	Human papillomavirus (HPV)
13–18 years	5th dose of diphtheria (low dose)/tetanus/polio (Td/IPV)
Adult	Boosters for tetanus and polio if less than 5 doses received
	Vaccines for occupational or lifestyle risks
65 years	Influenza
	Pneumococcus
Any age	Influenza, pneumococcus (medical risk groups)
	Travel vaccines

districts also vaccinate a significant proportion of their children much later than the target age; this further increases the pool of susceptibles allowing transmission to continue. A further consequence of late vaccination is the exposure of infants to pertussis and Hib at an age at which severity of disease is highest.

Contributing reasons for low or late immunisations may be as follows:
• Reduced public confidence in certain vaccines after media scares (e.g. MMR and pertussis). Concern may be highest in higher social class parents.
• Confusion amongst health professionals as to safety and true contraindications of vaccines, particularly pertussis.
• Factors related to social deprivation, particularly high population mobility, lone parenthood and large family size.
• Factors relating to religion (particular problem in the Netherlands), lifestyle and ethnicity. Immigrant children are often not up-to-date with vaccination.
• Problems with the way programmes are organised, delivered and remunerated.

Surveillance of vaccine safety and vaccine failures

Vaccine safety reporting schemes vary across Europe; however, in most countries there is a requirement to report specific adverse events following vaccination, particularly for new vaccines (such as human papillomavirus and pandemic influenza). If a cluster of adverse events occurs, the public health department will be involved in the investigation. A single serious event following vaccination is also likely to generate significant workload as anxiety will be high.

Clusters should be investigated to determine whether they are programme-related (e.g. due to faulty administration technique), vaccine related (e.g. due to a contaminated batch) or co-incidental. Control measures for programme-related cluster will involve re-education of staff giving vaccines. If a defective vaccine is suspected, this should be reported to the national regulatory agency, including details of the vaccine name, manufacturer, batch number, expiry date and nature of defect. The decision to undertake a

---

Box 4.7.1 NICE recommendations to improve immunisation uptake

Immunisation programmes
- Ensure national guidance and updates disseminated to professionals and implemented.
- Monitor vaccination uptake.
- Identified professional responsible for each local programme.
- Improve access to immunisation services.
- Ensure enough immunisation appointments available.
- Send tailored invitations for immunisation. Send tailored reminders and recall invitations to non-attenders and follow up by telephone or text.
- Provide tailored information, advice and support to parents and young people, including in appropriate minority languages.
- Ensure concerns can be discussed with healthcare professional.
- Ensure young people informed and, when appropriate, can give consent.
- Ensure young people and their parents know how to access services.
- Consider home visits for discussion with non-attenders and possible home vaccination.
- Check immunisation status at all other clinical appointments: discuss and offer immunisation where needed.
- Specific co-ordination and process for targeted neonatal hepatitis B vaccine programme.

Information systems
- Ensure local health organisation and medical practices have adequate methods for recording, maintaining and transferring accurate data on vaccination status of all children.
- Encourage and enable private providers to pass on details of all vaccines given.
- Record any factors that may make missed vaccinations more likely.
- Regularly maintain and update child health databases.
- Ensure up-to-date information available to all staff involved in immunisation.
- Use uptake and surveillance data to inform local needs assessment and equity audit.
- Monitor age structure of practice to ensure adequate capacity provided.

Training
- Ensure all staff trained and updated. Professional staff to be trained to national minimum standards.
- Ensure staff trained to document vaccinations accurately.

Nurseries, schools and colleges
- Attached healthcare staff should check immunisation status on enrolment/transfer.
- Attached healthcare staff to discuss with parent or young person and facilitate immunisation.
- Schools to become venues for immunising children.

Targeting groups with low uptake
- Improved access for those with difficulties with transport, language or communication and learning or physical disabilities (e.g. longer appointments, walk-in clinics, extended hours, mobile/outreach services).
- Provide information in variety of formats and translation services.

Box 4.7.2 (*Continued*)

• Provide information in other settings (e.g. pharmacies, libraries, shops, community venues).
• Check vaccine histories of new migrants, asylum seekers, young offenders and children in care on admission/registration.

Source: National Institute for Health and Clinical Excellence (NICE). *NICE Public Health Guidance 21: Reducing differences in the uptake of immunisations (including targeted vaccines) among children and young people aged under 19 years*. London: NICE, 2009. Available at: http://guidance.nice.org.uk/ PH21/Guidance/pdf/English.

---

vaccine recall or quarantine should only be made in consultation with the national regulatory agency.

Vaccine failures should be investigated to ensure laboratory confirmation and reported to the national public health institute, who should be involved in the investigation. Vaccine failures may be programme-related (e.g. inadequate cold chain), vaccine-related or coincidental. Control measures will depend on the cause, and may include education on handling, storage and administration.

4.8 Services for sexual health and HIV infection

Sexual health is an important part of physical and mental health and a key human right. To maintain and improve sexual health and avoid the risks of unintended pregnancy, illness or disease, the population requires access to accurate information and high quality sexual health services. Healthcare commissioning organisations are responsible for ensuring that there is a full range of screening, treatment, care and prevention services (these responsibilities may be split between organisations in some countries). This can be delivered through the appointment of a sexual health co-ordinator to oversee this work, as is usually the case in the UK. Services are delivered by a range of providers including specialist hospital-based infectious disease services, genitourinary medicine (GUM) clinics, GPs, community-based sexual health services, health promotion services, social services departments and voluntary organisations. Investment in services should be based on sound evidence and epidemiological data, which may be available from relevant national organisations. In England, the Department of Health published a National Strategy for Sexual Health and HIV in 2001 and followed this with an Action Plan in 2002, much of which is applicable to other similar areas of Europe. An Independent Advisory Group for Sexual Health and HIV monitors progress towards implementation of this plan and published a review on progress in 2008. Progress has been made and there have been significant improvements in sexual health and service provision: falling teenage pregnancy rates, improvements in access to state-funded abortions, improved GUM services and better access to testing and treatment including *Chlamydia* screening. However, there were still areas of concern such as increasing diagnoses of HIV and STIs and increasing demand for abortion. Despite the acceptance of a holistic view of sexual health and integrated care based on patient need, the wider determinants of sexual health such as social exclusion, poverty, stigma and substance abuse have been neglected and there has been under-investment in services for contraception and reproductive health, psychosexual problems and sexual assault. The continuing drive for sexual health improvement demands action in five priority areas (Table 4.8.1).

Table 4.8.1 Priorities for sexual health improvement (UK example)

Priority area	Details
Leadership at local, regional and national levels	Appoint designated local sexual health champions
	Carry out comprehensive sexual health needs assessments
Building strategic partnerships	Joint planning between health services, local government services and voluntary agencies
Commissioning for improved sexual health	Develop commissioning skills
	Adopt a holistic service commissioning model
	Strengthen the public voice in commissioning
	Base commissioning on best evidence and best practice
Investing in prevention	Ensure effective sexual health promotion
	Ensure prevention is an integral part of sexual health service provision
	Intensify efforts to tackle stigma
	Improve dissemination of evidence about effective interventions in relation to African communities, men who have sex with men and young people
	Embed sexual and relationships education in school curriculum
Deliver modern sexual health services	Ensure sexual health and HIV services are included in primary care centres/polyclinics
	Increase quality of and access to services
	Link workforce planning and training to changing models of care
	Ensure access to the full range of contraceptive methods
	Improve access to early medical and surgical abortion
	Improve STI and HIV incidence data
	Increase HIV testing in a range of existing and new settings
	Facilitate prompt testing and treatment for STIs
	Improve health and social care for people living with HIV

4.9 Services for tuberculosis control

In 2008, 461,645 tuberculosis (TB) cases were reported in the WHO European Region (about 6% of the TB cases reported worldwide), of these 82,611 cases were from the EU/European Economic Area. Although cases continue to decline, the rate of decline has slowed. Over the past 5 years, there has been no significant improvement in the TB treatment success rate in the EU. Reports of TB in UK increased by 22% from 6717 in 2000 to 8655 in 2008, crude rates increased from 11.4 per 100,000 population to 14.1. Some of this increase is due to more complete surveillance (particularly very recently with the introduction of web-based reporting), but most is due to inward migration of persons born in endemic countries who have latent TB that reactivates 2–3 years after their arrival. To tackle this increase there is a need to strengthen TB control services which in turn requires public health leadership and advocacy. In England in 2004 the Chief Medical Officer published a TB Action Plan with the aim of reducing and ultimately eliminating TB by reducing new infections, providing high quality treatment and care, and maintaining low levels of drug resistance. The key priorities for TB prevention and control are summarised in Table 4.9.1.

Table 4.9.1 Priorities for the prevention and control of tuberculosis (TB)

Policy area	Details
Surveillance	A detailed data set should be collected on all cases of TB including drug resistance and treatment outcomes. A computerised register should be maintained. Regular reports should be made to national surveillance centres. A local TB annual report should be published.
Commission high quality services	Responsibility for commissioning services should be clear and the commissioning organisation should have a designated TB lead. The local public health team should assist with the commissioning process. Service users should be involved. A multidisciplinary team approach is commended comprising a TB (thoracic medicine or infectious disease) physician and a TB nurse specialists with support from a microbiologist, the hospital infection control team, the CCDC and the HIV or GUM physician as required. TB clinical networks are encouraged. TB services should be adequately resourced.
Diagnosis	All isolates must be sent to a designated TB reference laboratory (e.g. regional centres for mycobacteriology in UK). HIV testing should be offered where appropriate. Genotyping should be available to assist in identifying linked cases. The proportion of cases with culture confirmation should be improved.
Notification	All cases of TB (including those associated with HIV infection) must be reported to local public health authorities.
High quality services for the management of cases	Treatment of all cases must be supervised by a TB physician and specialist TB nurse. A TB key worker should be identified for each case. Delays in diagnosis should be avoided and compliance with treatment should be a priority to minimise the spread of infection and emergence of drug resistance. Accurate prescribing is important. There should be early recognition and management of drug-resistant TB. Particular skills and tactics are needed with patients who are non-compliant or who have disorganised lifestyles (hard-to-reach patients), homeless persons and problem drug users. DOT should be used if necessary. Compulsory admission to hospital for treatment is not usually practicable.
Contact tracing	Contact tracing should be undertaken promptly to minimise the risk of continuing transmission. Contacts are managed according to national guidelines.
Control of infection	All hospitals that may admit patients with TB should have a TB control plan drawn up in conjunction with the infection control team covering assessment of risk of infection and transmission including HIV-related and drug-resistant TB, isolation room requirements, measures for the protection of healthcare workers and other contacts, including use of masks and disinfection of equipment. When patients in a hospital have been exposed to a healthcare worker or another patient with infectious TB, the infection control team, TB physician, occupational health department and the CCDC should work jointly to agree appropriate control measures.
Case finding	Case finding should be carried out by screening population groups at risk of infection and offering chemoprophylaxis and BCG where appropriate. High risk groups include contacts of TB cases, new immigrants, refugees and asylum seekers, rough sleepers, hostel dwellers and those with HIV infection. IGRA tests should be available for the diagnosis of latent TB in persons who may benefit from preventative therapy.

(Continued on p. 324)

Table 4.9.1 (*Continued*)

Policy area	Details
BCG immunisation	Local immunisation policies should follow national guidelines. In the UK, immunisation is recommended for high risk neonates, contacts of cases with active pulmonary TB, new immigrants from high-prevalence countries, those at risk of occupational exposure and those planning to travel to and stay in a high prevalence country for more than a month.
Occupational health	Employers are required to assess the risk of TB for their employees and select appropriate control measures. These may include pre-employment screening and use of BCG. Staff should be made aware of the symptoms of TB so that they can seek advice early if problems arise. This is particularly important for agencies that deal with vulnerable groups (e.g. health and education).
Prisons and other institutions where residents may be at higher risk of TB	The local health protection unit should liaise with medical staff at prisons and other relevant institutions where residents may be at higher risk of TB to agree appropriate policies for staff and prisoners
Arrangements for outbreak, recognition and investigation	The identification of a single case of TB in a school or hospital or a cluster of cases of TB in a community setting requires a co-ordinated response, as with any other infectious disease incident or outbreak. The health protection team should support local TB services.
Education and training	There should be appropriately targeted educational material for the general public and healthcare staff and others at higher risk of TB. This should recognise the high rates of TB in people from the Indian subcontinent and sub-Saharan Africa.
Monitoring and audit	Performance targets should be set. There should be an audit of completeness of notification.
Research needs	Research priorities include new drugs for the treatment of TB, new vaccine development and new diagnostic tests, the effectiveness of interventions for hard to reach groups and TB transmission within individual European countries.
Global TB	Nations should support international efforts to tackle TB especially where TB is associated with HIV infection.

BCG, bacille Calmette–Guérin: CCDC, Consultant in Communicable Disease Control; DOT, directly observed treatment; GUM, genitourinary medicine; IGRA, interferon-gamma release assay.

4.10 Travel health

There are over 850 million international tourist arrivals each year, at least 50 million to developing countries; half those travelling to the less-developed world for 1 month will have a health problem associated with the trip. These are mostly minor and less than 1% require hospitalisation.

Individuals carry their epidemiological risk with them; hence cardiovascular disease is the most common causes of death in trav-ellers from Europe. Injury and accidents (particularly motor vehicle) are the next most common cause of serious morbidity and mortality. Infection contributes substantially to this morbidity in travellers, particularly diarrhoeal disease, but only about 3% of deaths.

Infectious disease complications of travel depend on pre-existing disease, destination and risk behaviour, and underlying disease. Ever more exotic locations and activities increases contact with, and susceptibility to, organisms one would not routinely meet.

Prevention of ill health in travellers

Travel health clinics can, through providing up-to-date advice on risk and risk reduction, prevent ill health by simple precautions and interventions. Travel clinics must have access to up-to-date information and recommendations as the epidemiology of travel-related infection risk changes rapidly and continuously. Giving appropriate advice to those with complex itineraries and/or pre-existing conditions may be a difficult task. Opportunities should be taken to ensure that those who travel at short notice have their vaccination status reviewed regularly.

Advice should cover the following:
• Basic food, water and personal hygiene.
• Avoiding insect vectors (advice about bed nets, avoiding tick bites).
• Safe sex and avoidance of potential blood-borne virus exposure.
• Malaria prophylaxis.
• Vaccination against specific diseases as appropriate.
• Avoiding dog bites and other potential rabies exposures.

Travellers' diarrhoea

Diarrhoea, usually short-lived and self-limiting, is a major cause of illness in travellers; 20% of cases are confined to bed. The main risk factor is the destination; incidence rates vary from less than 10% per 2-week stay in industrialised countries to over 50% in parts of Africa, Central and South America and South-East Asia. Infants and young adults are at particularly high risk.

The likelihood of diarrhoea is related to dietary indiscretions. The risk of travellers' diarrhoea and other faeco-orally transmitted disease (e.g. hepatitis A and typhoid) in those who travel to developing countries can be reduced by the following measures:
• Washing hands after toilet and before preparing or eating food.
• Using only sterilised or bottled water for drinking, cleaning teeth, making ice and washing food (e.g. salads).
• Avoiding uncooked food (unless you can peel it or shell it yourself), untreated milk or milk products (e.g. ice cream), uncooked shellfish, food that may have been exposed to flies and any other potentially contaminated food.
• It is usually safe to eat freshly cooked food that is thoroughly cooked and still hot; hot tea and coffee; commercially produced alcoholic and soft drinks.
• Antibiotic chemoprophylaxis is not recommended for most travellers.

Malaria

Over 1500 cases of malaria are imported in the UK annually, with 5–15 deaths per year (see Chapter 3.48). The risk varies by season and place; it is highest in sub-Saharan Africa and Oceania (1 : 50 to 1 : 1000).

Compliance with antimalarial chemoprophylaxis regimens and use of personal protection measures are key to the prevention of malaria. However, fewer than 50% of travellers at risk adhere to basic recommendations for malaria prevention.

Measures to reduce the risk of mosquito bites include the following:
• Sleep in screened rooms, use knockdown insecticide in the evening and use an electrical pyrethroid vaporiser overnight.
• If the room cannot be made safe, use impregnated bed nets.
• Wear long-sleeve shirts and long trousers in evening. Use insect repellent.

Advice on chemoprophylaxis has been made more difficult by the increase in chloroquine and multidrug-resistant falciparum malaria, and primaquine and chloroquine-resistant strains of *Plasmodium vivax*. The recommended regimen will depend upon the proposed itinerary: most situations will be covered by the latest published guidance (http://www.hpa.org.uk/infections/topics_az/malaria/guidelines.htm).

Travellers to endemic countries should be aware of the symptoms of malaria and the need to seek urgent medical attention. Those who will be out of reach of medical services can be given stand-by therapy.

Immunisation and travel

Many countries and the WHO produce recommendations for vaccination of travellers (see Appendix 2); these should be consulted.

Diphtheria, tetanus and polio

Foreign travel is an ideal opportunity to have these immunisations updated. Diphtheria is a problem worldwide, with large outbreaks in the early 1990s in the Russian Federation and more recently in Haiti. There are low levels of tetanus antitoxin and immunity to polio serogroups in many adults. Polio outbreaks have occurred recently in Tajikistan and Angola and polio is still endemic in parts of India, Nigeria, Afghanistan and Pakistan

Hepatitis A

Hepatitis A is a common vaccine-preventable infection in travellers. It is endemic in many parts of the world, including Southern Europe. The risk is especially high for those who leave the usual tourist routes. Immunisation is recommended for travellers to countries in Africa, Asia, Central and South America and the Caribbean, where hygiene and sanitation may be poor, and for some countries in Eastern Europe, although it may be less important for short stays in good accommodation.

Hepatitis B

Immunisation against hepatitis B virus should be given to all those who may come into contact with body fluids (e.g. those planning to work as healthcare workers). The incidence also appears raised in other long-stay overseas workers, perhaps as a result of medical and dental procedures received abroad or sexual transmission. Immunisation is not necessary for short-term business or tourist travellers, unless their sexual behaviour puts them at risk.

Typhoid

The risk of typhoid is especially high for those leaving the usual tourist routes, or visiting relatives or friends in developing countries. A total of 16–33 million cases occur worldwide annually, almost 500 cases of enteric fever were reported in the UK in 2006. Typhoid vaccine is recommended for the same groups as hepatitis A vaccine. Vaccination against paratyphoid is not recommended.

Cholera

The risk of cholera is extremely low; cholera vaccine is not indicated for travellers. No country requires proof of cholera vaccination as a condition for entry.

Yellow fever

A yellow fever vaccination certificate is required for entry into most countries of sub-Saharan Africa and South America in which the infection exists. Many countries require a certificate from travellers arriving from or who have been in transit through infected areas. Some countries require a certificate from all entering travellers.

As the areas of yellow fever virus circulation exceed the officially reported zones, vaccination is strongly recommended for travel to all countries in the endemic zone (particularly if visiting rural areas), even if these countries have not officially reported the disease and do not require a vaccination certificate.

The vaccination has almost 100% efficacy, while the case fatality rate for the disease is more than 60% in non-immune adults. In recent years, fatal cases of yellow fever have occurred in unvaccinated tourists visiting rural areas within the yellow fever endemic zone.

Rabies

Rabies vaccination should be considered in those who are likely to come into contact with animals where the disease is present (e.g. veterinarians), and those undertaking long journeys in remote areas.

Japanese B encephalitis

Immunisation should be considered in those staying for a month or longer in rural areas of endemic countries and those whose itineraries take them to rural areas of wetland (marsh, rice fields) in the transmission season.

Meningococcal disease

Immunisation should be considered in those going to areas of the world where the incidence is high (e.g. the 'meningitis belt' of sub-Saharan Africa, and areas in the north of the Indian subcontinent). Pilgrims travelling to Saudi Arabia for the Hajj must have proof of vaccination.

Tick-borne encephalitis

Vaccination is recommended for those who are to walk, camp or work in late spring and summer in warm, heavily forested parts of Central and Eastern Europe and Scandinavia. They should also cover arms, legs and ankles and use insect repellent.

Pregnancy, infection and travel

Pregnant travellers should be helped to balance the benefits and risks of travel during pregnancy. Dehydration resulting from diarrhoea can reduce placental blood flow, therefore pregnant travellers must be careful about their food and drink intake; infections such as toxoplasmosis and listeriosis have potentially serious sequelae in pregnancy. Women should be encouraged to breastfeed if travelling with a neonate. A nursing mother with travellers' diarrhoea should not stop breastfeeding but should increase her fluid intake.

Malaria during pregnancy carries a significant risk of morbidity and death. Pregnant women should be advised of this increased risk if intending travelling to endemic areas. If travel is essential, then chemoprophylaxis and avoidance of bites are essential (take specialist advice).

The HIV infected traveller

The HIV infected traveller may be at risk of serious infection. Those with AIDS, CD4$^+$ counts of less than 200/L and those who are symptomatic should seek specialist advice, particularly before going to the developing world. Those with a CD4$^+$ cell count above 500 probably have a risk similar to a person without HIV infection.

Gastrointestinal illness

The HIV infected traveller needs to be particularly careful about the foods and beverage consumed. Travellers' diarrhoea occurs more frequently, is more severe, protracted and more difficult to treat when in association with HIV infection. Infections are also more likely to be accompanied by bacteraemia. Organisms particularly associated with severe chronic diarrhoea in HIV positive travellers include *Cryptosporidium* and *Isospora belli*.

Immunisation

All of the HIV infected traveller's routine immunisations should be up-to-date. In general, live attenuated vaccines are contraindicated for persons with immune dysfunction. Live oral polio vaccine should not be given to HIV-infected patients or members of their households. Inactivated polio vaccine (IPV) should be used. Live yellow fever vaccine should not normally be given to HIV infected travellers; however, if travel in an endemic area is absolutely necessary, vaccination may be considered after a risk assessment and consideration of the CD4 count. Bacille Calmette–Guérin (BCG) should not be given because of disseminated infection in HIV infected persons.

4.11 Pandemic preparedness and the influenza A H1N1 2009 pandemic

Influenza pandemics

Immunological basis for pandemics

Of the three types of influenza viruses (A, B and C), only influenza A has pandemic potential. Influenza A viruses originate from birds, but many strains are able to successfully infect both pigs and humans.

The basis for the epidemiology of influenza A is population immunity to circulating viruses. Influenza A has two main surface proteins: haemagglutinin (H) and neuraminidase (N). Of the 16 known haemagglutinins and 9 known neuraminidases, H1, H2, H3, N1 and N2 have been successfully transmitted in seasonal and pandemic influenza, while the rest are only seen in epizootic disease.

Pigs can be infected by influenza A from birds and humans as well as from other pigs. In an animal infected by two or more influenza strains, the Hs and Ns can mix (recombine) to create a 'new' virus (antigenic shift). This virus can then spread among other pigs, but also infect humans. If there is little immunity in the human population to this virus, and it has the ability to easily transmit between humans, there is a potential for a new influenza pandemic.

In 2005, the World Health Organization (WHO) defined an influenza pandemic as the emergence of an influenza A virus significantly different genetically from circulating human influenza A viruses (i.e. many or most of the population are non-immune to the new virus) with the following three characteristics:
- able to infect humans;
- able to cause disease in humans; and
- able to spread from human to human quite easily.

It is noteworthy that severity is not part of the definition.

The most favourable environment for the emergence of a new pandemic virus is East and South-East Asia, where birds, pigs and humans are in close contact with each other.

After the first wave(s) of a pandemic the virus becomes gradually more adapted to humans, and normally establishes itself as a seasonal (inter-pandemic) strain, circulating for many years. While immunity due to influenza infection typically lasts for many years, small mutations in the H and N proteins (antigenic drift) allow the viruses to escape vaccine-induced immunity, causing new waves of seasonal infections every winter.

Previous pandemics

Large epidemics most likely due to influenza were described in Ancient Greece and since the late sixteenth century some 30 pandemics may have occurred. The twentieth century saw three pandemics: the H1N1 Spanish flu (1918–1919), the H2N2 Asian flu (1957–1958) and the H3N2 Hong Kong flu (1968–1969). Additionally, two new subtypes have been transmitted between humans, but not given rise to pandemics: an H1N1 swine flu causing an outbreak in a US military camp in 1977 and single cases of H5N1 avian flu since 1997.

Of the recorded pandemics, Spanish flu has surpassed all others in severity. Between 20 and 50 million people died in this pandemic (2–3% case fatality rate), which is more than the total number of lives is lost in the First World War. The two subsequent pandemics were less severe and had an estimated attributable excess mortality of 2–3% (<0.2% case fatality rate). Each of these three pandemics had its own age profile, with Spanish flu mainly affecting young adults, Asian flu small children and Hong Kong flu all age groups. Spanish flu and Hong Kong flu both had severe waves over two seasons, and for the former a substantially increased severity during the second seasonal wave.

Pandemic preparedness

The potentially devastating consequences of an influenza pandemic has made pandemic preparedness a public health priority. When the H5N1 highly pathogenic avian influenza (HPAI) first appeared in Hong Kong in 1997, an influenza pandemic was believed by many to have been adverted only by the immediate culling of all poultry in the city (1.5 million birds in 3 days). The subsequent large-scale H5N1 panzootic among poultry and fowl, with its rare spillover of fatal disease to humans, has put pandemic preparedness on the public health agenda since late 2003.

The fear has been a human adaptation of this virus with increased transmissibility but retained virulence, potentially causing a pandemic of the same magnitude as Spanish flu. This could happen either from adaptive mutations or through a combination of genes from avian and human influenza (re-assortment) in a human or a porcine host infected with both avian H5N1 and human influenza A viruses. Because re-assortment may also take place in a human host, all people that might be in contact with live or dead birds infected with avian influenza, or healthcare workers involved in the care of patients infected with the disease, have been strongly advised to be vaccinated against human influenza and take prophylactic antiviral drugs, such as oseltamivir.

In 1999, the WHO published an influenza pandemic plan to support national and regional planning. This was updated in 2005 as a global influenza preparedness plan. A cornerstone in the planning was the definition of six pandemic phases (Box 4.11.1).

Triggered by the worldwide spread of the avian H5N1 virus (with its first outbreaks in Europe in 2005), all EU countries have developed detailed national preparedness plans. The work to develop these plans has been facilitated by a methodology for preparedness

---

Box 4.11.1 WHO global pandemic phases

Interpandemic period

Phase 1: no new influenza virus subtypes have been detected in humans. An influenza virus subtype that has caused human infection may be present in animals. If present in animals, the risk of human infection or disease is considered to be low.

Phase 2: no new influenza virus subtypes have been detected in humans. However, a circulating animal influenza virus subtype poses a substantial risk of human disease.

Pandemic alert period

Phase 3: human infection(s) with a new subtype but no person-to-person spread or at most rare instances of spread to a close contact.

Phase 4: small cluster(s) with limited person-to-person transmission but spread is highly localized, suggesting that the virus is not well adapted to humans.

Phase 5: larger cluster(s) but person-to-person spread is still localized, suggesting that the virus is becoming increasingly better adapted to humans but may not yet be fully transmissible (substantial pandemic risk).

Pandemic period

Phase 6: pandemic phase: increased and sustained transmission in the general population.

Postpandemic period

Return to the interpandemic period.

Source: adapted from WHO/CDS/CSR/GIP/2005.5. WHO global influenza preparedness plan: http://www.who.int/csr/resources/publications/influenza/WHO_CDS_CSR_GIP_2005_5.pdf.

assessments developed by the European Centre for Disease Prevention and Control (ECDC) and the WHO Regional Office for Europe. Since 2005, ECDC has visited all EU countries to review their plans and support further refinements – a number of planning and guidance documents as well as indicators for self assessments are available on the ECDC web portal (www.ecdc.europa.eu).

A critical issue in national planning has been to move from paper plans via practice to full preparedness. This means involvement not only of the health sector but of society as a whole and efficient outreach to local level. Key features in pandemic preparedness are as follows:

• Planning, coordination and maintaining essential services.
• Surveillance, situation monitoring and assessment.
• Prevention and reduction of transmission.
• Health service response.
• Antivirals for therapy and prophylaxis.
• Communication.
• Co-operation between countries.

Many countries in Europe have developed nationally based planning assumptions, including 'worst-case scenarios', based on influenza A H5N1. Unfortunately, these scenarios have often been perceived as 'predictions'. When the reality during the A H1N1 2009 pandemic was more favourable than these assumptions, many countries experienced mistrust and severe communication challenges.

A H1N1 2009 pandemic

Origin of the pandemic

The recent A H1N1 2009 pandemic (henceforth, the 2009 pandemic) defied all predictions. It had its origin in swine influenza, rather than in an avian influenza, it first appeared in North America, not in East Asia, and it showed many new features.

The first reports came from children in Southern California in April 2009, but it was soon clear that the pandemic had originated in Mexico in early March. Outbreaks in other parts of the USA were soon identified, and

on 29 April the Director General of WHO declared a shift to pandemic phase 5. Following outbreaks in more than 70 countries, pandemic phase 6 was declared on 11 June.

The new virus harboured a unique combination of eight gene segments from three different sources a human influenza A virus, an avian influenza virus seemingly of North American lineage, and a North American triple-reassortant swine virus strain. The H1N1-coding genes have the same lineage as the Spanish flu virus, and have likely passed over to pigs and been circulating among them for decades. The relatedness to the 1918 H1N1 virus strain (being the ancestor of the seasonal H1N1 viruses circulating until the 1957 Asian flu), have been shown in the protective immunity to the 2009 pandemic virus observed in many people born before 1957.

Epidemiology and clinical features

The first European cases were identified in late April in travellers returning from Mexico. A distinct first wave of local transmission was observed in most European countries in late spring and early summer, especially in Spain and the UK. This first wave died out as schools closed, but resumed in the early autumn following a west-to-east progression, and by mid-February 2010 most countries had passed the peak.

As in other parts of the world, around half of cases were children below the age of 19 years, with a male preponderance in the younger age groups. The oldest age groups were heavily under-represented compared to seasonal influenza epidemics. A striking feature of the 2009 pandemic was a very large proportion of mild and asymptomatic cases. At the same time the severe cases often had a dramatic clinical picture with primary viral pneumonitis leading to acute respiratory distress syndrome, in many cases necessitating prolonged intesive care unit (ICU) treatment, including extracorporeal membrane oxygenation – a situation very rarely seen during seasonal influenza. Early in the course of the pandemic, pregnancy and obesity were recognised as specific risk factors, but many of the most severe cases were young, previously healthy adults.

While during seasonal influenza, 90% of the deaths are normally seen in patients over the age of 65 years, some 80% of the deaths in the 2009 pandemic were seen in patients under the age of 65 years. It is important to take this into account when judging the severity of the 2009 pandemic. While the number of deaths may not seem to be dramatic, the number of years of life lost was substantial and likely somewhere between a 'bad' seasonal influenza with the aggressive H3N2 virus and the 1968 Hong Kong flu pandemic.

During the 2009–2010 influenza season, the novel H1N1 pandemic virus, more or less totally replaced the two previously dominating seasonal influenza A strains (H3N2 and H1N1), while influenza B could be identified all through the pandemic autumn–winter wave. A small minority of tested strains (2.5%) were resistant to oseltamivir, none to zanamivir and all strains were resistant to the old M2 inhibitors. A specific genetic variant (D222G substitution) was isolated from patients with severe disease in Norway and some 20 other countries globally, but the overall significance of this finding is unclear.

The overall epidemiological picture of the 2009 pandemic will only be evident once sero-epidemiological studies are completed and overall mortality data have been analysed.

Countermeasures

The initial response to the pandemic in many countries was an attempt to contain the disease through vigorous case detection, isolation, contact tracing and treatment. This very resource-intense countermeasure was abandoned in all European countries by the end of June or early July with subsequent emphasis on mitigation. With some variations, the use of antivirals in most countries was restricted to prescription-only, and the overall consumption in Europe outside the hospitals was surprisingly low.

It was soon evident that the H1N1 component in the existing seasonal vaccines did not confer any immunity to the new 2009 pandemic virus, meaning that new monovalent vaccines had to be developed urgently. By the end of September and early October, three adjuvanted pandemic vaccines received market authorisation in the EU through a fast-track 'mock-up' procedure. An initial two-dose regime was soon changed to one-dose. In addition to the three centrally authorised vaccines, a number of other vaccines have been authorised by national authorities. A very ambitious system to register and analyse adverse events following immunisation has been set up by the European Medicines Agency together with national authorities. Based on existing data the vaccines have been very safe.

The access to and utilisation of the pandemic vaccines have varied considerably between the EU countries. Also even in the countries with the most efficient vaccination campaigns, mass vaccination most likely came too late to have a major impact on the epidemiology of the pandemic autumn–winter wave.

Conclusions

The first pandemic of the twenty-first century had a number of striking novel clinical and epidemiological features. While the overall impact on society was limited, the communication challenges were immense. It is likely that the experiences from the pandemic will result in a more flexible planning approach in the future.

4.12 Non-infectious environmental hazards

Environmental health comprises aspects of human health and quality of life that are determined by physical, biological and social factors in the environment. Some physical and chemical factors in particular have the potential to adversely affect health and are described as environmental hazards (Table 4.12.1). However, there are other equally

Table 4.12.1 Environmental hazards

Hazard	Notes
Factories and industrial processes	These may cause nuisance as a result of soiling of the environment, noise, odour or road traffic. Potential health effects may arise from chemical releases, fumes and particulates. In the UK, Environmental Permits regulate the environmental effects of industrial activities including emissions. Such regulation requires that there is local and open consultation. Public health professionals should be involved in this consultation process as they are can offer the Regulator independent advice on both the impact of emissions and the health of the local population. In the UK, primary care trusts (PCTs) and the HPA are consulted on the potential health effects of industrial activities. These arrangements will change as a result of the 2010 proposed health service changes. A similar process of consultation on infrastructure developments that may have an effect on health is required by the Planning Act 2008.
Hazardous sites	Factories and other installations may store hazardous materials that in the event of an accident could threaten public health. Across Europe, the regulation of sites storing large quantities of hazardous materials falls under the Seveso II Directive. In the UK, this Directive is implemented through the Control of Major Accident Hazard Regulations 1999 (COMAH).
Chemicals	Chemicals either exist naturally in the environment or will have been manufactured. There are many million known chemicals of which it is estimated 70,000 are in regular use and several hundred new chemicals enter the market place each year. Chemicals may have beneficial, harmful or no effect on health. Most chemicals have had little or no toxicological assessment. Large-scale industrial releases with serious effects are rare but smaller scale events do occur including leaks and fires. It is helpful to identify local sites that may represent sources of major chemical hazard. This will allow action to be taken in the event of an accidental release. The Control of Substances Hazardous to Health Regulations 1999 (COSHH) are made under the Health and Safety at Work, etc. Act 1974. They require employers to control exposure to hazardous substances to prevent ill health. Increasingly, people are adopting a precautionary approach and limiting unnecessary exposure to chemicals that may be found in commercial products sold for home or workplace use.
Outdoor air quality	Concentrations of outdoor air pollutants vary from region to region and from day to day. It is accepted that exposure to current levels of common air pollutants damages health. Both long-term and short-term increases in the concentrations of air pollutants can have measureable health effects. Long-term exposure to particles is associated with increases in cardiovascular disease and lung cancer while short-term increases in particles can increase death due to heart attacks and from respiratory disease and increase admissions to hospital. Air pollution may have a long-term effect on children's lung function. European and US studies have shown that air pollution (measured as particles) may reduce lung development in children from the ages of 10 to 18 years old. For some pollutants, there is no threshold of effect and any concentration should be assumed to be associated with some effect on health. The WHO for Europe publishes health-based air quality guidelines for a range of pollutants. These represent concentrations at which there should be little or no threat to human health at a population level. Air quality improvement targets have been published. There is an extensive network of air quality monitoring stations throughout the UK and

Table 4.12.1 (*Continued*)

Hazard	Notes
	real-time data from this can be found in the national archive of UK air quality data (http://www.airquality.co.uk/archive/index.php). Pollutants such as benzene and 1,3-butadiene are carcinogens. Particulate matter, ozone and sulphur dioxide may have acute effects on susceptible members of the population, leading to premature mortality and hospital admissions in those with pre-existing respiratory disease. Other air pollutants may have an effect on life expectancy as a result of long-term exposure throughout life.
Indoor air quality	Rates of respiratory disease and incidence of allergic responses such as asthma have increased in recent years, and there is concern that some of this increase may be linked to changes in the indoor environment, including allergens, tobacco smoke, oxides of nitrogen and formaldehyde.
Drinking water	Over 99% of the population in the UK receives mains water supplies; the quality of these supplies is very high and all are safe to drink. The basic unit of water supply is the water supply zone, which is designated by the water company, normally by reference to a source of water, and which covers a population of about 50,000 people. There are water quality standards, which include microbiological, chemical, physical and aesthetic parameters. Water in some water supply zones is temporarily permitted to exceed these statutory standards for certain chemicals such as lead, polycyclic aromatic hydrocarbons and pesticides. The most important source of lead in tap water in the UK is dissolution from household plumbing systems. Private water supplies are regulated by the local authority, but are subject to a much reduced sampling regime.
Sewerage systems	In Northern European countries most households are connected to wastewater treatment plants which efficiently remove nitrogen, phosphorus and organic matter. In Central European countries more than half of the wastewater is treated in this way. In Southern and Accession countries only around half of the population is connected to wastewater treatment plants.
Water resources management	Under the Water Resources Act 1991 in England and Wales, the Environment Agency regulates any discharges to water to improve the quality of bathing waters.
Solid waste	In the EU use of materials averages 15–16 tonnes per capita per year (Italy 12, Finland 38) and results in 4–5 tonnes of waste per capita each year. Waste is sent to landfill (45%), recycled or composted (37%), or incinerated with energy recovery (18%). Healthcare waste refers to any waste produced as a consequence of healthcare activities and this may also be offensive or hazardous waste. There are EU regulations governing the management of waste, its storage, carriage, treatment and disposal, and health and safety aspects.
Contaminated land	In the UK, a long industrial history has resulted in a substantial legacy of land contamination. In the UK, the legal definition of contaminated land explicitly links land with the potential to cause significant harm. Contaminated land is defined in Part 2A of the Environmental Protection Act 1990 as land where by virtue of contamination there is a *significant possibility of significant harm* or where there may be water pollution. The local authority is the main regulator of contaminated land and they may be assisted by the HPA and local health protection team with interpreting human health risk assessments and communicating the results to the community.

(*Continued on p. 334*)

Table 4.12.1 (*Continued*)

Hazard	Notes
Ionising and non-ionising radiation	Radioactivity occurs naturally and various medical, scientific, commercial and educational activities involve the use of radioactive material and result in radioactive waste. In recent years there have been incidents involving the accidental and deliberate release of radioactive materials in the environment. There is a need for an expert service to protect public health from the harmful effects of radiation through surveillance, monitoring, advice and intervention. In the UK, the Radiation Protection Division (formerly the National Radiological Protection Board) of the HPA fulfils these functions. The body that advises on standards of protection against ionizing radiation is the International Commission on Radiological Protection (ICRP). In the UK there are regulations that govern workplace exposure. Exposure to manmade radiation gives rise to great public concern, although natural sources, such as radon, have greater health effects. A national survey of exposure to radon in homes has shown that while radon exposure in most homes is low, there are some in which it can pose a risk to health. Monitoring should identify homes above the radon action level so that appropriate remedial action can be taken.
Noise	Noise has an important effect on the quality of life. Prolonged exposure to very loud noise can cause permanent hearing damage, but the relationship between noise and other aspects of health is complicated. Road traffic noise is the most widespread form of noise disturbance, but people object most to neighbour noise. Annoyance is the most frequently reported personal consequences of exposure to noise in the home. In the UK, although levels of environmental noise do not reach the intensities needed for damage to hearing, a significant number of people live in areas where the levels exceed the WHO guidelines of 55 dB for average daytime noise.

important environmental determinants of health, including regeneration, transport policy, sustainable development, energy policy, housing policy, social inclusion, planning policy, food policy and industrial accidents and occupational health and safety. Other determinants are natural disasters such as flooding, weather, climate change, war and famine. Environmental health practice is concerned with assessing, controlling and preventing environment factors that can adversely affect health now or in the future. Of relevance to the work of the local health protection team are surveillance of disease and the environmental determinants of disease to identify unusual or novel patterns; a disease cluster or a longer term increase in the incidence of a disease in a particular area that may be associated with a point source of pollution or contamination, and the response to an acute incident or other accident.

Investigating the health effects of environmental hazards

Communities living near potential sources of pollution such as industrial sites, contaminated land and other environmental hazards are often concerned about possible effects on health. They may link locally observed health effects with exposure at these sites. Clusters are defined as the aggregation of a number of similar illnesses in space and time and the perception that the number is excessive. Most types of health event may cluster, but cancer clusters receive the most attention. Greater significance is attached to a cluster when a site of industrial pollution is involved. The local health protection team may be asked to investigate possible clusters and other health problems associated with environmental hazards. The methodology is similar to that used for the investigation of

Table 4.12.2 Investigation of clusters of disease

1. *Initial enquiry*	
Initial report	Use standard form to record details
Initial case definition	What is the disease/health event or symptoms?
Define the problem	Where is the affected area/population?
	Who are the index cases?
	When did the particular health event occur?
	What are the suspected exposures?
Follow up with the informant	The investigation may be resolved at this stage. The disease may be common, affected persons may only recently have moved to the area, there may not be a single plausible environmental factor, there may be no data on exposure, the increase in cases may be a chance occurrence.
Review	Further investigation may be indicated if there is an unusually high number of cases, a biologically plausible exposure(s) or community concern. As a minimum a report should be written and the results disseminated.
2. *Confirm diagnosis and exposure*	
Confirm diagnosis	Involve informant, clinicians and others. Examine records such as
Specific case definition	death certificates, birth certificates, hospital case notes, cancer and
Assess exposure	birth defect registries, occupational health records, GP records. Consent of the index case may be needed.
	Exposure via personal contact, food, water or drug consumption can be assessed by questionnaire. Exposure via water, air, soil or dust is more difficult to assess.
	Company records, aerial photographs, maps, records of water, soil and air quality monitoring, meteorological data and planning records about previous industrial sites and property uses may be used.
	The assistance of an environmental health specialist or an occupational hygienist may be needed but measurement of exposure is usually not necessary at this point.
Review the literature	Review previously reported clusters of the disease, known associations with environmental exposure and any other epidemiological and toxicological information.
Review	On review, there may not be an excess number of cases, the apparent excess may be due to inward migration to an area or the cases may have different diagnoses. The cluster may be explained because it involves a common disease or because of the characteristics of the local population. The nature of the disease and exposure, the size of the cluster and the plausibility of a disease/exposure relationship may require further investigation.
3. *Intensive case finding*	Identify further cases by examining the following data sources: hospital episode statistics, death certificates, cancer and birth defect registrations, occupational health records.
	Collect a minimum dataset on each case: name, date of birth, ethnic group, sex, age at diagnosis, residence and length of residence at diagnosis, past residence, diagnosis, family history, exposures, confounding factors such as smoking, occupational history.
	Ethical approval may be required.

(*Continued on p. 336*)

Table 4.12.2 *(Continued)*

Analyse data	Use population data to calculate expected numbers of cases and compare with observed cases. Mapping the data may be helpful; a geographical information system (GIS) can be used. Plume dispersion modelling may be helpful. Allow for confounding factors such as smoking and socio-economic factors. Statistical significance may not be aetiologically important.
Review	If there is an excess of cases, further investigation may be needed if there is continuing concern, if the exposure is biologically plausible, if there has been a recent increase in cases or if the cases are concentrated around suspected environmental hazards or in particular occupational groups. As a minimum a report should be written and the results disseminated.
4. *Surveillance or epidemiological study*	A surveillance programme over several years will allow the epidemiology to be described. A registry or reporting system may have to be established. A case–control, cohort or cross-sectional study may be feasible.

infectious disease incidents but, as a general rule, site-specific epidemiological studies are not recommended because they often have insufficient statistical power to confirm or refute hypotheses. Similarly, small area level data in the context of single sites or events can be difficult to interpret. When investigating health problems that may be associated with environmental hazards a systematic approach should be adopted (Table 4.12.2).

Dealing with the concerns of the public and media is fundamental to investigating clusters. Risk communication, risk perception and skills in handling enquiries from the public and the media are all important. From a public health perspective, addressing the community's perception of a cluster may be more important than epidemiological or statistical arguments.

4.13 Managing acute chemical incidents

An acute chemical incident is defined as an unforeseen event leading to:
• exposure of people to a non-radioactive substance resulting in illness;

• two or more individuals suffering from a similar illness, which might be due to exposure to toxic substances; and
• a potential threat to health from toxic substances.

Potentially harmful chemicals may be released into the environment as a result of leakage, spillage, explosion, fire or inappropriate disposal. Deliberate release may be part of a criminal or terrorist activity. Exposure by swallowing, inhalation or contact with skin and mucous membranes may be direct or indirect, via contaminated air, food, water or soil. Chemicals can be dispersed from the site of an accident as gas, vapour or particulate cloud, by water and on clothing, equipment, livestock or vehicles (including on human casualties, emergency service personnel and equipment). Exposure to a harmful chemical may result either in acute injury or poisoning, or in longer term health effects. Following a chemical incident, public health interventions include shelter, evacuation, decontamination, supportive treatment, specific treatment with antidotes, short-term and long-term follow up of those affected with clinical and biological monitoring if necessary and population studies. Various agencies are involved in the management of an acute chemical incident (Table 4.13.1). In the UK, the Consultant in Communicable Disease

Table 4.13.1 Agencies involved in the response to an acute chemical incident

Police	Co-ordinate response of emergency services
	Save lives, protect and preserve the scene
	Advice to the public on sheltering, evacuation
	Investigation of the incident
	Casualty information
	Media enquiries
Fire and rescue services	Control, fight and prevent fires
	Urban search and rescue
	Save life
	Manage hazardous materials
	Safety of staff
	Minimise effect of incident on environment
	Decontamination of casualties and exposed persons
	Clean up spillage
	Arrange with contractor to remove substance, etc.
Ambulance service	Co-ordinate all health service activities on site
	Immediate care and treatment of casualties
	Transport to hospital
	Assist with casualty decontamination (with fire service)
PCTs* supported by local health protection team	Planning for chemical incidents
	Leads and co-ordinates health service response
	Assessing health risk
	Sampling
	Health advice to the public
	Monitoring and follow up of affected persons
	Mobilises resources to ensure provision of healthcare (resuscitation, decontamination, treatment with antidotes, intensive care, supportive care, community response)
HPA CRCE	24-hour advice and support to PCTs and health professionals on managing chemical incidents, toxicology, personal protective equipment, decontamination and evacuation, health effects, industrial processes, antidotes and medical treatment, chemical incident surveillance, emergency planning, training, research
NHS hospitals	Support the ambulance service
	Treatment and care of casualties
	Decontamination
Local authority departments	Support the emergency services
	Open emergency rest centres if necessary
	Co-ordinate response of other organisations including voluntary agencies
	Restore environment
	Lead the long-term recovery process
Health and Safety Executive	At sites at which chemicals are manufactured or used:
	• inspect workplaces
	• investigate accidents and cases of ill-health
	• enforce good standards and legislation
Environment Agency	Advises on environmental impact and disposal of contaminated water and other materials
Local water company	Advises on disposal of contaminated water via sewers and impact on water sources

(*Continued on p. 338*)

Table 4.13.1 (*Continued*)

Food Standards Agency	Advises on chemical contamination of the food chain
Meteorological Office	Forecast behaviour of chemical plume according to prevailing weather conditions
NPIS	UK-wide clinical toxicology service for healthcare professionals. Advice on diagnosis, treatment and management of patients who have been poisoned. Six UK centres. Online TOXBASE database at http://www.toxbase.org/

CRCE, Centre for Radiation, Chemical and Environmental Hazards; NPIS, National Poisons Information Service; PCT, primary care trust.
*Arrangements will change as a result of the 2010 proposed changes to the NHS in UK.

Table 4.13.2 Checklist for local public health officer in acute chemical incidents

Action	Notes
Details of incident: • What type of incident • Where and when • What medium is affected • Source of contamination • What chemical(s) are involved	Initial report may come from HPA CRCE, emergency services, public, media.
Adverse health effects or complaints: • How many people exposed • How many affected • What symptoms • How serious • Decontamination • Antidotes, first aid • Weather conditions	Information from ambulance service, GPs, accident department, water company, NHS Direct.
Initial response: • What agencies are involved • What are the command and control arrangements • Should other agencies be called • Is the site secure • Has sheltering or evacuation been advised • What has been said to media	Consider implementing PCT chemical incident plan, convening response team and setting up incident room.
Assessing risk to health: • Review health effects and exposure pathways • Define affected population • Establish register of exposed/symptomatic persons	Obtain toxicological advice. Map plume. Consider sampling cases, other exposed persons, animals, environment. Collect dataset on those affected by the incident or exposed to the chemical(s).
Communications: • Partner agencies (local and national) • Professionals • Media • Public	Set up telephone helpline, use NHS Direct.

Table 4.13.2 (*Continued*)

Action	Notes
Post acute-phase response: • Site clean-up • Environmental effects • Epidemiological study • Long-term surveillance	Those affected may require examination, testing, advice, treatment or follow-up, normally carried out by local clinicians Counselling may be considered to avoid stress-related illness. As a minimum there should be a descriptive study, but there may be an opportunity for an analytical study to determine the strength of any association between the chemical exposure and its health effects.
Post incident: • Written report • Audit of response	Incident documented, report prepared and circulated.

Control (CCDC) on behalf of the NHS has particular responsibilities for the health aspects of chemical incidents: Table 4.13.2 gives a useful checklist for local public health staff involved in acute chemical incidents.

Surveillance of chemical incidents

In the UK, data on chemical incidents is collected by the Health Protection Agency (HPA) and work is in progress to integrate incident data into an environmental public health tracking system, which aims to routinely link data on chemical exposure and health impacts. Catastrophic chemical incidents are rare. The HPA recorded over 6000 incidents in the UK between 1999 and 2004, an average of 1200 incidents per year. The most commonly identified chemicals were asbestos, carbon monoxide, chlorine, petroleum products, acids and mercury.

4.14 Managing acute radiation incidents

Major radiation incidents, such as accidents involving nuclear reactors, military operations and nuclear powered satellites crashing to earth, are uncommon. However, because of the widespread use of radioactive materials in medicine, science and industry, small-scale incidents following transportation accidents, leaks and the loss or theft of sources do occur.

In a radiation incident, radioactive material may be released into the atmosphere as a gas or particles (Box 4.14.1). This forms a windborne plume, which is dispersed and diluted. Some material will fall to the ground, particularly if there is rain. People may be exposed by direct radiation from the plume, by inhalation, by contamination of the environment leading to direct radiation or by consumption of contaminated food or drink.

In the UK, health services do not normally take the lead in responding to releases of radioactive materials, but they do have a role in dealing with their health effects and allaying public anxiety (Box 4.14.2; Table 4.14.1). They must have a written plan to cover this and a named person to take overall responsibility who is usually the Director of Public Health (DPH). The DPH can ask for advice and practical assistance from the Health Protection Agency (HPA), which has a specialist Radiation Protection division.

Countermeasures

Intervention after a radiation accident is based on countermeasures that aim to do

Box 4.14.1 Ionizing radiation

Ionizing radiation is released when an unstable element or radionuclide decays. It is either electromagnetic radiation (X-rays and gamma-rays) or fast-moving particles (alpha particles, beta particles). Ionising radiation releases energy as it passes through biological tissues, resulting in damage. The amount of radioactivity is measured in Bequerels (Bq), the energy deposited by radiation is measured in Grays (Gy) and the effective dose of the radiation is a measure of radiation-induced harm and is measured in sieverts (Sv) or millisieverts (mSv). The average annual exposure in the UK is 2.5 mSv. Of this, 87% comes from natural background radiation (cosmic rays, granite), 12% comes from medical X-rays, 0.1% from nuclear discharges and 0.4% from fallout. The maximum permitted radiation from artificial sources is 1 mSv. A person will be exposed to ionising radiation by being in close proximity to a radioactive source in their surroundings. Prolonged exposure will follow contamination of skin, clothing and wounds and ingestion. Cells that divide frequently are most sensitive to the effects of ionising radiation. The effects of rapid whole-body radiation exposure are summarised in Table 4.14.2. Any dose of radiation increases the risk of cancers and hereditary diseases. An average individual exposed to 5 mSv as a result of eating contaminated food in the first year after a radiation accident has an additional lifetime risk of about 1 in 4000 of developing fatal cancer (the lifetime risk of dying in a fire is about 1 per 1000 and the lifetime risk of dying in a road traffic accident is 10 per 1000). The average person in the UK received 0.1 mSv from the Chernobyl accident in 1986. In the event of a nuclear accident, sheltering or evacuation would be recommended to prevent a whole-body dose of 30 mSv (the ERL). This is well below the dose that could lead to physical symptoms.

Non-ionising radiation includes ultraviolet radiation, light, infrared radiation and radiofrequency radiation. These radiations do not produce ionization in matter and when they pass through living tissue they do not have sufficient energy to damage DNA directly.

more good than harm. Countermeasures include sheltering, evacuation, iodine prophylaxis and banning contaminated foodstuffs. In an accident involving radioactive iodine-131, 60–70% of uptake can be blocked if potassium iodate tablets are given within 3 hours and 50% at approximately 5 hours. In the UK, potassium iodate tablets are part of the UK National Reserve Stock for Major Incidents. However, local accident and emergency departments are advised to maintain stocks for small-scale local incidents. Criteria

Box 4.14.2 Check-list for CCDC in acute radiation incidents

- Enquire about:
  (a) nature and scale of the incident;
  (b) whether anyone has been exposed to radiation as a result of the accident;
  (c) whether they can be traced;
  (d) the likely clinical effect of exposure to the source of radiation;
  (e) the extent and nature of any environmental contamination; and
  (f) the wider population that might have been exposed.
- Carry out an initial risk assessment.
- Consult with local, regional or national sources of expert advice (keep up-to-date contact details in written plan).
- Agree countermeasures, public information, follow-up.

Table 4.14.1 Radiation incidents: responsibilities in the UK

Department of Trade and Industry	Civil nuclear installations.
	Site operators must consult with local agencies and draw up emergency plans including plans for an off-site facility. Radiation (Emergency Preparedness and Public Information) Regulations 2001 (REPPIR) require site operators, local authorities and fire services to provide information for the public living near nuclear installations on the action to be taken should an emergency arise.
Department of Transport	Accidents that occur during transportation of civil radioactive material.
	Operators are regulated by the Radioactive Material (Road Transport) Regulations 2002. They must prepare a plan. Operators subscribe to RADSAFE scheme.
Ministry of Defence	Incidents at defence nuclear installations and transport accidents involving nuclear materials.
Department of Environment, Food and Rural affairs (DEFRA)	Incidents at nuclear installations overseas
	DEFRA operates the UK's Radioactive Incident Monitoring Network (RIMNET) consisting of some 92 continuous radiation monitoring stations. These automatically raise an alarm if abnormal increases in the levels of radiation are detected at any of the sites.
HPA Centre for Radiation, Chemical and Environmental Hazards (CRCE)	Advice to government, other agencies and the public on all aspects of protection from radiological hazards.
	The National Arrangements for Incidents Involving Radioactivity (NAIR) covers radiation incidents in public places. NAIR is usually activated by the Police and is co-ordinated by HPA CRCE. First-stage assistance comes from local radiation staff and second-stage assistance comes from radiation staff from nuclear power stations or other similar establishments.
Health and Safety Executive	Industrial sites with large amounts of nuclear material.
Health services including PCTs, ambulance service and hospitals	Prepare emergency plans. Reception, treatment and decontamination of casualties at designated hospitals, monitoring people and their personal belongings following exposure, by local medical physics departments, distribution of potassium iodate tablets, information to the public and the media on health aspects of the accident, collating advice from expert sources, telephone advice line, long-term follow-up of exposed persons for clinical or epidemiological purposes.
Food Standards Agency	Advice on what food and drink can be consumed
Environment Agency/water company	Advice on whether radioactive material can be flushed into the drains.
Home Office	Nuclear-powered satellite accidents. Terrorism.

for countermeasures are based on Emergency Reference Levels (ERLs). ERLs are expressed in terms of the radiation dose to an individual that could be averted if the countermeasure is implemented. For each countermeasure a lower and an upper ERL is recommended. The lower ERL is the smallest reduction in dose likely to offset the disadvantages of the countermeasure. If the estimated averted dose exceeds the lower ERL, then implementation of the countermeasure should be considered, but is not essential. The upper ERL is the reduction in dose for which the countermeasure would be justified in nearly all situations.

Table 4.14.2 Effects of rapid whole-body radiation exposure

Less than 1 sievert (Sv)	Usually asymptomatic
Whole-body doses less than 0.5 Sv are unlikely to cause acute symptoms	Mild gastrointestinal symptoms in first 48 hours in 1–10%
	Low WBC at 2–4 weeks
	No fetal effects if effective dose less than 100 mSv
	Counselling needed if pregnant and effective dose more than 100 mSv
1–8 Sv	Haematopoietic syndrome
Partial-body exposure causes localised effects (e.g. skin damage, burns, ulcers)	Gastrointestinal symptoms 1–4 hours after exposure
	After 2 days–4 weeks: bone marrow depression, bleeding, bruising
	3–4 Sv: hair loss at 2–3 weeks
	$LD_{50/60}$ is around 4.5 Sv without treatment
6–20 Sv	Gastrointestinal syndrome
	Early gastrointestinal symptoms
	In first week severe gastrointestinal symptoms
	LD100 is about 10 Sv, death usually within 2 weeks
More than 20 Sv	CNS/CV syndrome
	Immediate severe gastrointestinal symptoms
	Convulsions, coma, hypotension, shock
	Death within 2–3 days

CNS, central nervous system; CV, cardiovascular; LD, lethal dose; WBC, white blood cell count.

4.15 Deliberate release of biological, chemical or radiological agents

Deliberate release of biological, chemical or radiological agents may be overt or covert. An overt release may be preceded by a warning, there may be an obvious release in a public place or a number of individuals may present with contamination by an unknown substance. Those exposed may or may not be acutely ill and a sample of the agent may be available for analysis. The health service may be alerted by the police. Should those exposed develop symptoms within the first few minutes or hours the most likely cause is a chemical agent, followed by a biological toxin or hysteria. Slightly longer incubation periods suggest that an infectious or radiological hazard may be responsible. Many incidents will turn out to be a hoax or a misinterpretation of a normal event (e.g. the use of powdered silica in packaging triggering a 'white powder' incident). The principles of dealing with these incidents build on those followed when managing accidental releases.

A covert incident (e.g. a substance introduced into food or the water supply) may only become apparent when ill patients present to health services. This may be some time after exposure, depending on the nature of the agent. Cases may not occur in an obvious geographical area or in people with an obvious common exposure. Potential indicators of a covert release are given in Box 4.15.1. It is likely that the health services will be the first agency to discover a covert release and will have to inform other agencies of their suspicions. The principles of investigating such incidents build on those used in controlling outbreaks or other longer term incidents (see Chapter 4.2).

Advance preparation is the key to success in organising a response and consists of the following:
• multi-agency contingency plans;
• ensuring access to equipment (e.g. personal protective clothing, decontamination facilities and therapeutic countermeasures); and
• training of staff and multi-agency exercises.

Box 4.15.1 When to consider possibility of a deliberate release

- Number of ill people with similar disease or syndrome presenting around the same time.
- Number of cases of unexplained disease, syndrome or death.
- Single case of disease caused by an uncommon agent.
- Recognised illness occurring in an unusual setting or key sector within a community.
- Failure of a common disease to respond to usual therapy.
- Disease with unusual geographical or seasonal variation.
- Multiple atypical presentations of disease agents.
- Similar typing of agents isolated from temporally or spatially distinct sources.
- Unusual, atypical, genetically engineered or antiquated strain of agents.
- Simultaneous outbreaks of similar illness in non-contiguous areas.
- No local cause for unexpected acute event with syndrome of confusion, nausea, vomiting, respiratory, eye and skin irritation, collapse, difficulty seeing, frightened and possible delayed effects. May be smell or plume without explained cause.
- Deaths or illnesses among animals that precedes or accompanies illness or death in humans.
- Suspected or known deliberate release in other countries.

Organisational response to acute and overt incidents

Co-ordination, command and control of acute deliberate release incidents follow the same principles as those adopted for the emergency response to any incident (e.g. explosion, plane crash or flooding) and comprise three levels:

- *Bronze* (operational): usually located at the scene and operating at 'activity' level (e.g. individual patient care).
- *Silver* (tactical): usually located near the scene and operating at function or range of activities level.
- *Gold* (strategic): usually off-site at a headquarters office and is responsible for multi-agency strategic co-ordination.

In the case of suspected deliberate release incidents, an overall lead agency is required to co-ordinate the response. In the UK, this is the police. The multi-agency strategic (gold) group will be supported by a team to provide health advice (called a Scientific and Technical Advice Cell (STAC) in the UK) which:

- takes advice on the health aspects of the incident from a wide range of sources;
- provides advice to the Gold Commander on the health consequences of the incident, including the consequences of any evacuation or containment policies;

- agrees the advice to be given to the public on health aspects of the incident with the Gold Commander;
- liaises with the national Department of Health and other national and local health agencies;
- formulates advice to health professionals in hospitals, ambulance services and primary care; and
- formulates advice on strategic management of the health service response (but does not actually do the strategic management).

The STAC is chaired by the local Director of Public Health or health protection consultant and has multi-agency membership similar to that for an accidental incident or outbreak, plus national experts made available via national arrangements.

Technical aspects of response

In chemical and biological incidents, the actions in order of priority are containment, decontamination, resuscitation, primary treatment, definitive care and follow up. A schematic illustration of how this might be organised at the scene is given in Figure 4.15.1. In general, only simple life-saving treatment can be carried out in the 'warm zone' before decontamination. This

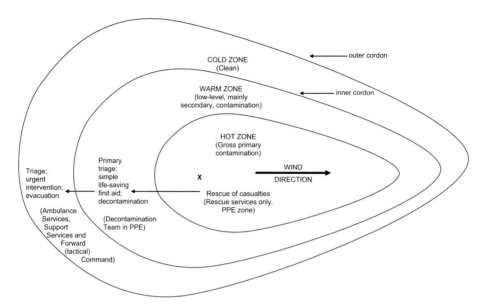

Fig. 4.15.1 Organisation of on-scene response.

comprises simple airway opening manoeuvres, bag-valve-mask ventilation and pressure on 'bleeding wounds'.

Advice should be taken on decontamination, but, in general:
• Remove exposed person from scene of contamination.
• Remove all clothing (80% reduction in contamination).
• General decontamination: the decontaminant of choice for most chemicals is water and detergent using the 'rinse-wipe-rinse' method (water or saline only for eyes and mucus membranes).
• Liquid chemical contamination must be removed as soon as possible.
• Water and hypochlorite are preferred for biological contamination of small numbers of casualties.
• Biological contamination of large numbers can usually wait for mass decontamination facilities to be set up.
• Contaminated clothing, equipment and effluent, where possible, to be stored in safe area, awaiting disposal (or evidence collection).
• For radiation, external decontamination is similar to that for non-radioactive chemicals, but extra care is taken with clothes, etc.
• Decontamination team must wear personal protective equipment (PPE).
• Ensure that decontaminated persons are kept separate from those awaiting decontamination (and moved away from contamination).

Following decontamination, triage will separate exposed into priority groups for treatment and evacuation. Advanced life support procedures and other generic interventions can then be deployed.

It may be possible to identify the causal agent, based on the symptom profile of those who become ill or the results of screening of samples from the environment and patients. This will allow specific countermeasures or antidotes to be deployed (for symptoms and antidotes of main chemical threats see Table 4.15.1).

Table 4.15.1 Potential chemical terrorism agents

	Symptoms	Speed of action	Antidotes and treatment
Nerve agents (organophosphates and related agents e.g. Sarin, VX)	Mild: headache, nausea, small pupils, visual difficulties, painful eyes, running nose, excess salivation, mild weakness and agitation Moderate: dizziness, disorientation, confusion, sneezing, coughing, wheezing, drooling, excess phlegm, vomiting, diarrhoea, marked weakness, difficulty breathing Severe: respiratory difficulty, convulsions, arrhythmias	Unconsciousness and convulsions within seconds; death in minutes	Atropine Oximes Diazepam
Mustard	Early: nausea, vomiting, retching, eye irritation, erythema Hours: nausea, fatigue, headache, painful eyes, lacrimation, blepharospasm, photophobia, runny nose, erythema, sore throat, hoarseness, tachycardia, tachypnoea, oedema Days: inflammation, blistering, pus, necrosis, coughing	$^1/_2$–2 hours 2–6 hours 13–72 hours	Decontaminate ASAP No specific antidote Symptomatic and supportive care only. May need ICU facilities
Chlorine	Inhalation: irritation of eyes, nose and throat, followed by coughing, wheezing, dyspnoea, sputum, bronchospasm, chest pain. Metabolic complications from mild alkalosis to severe acidosis and hypoxaemia. Cardiorespiratory arrest due to hypoxia may occur Dermal: skin irritation with burns at high concentration	Irritation occurs rapidly Chemical pneumonitis and pulmonary oedema can take 12–24 hours	Removal from contaminated area No specific antidote Symptomatic and supportive care only. May need ICU facilities
Hydrogen cyanide	Low dose: dyspnoea, headache, dizziness, anxiety, tachycardia, nausea, drowsiness, possibly metallic taste High dose: hyperventilation, unconsciousness, convulsions, fixed dilated pupils, cyanosis, death	Unconsciousness and convulsions in seconds. Death in minutes	Removal from contaminated area and resuscitation Dicobaltedetate or sodium nitrite

(Continued on p. 346)

Table 4.15.1 (Continued)

	Symptoms	Speed of action	Antidotes and treatment
Phosgene	Initial phase: eye irritation, lacrimation, nausea, vomiting, chest tightness, retrosternal discomfort, bronchoconstriction, hypertension, brady or tachycardia. Severe exposure can lead to haemolysis and rapid death Latent phase: may appear well, symptoms precipitated by exercise Oedema phase: pulmonary oedema, dyspnoea, bronchospasm, frothy sputum, hypotension, tachycardia, hypoxia, ARDS, death (severity of initial phase not related to severity of oedema)	Major effects usually take hours, but may be immediate pain at exposed sites	Decontaminate ASAP Symptomatic and supportive No specific antidote May need ICU facilities
Ricin	Fever common Ingestion causes irritation of oropharynx and oesophagus plus gastroenteritis Bloody diarrhoea, vomiting, abdominal pain, conjunctivitis, miosis, mydriasis, pulmonary oedema, pneumonia, ARDS, seizures, CNS depression, multiorgan failure, death. Abnormal LFTs, haematuria, proteinuria, high creatinine	Delayed	Symptomatic and supportive No specific antidote
Lewisite (arsenical compound)	Early: very irritating, pain on contact Damage to eyes, skin, airways. Similar to mustard	Minutes	Decontaminate ASAP British-Anti-Lewisite
Saxitoxin	Paralytic shellfish poisoning (see Chapter 3.91.6) May be confused with nerve agents	10–120 minutes	Induce vomiting May need ICU Avoid atropine!
Tricothecene mycotoxins ('Yellow rain')	Burning skin, redness, tenderness, blistering, necrosis Dyspnoea, wheezing, coughing, weakness, prostration, dizziness, ataxia Tachycardia, hypothermia, hypotension	Minutes	Decontamination of skin No specific antidote

ARDS, acute respiratory disease syndrome; ASAP, as soon as possible; ICU, intensive care unit; LFT, liver function test.

Suspicious packages or materials

A package may be considered suspicious if:
• suspicious or threatening messages are written on it;
• envelope is distorted, bulky, rigid, discoloured, has an oily stain, has an obvious odour or feels like it has powder inside;
• unexpected envelope, particularly from a foreign country;
• no postage stamp, no franking or cancelling of stamp;
• incorrect spelling of common names, places or titles;
• handwritten envelope from unknown source, particularly if addressed to an individual and marked personal or addressee only; or
• on opening, suspicious power or material is found.

The immediate response should be not to open the package and to call the police immediately for advice. If the package has been opened or suspect material is found then, in addition:
• shut the windows and doors to the room and switch off any air-conditioning;
• the room occupants should move to an unoccupied adjacent room away from the hazard;
• seek medical advice for anyone showing symptoms;
• notify the building manager to switch off air-conditioning, close fire doors and close all windows in the rest of building; and
• do not touch or attempt to clean up any suspect material.

The police should then perform a risk assessment, to decide whether the threat is credible. Figure 4.15.2 gives details of action to be taken in response to their assessment. A number of agencies will need to be involved if a credible threat is declared and specialist advice should be taken.

Investigation of incidents of unusual illness

A cluster of an unusual or unknown illness, a single occurrence of an unexpected illness for that community or illness that fails to behave as expected should be investigated according to standard epidemiological and public health practices (see Chapter 4.2). However, there may be some features that should raise the suspicion of a deliberate release (Box 4.15.1). Infectious agents that are considered to have bioterrorist potential are given in Table 4.15.2. Of note is that in deliberate release scenarios, the presentation may be more sudden, more severe and involve larger numbers than in natural outbreaks, particularly if aerosol dispersion has been used. Fortunately, most such agents do not spread onwards from person to person, although smallpox and pneumonic plague are important exceptions.

In addition to notifying local, regional and national public health authorities, a suspected deliberate release must also be reported to the police, who will have their own investigative needs. As always, meticulous record keeping is essential.

In addition to standard outbreak and incident investigation steps (case-definitions; case finding; data collection and recording; laboratory investigations; descriptive epidemiology; hypothesis generation and testing), particular issues for management include:
• defining those 'exposed but not ill' and collecting data on them;
• guidance on investigation and best treatment of rare illnesses or variant organisms;
• risk to contacts, including healthcare staff;
• information for the public;
• communications arrangements; and
• environmental contamination.

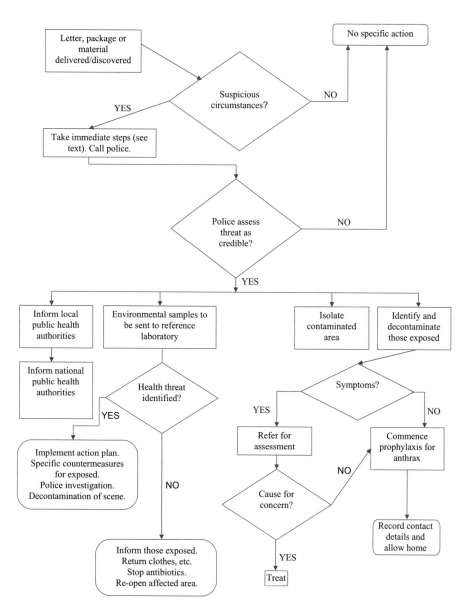

Fig. 4.15.2 Response to suspicious package or material.

Table 4.15.2 Potential bioterrorism organisms and toxins

Agent (disease)	Potential source	Ability to cause disease	Incubation period	Ability to spread from person-to-person	Chemoprophylaxis	Further details
Bacillus anthracis (anthrax)	Aerosol (spores)	Moderate	1–6 days	None	1. Ciprofloxacin 2. Doxycycline 3. Amoxicillin	Chapter 3.2
Brucella sp (brucellosis)	1. Aerosol 2. Food	High	Days to months	None	1. Ciprofloxacin 2. Doxycycline	Chapter 3.5
Burkholderia mallei (glanders)	Aerosol	High	Days to weeks	Low	1. Doxycycline 2. Ciprofloxacin	Chapter 3.6
Burkholderia pseudomallei (melioidosis)	Aerosol	High	1–7 days	Negligible	1. Ciprofloxacin 2. Doxycycline	Chapter 3.6
Chlamydia psittaci (psittacosis)	Aerosol	Moderate	Range from 4–28 days to (usual) 5–15 days	Negligible	Doxycycline	Chapter 3.11
Clostridium botulinum toxin (botulism)	1. Food/water 2. Aerosol	High	Ranges from a few hours to 8 days (usually 12 hours–3 days)	None	None Antitoxin available	Chapter 3.4
Coccidioides immitis (coccidioidomycosis)	Aerosol	High	1–2 weeks	None	Fluconazole	Stable agent of low lethality
Coxiella burnetii (Q fever)	1. Aerosol 2. Food supply	High	9–33 days (median 20 days)	Negligible	1. Doxycycline 2. Erythromycin	Chapter 3.61
Ebola/Lassa/CCHF (viral haemorrhagic fevers)	Aerosol	High	3–15 days	Moderate (body fluids)	None available	Chapter 3.85
Francisella tularensis (tularaemia)	Aerosol	High	2–10 days	None	1. Ciprofloxacin 2. Doxycycline	Chapter 3.81

(Continued on p. 350)

Table 4.15.2 (Continued)

Agent (disease)	Potential source	Ability to cause disease	Incubation period	Ability to spread from person-to-person	Chemoprophylaxis	Further details
Hantavirus	Aerosol	High	4–42 days	None	None available	Chapter 3.29
Histoplasma. capsulatum (histoplasmosis)	Aerosol	High	1–2 weeks	None	Fluconazole	Can persist in soil, but low lethality
Influenza virus	Aerosol	High	7–67 hours	High (respiratory)	1. Oseltamir 2. Zanamivir	Chapter 3.40
Junin virus	Aerosol	Moderate	7–16 days	Low	None (ribavirin if fever)	Chapter 3.91.4
Machupo virus	Aerosol	Moderate	7–14 days	Low	None (ribavirin if fever)	Chapter 3.91.4
Rickettsia prowazekii (typhus)	1. Aerosol 2. Infected vectors	High	6–16 days	None	Doxycycline	Chapter 3.83
Rickettsia rickettsii (Rocky Mountain spotted fever)	1. Aerosol 2. Infected vectors	High	3–10 days	None	Doxycycline	Not very stable but high lethality
Rickettsia tsutsugamushi (scrub typhus)	1. Aerosol 2. Infected vectors	High	4–15days	None	Doxycycline	Not very stable and low lethality
Rift Valley fever virus	Aerosol	Moderate	2–12 days	None	None (ribavirin if fever)	Chapter 3.91.4 Would also cause disease in sheep and cattle
Salmonella sp (gastroenteritis)	1. Food 2. Water	Low	4 hours–5 days (usually 12–48 hours)	Moderate (faeco-oral)	Ciprofloxacin	Chapter 3.68
Salmonella typhi (typhoid)	1. Food/water 2. Aerosol	Moderate	3–40 days (median 14 days)	Low (faeco-oral)	1. Ciprofloxacin 2. Ceftriaxone	Chapter 3.82
Shigella sp (dysentery)	1. Food 2. Water	High	12 hours–4 days (usually 1–3 days)	High (faeco-oral)	Ciprofloxacin	Chapter 3.71

Agent	Transmission	Infectivity	Incubation period	Person-to-person spread	Prophylaxis/treatment	Reference
Smallpox virus	Aerosol	High	10–17 days	High (aerosol)	None available / Vaccine for contacts	Chapter 3.72
Staphylococcal enterotoxin B	1. Sabotage 2. Aerosol		1–6 hours	None	None	Stable toxin of low lethality
Venezuelan equine encephalitis virus	Aerosol	High	1–6 days	None	None	Chapter 3.91.4
Vibrio cholerae (cholera)	1. Food/water 2. Aerosol	Low	1–5 days	Negligible	1. Ciprofloxacin 2. Doxycycline	Chapter 3.13
VTEC (haemorrhagic gastroenteritis)	1. Food 2. Water	High	6 hours–10 days (usually 2–4 days)	High (faeco-oral)	None	Chapter 3.26
Yellow fever virus	Aerosol	Moderate	3–6 days	None	None	Chapter 3.89
Yersinia pestis (plague)	1. Aerosol 2. Vectors	High	2–3 days	High (pneumonic)	1. Ciprofloxacin 2. Doxycycline	Chapter 3.58

CCHF, Congo–Crimean haemorrhagic fever; VTEC, verocytotoxin-producing *Escherichia coli*.

4.16 Media relations and crisis communication

The media should be considered as an ally in protecting the health of the public. They are one of the most powerful influences upon the public. Relationships with the media should be developed proactively; good routine relationships with the media will make dealing with them during emergency situations much easier.

Communicable disease issues arouse interest and anxiety in the public. The public have a right to be informed and the press is often the best route. Virtually all issues can be presented in a way that the public can understand. Professionals should not hide behind technical obfuscations. Do not expect to have any control over material that you provide, press releases can be selectively quoted and interviews can be edited. However, journalists are usually interested in accuracy.

Training

Anyone who is likely to deal with the media should undergo media training. This will help in understanding what the media needs. Journalists often have a similar agenda to public health workers, they wish to inform and educate the public. If they encounter a group of professionals who understand their needs, and are trying to help, then journalists are less likely to be antagonistic. Identify people within the organisation who are particularly good with the media – they may not be the most senior people.

Routine relationships

Develop regular contact with your local print and broadcast media. Be available to answer their questions, and treat your local reporters as friends. If they trust you and rely on you as an authoritative source it will make things much easier if a story is breaking.

Local papers may be willing to publish a regular column; this is a powerful way of getting health advice across. Use opportunities to publish in local papers, women's magazines, parents' magazines, etc. This will probably have a greater influence on health than publishing in the peer-reviewed medical press. Have basic information packs available for journalists. These should describe the clinical features and importance of an infection and the salient epidemiological features and recent trends.

Crisis (outbreak) communication

During outbreak or emergency situations it is important to maintain good relations with the press. Journalists have a job to do, they can become intrusive, but they will understand that you also have a job to do. Let the journalists know that they will be kept informed, that there will be regular briefings, daily or even twice daily. Ensure that the briefings do happen. Appoint a media spokesperson and ensure that all media briefings are done through that person. The outbreak control team should co-ordinate the local flow of information. Sometimes, several actors (at different levels) are involved, all with their own media contacts, it is then important to have coordinated messages and shared lines-to-take. If not, journalists will likely focus on the differences rather than on the main messages.

WHO has developed outbreak communication guidelines that could be used as a reference by anyone involved in outbreak communication. The main principles include the following:

• build, maintain and restore trust;
• announce early;
• aim at maximum transparency (taking into account privacy issues);
• understand the public; and
• plan in advance.

Messages

Decide beforehand what your key messages are; if possible discuss these with the journalist and discuss the questions that will be asked. Decide if there are any areas that you do not wish to be drawn into. Be honest, accurate and keep technical details to a minimum. Get the key message across first, then provide the reasoning behind it. Stress the facts and explain the context. Do not try to hide the truth or lie. If you are uncertain of the facts or some detail say so and offer to get the information. Do not be drawn into areas you feel you cannot or should not discuss, be firm and polite and say that you cannot discuss that issue. Try to avoid discussions of money and cost saving, stress public health action and your concern for safeguarding the public health. Avoid being drawn into speculation, or other criticisms of other groups. Behave as if you were always 'on the record'. Make sure that you know if a broadcast is live or recorded. Always ask to see the article before it is published in order to correct factual mistakes – most serious journalists appreciate that. However, do not expect to be able to change the direction or angle of the article, attempts to do that will likely just upset the journalist.

Press releases

Keep the press release short (8–10 paragraphs), make sure you have considered the message and the audience for the release, consult a press officer. Get the most important message into the first paragraph and support it with a quote from a senior official. In the introduction, describe who, what, where, when, why/how. In the middle, expand the story with supporting detail, conclude by summarising and identifying the next steps.

Internet, blogs and social networks

Information is increasingly disseminated through the Internet. Treat any Internet site as if it might be read by any member of the public. Do not write anything that you would not wish to see in the public domain. Internet interviews or Q&A sessions are an effective way of disseminating information; however, they can appear informal, so be careful that you are not drawn into a statement you would not make in conventional media.

Problems

The press might want access to cases or locations such as outbreak rooms for atmospheric pictures or interviews. These requests should be considered very carefully. Considerations of confidentiality and the smooth running of an investigation must come first. However, on occasion such photo opportunities might, by raising public awareness of an issue, be beneficial. If things go wrong remember that they can do in the best of relations. Developing good relations with the media takes time and effort. If errors of fact appear in an article, or you feel you have been misrepresented, contact the journalist and discuss them; if necessary talk to the editor.

4.17 Clinical governance and audit

Clinical governance provides a framework in which organisations involved in public health protection are accountable for continuously improving the quality of their services and safeguarding public health by creating an environment in which high standards of service are assured and excellence in health protection (HP) practice will flourish.

The main components for clinical governance are the following:
• clear lines of responsibility and accountability for the overall quality of the service provided;
• a comprehensive programme of quality improvement activities;

- clear policies aimed at managing risk; and
- procedures to identify and remedy poor performance.

The work of communicable disease control (CDC)/HP departments does not fit neatly into these compartments, but a suitable breakdown could be as follows.

Responsibility

Clinical governance emphasises that the organisational responsibility for quality lies at board level, which has a responsibility for encouraging an environment in which quality can flourish. The board of the organisation needs to set clear objectives for the service. It must also take a particular interest in the organisation's 'strategic capacity' to deliver a quality service and assess and control the risk to that capacity. This includes:
- workforce capacity (Box 4.17.1) and competence;
- leadership;
- culture or organisational behaviour;
- accountability for key elements of service;
- team working;
- adequate finance;
- information management and technology;
- partnerships;

- facilities and equipment; and
- policies and procedures.

The health commissioning organisation is also responsible for ensuring that other health services involved in CDC/HP (e.g. laboratories, chest clinics, STI clinics) have adequate clinical governance arrangements.

In practice, the executive lead for surveillance, prevention and control of communicable diseases (and other related functions) locally lies with the local health protection unit (HPU), whose director should therefore take the lead in assuring the quality of the district CDC/HP function. The HPU director is also responsible for ensuring that support staff provide a quality service by encouraging training, openness, teamwork, the seeking of advice where appropriate and performance review.

Quality improvement

CDC/HP teams should complete a baseline self-assessment of their strengths and weaknesses. This could cover the following areas:
- Service structure, personnel and skills.
- Arrangements for on-call and for covering leave.

Box 4.17.1 Suggested staffing levels for district CDC departments

Medical
- Minimum of 1.0 whole time equivalent (wte) consultants per 400,000 population.
- Minimum 0.5 wte allocated time and available throughout office hours.
- Extra consultant sessions in districts with more complex workload and for any non-CDC duties.

Nursing
- Minimum of 1.0 per 400,000 population.
- Extra nurse sessions in districts with large number of community settings (e.g. care homes).

Information scientist
- 0.2–0.5 per 400,000 population.
- Minimum of 1 session per week.

Secretarial/clerical/data entry
- Minimum of 1.5 wte per 400,000 population.
- Must be telephone cover during working hours.

Source: Report to NHS Executive, England, 1997.

- Access to operational support and infrastructure within healthcare and health protection organisations (e.g. administrative, IT, statistical expertise, communications, public relations).
- Access to specialist advice, library services and relevant Internet sites (e.g. Medline, Cochrane).
- Arrangements for multi-agency working, particularly with environmental health departments and hospital control of infection teams. Should include relevant operational support from other health organisations (e.g. healthcare commissioning and provider organisations) for activities such as surveillance, contact tracing and incident control.
- Clarity of roles and responsibilities of different organisations and individuals.
- How well the unit functions as a team.
- Adequacy of surveillance: data access (timeliness, quality), analysis and dissemination.
- Completeness and updating of policies and plans.
- Use of evidence-based practice and mechanisms for disseminating good practice.
- Support to prevention and control in community settings.
- Mechanisms to maintain patient confidentiality.
- Multi-agency fora and committees (e.g. district control of infection, immunisation) for agreeing policies and procedures.
- Patient, service user, carer and public involvement.
- Audit and evaluation (see below).

Departments may also wish to invite an external peer reviewer to comment on how their services compare with standard/best practice elsewhere.

The HPU director should formulate a risk register in the light of the baseline assessment, with a prioritised action plan with clearly assigned responsibilities and timescales. This should then be discussed with the appropriate clinical governance lead for the organisation. Progress on the action plan needs to be regularly reviewed.

One important element of quality improvement will be continuing professional development (CPD) for CDC/HP staff. Each staff member should have a personal development plan, which should be discussed with their line manager. This could include training and updating in the following areas:

- Epidemiology and control of communicable diseases.
- Epidemiological methods and statistics for surveillance, outbreaks and research.
- Information technology.
- Infection control and environmental health.
- Management methods such as leadership, organisation, supervisory skills, team working, time management, presentation and media skills.
- New governmental, organisational or professional priorities.
- Non-communicable risks to health (if relevant).

Departmental CPD should include training and updating in on-call issues for all staff on the out-of-hours rota. Those whose routine work does not include a large component of CDC/HP would benefit from attendance at a specialist course at least every 3 years. In UK, the role of the General Medical Council and Royal Colleges in revalidation will mean that doctors will need to be able to demonstrate regularly that they are keeping themselves up-to-date and remain fit to practise in their chosen field.

Policies for managing risk

Such policies should include the following:
- Incident response plans for:
  (a) community outbreaks;
  (b) hospital outbreaks;
  (c) water-borne diseases;
  (d) instances requiring patient tracing, notification and helplines;
  (e) chemical incidents;
  (f) radiation incidents;
  (g) major emergencies; and
  (h) deliberate release.

These plans need regular revision. If used in an incident, a written report should be produced. If not recently used, consideration should be given to a simulation exercise:

• Policies and procedures for dealing with common or serious diseases.
• A regularly updated on-call pack, which includes relevant policies and contact details for staff and other organisations.
• Good documentation of incidents and requests for advice.
• A system for reporting and learning lessons from complaints, problems encountered in delivering service, or poor outcomes. The system should include a mechanism for ensuring that action is taken in response to lessons learned.

Rectifying poor performance

In CDC/HP this primarily revolves around clinical audit and CPD (there is obvious overlap with quality improvement processes).
• Clinical audit involves:
  (a) setting standards;
  (b) comparing actual performance to standards; and
  (c) rectifying identified deficiencies.
• Audit should involve an element of peer review. One useful mechanism is to involve staff in neighbouring teams, perhaps as part of a Regional Audit Group. Where national standards do not exist, this group can devise regional ones on which to base audit.
• Suitable topics for audit might be:
  (a) adequacy of contingency plans;
  (b) adequacy of district surveillance systems for spotting outbreaks and analysing trends;
  (c) response of on-call staff (including partner organisations);
  (d) review of management of an actual outbreak;
  (e) review of response to (randomly selected) cases of meningococcal disease;
  (f) immunisation uptake rates and methods used to improve them; and
  (g) appropriateness of HIV prevention strategy.
• A report should be written on all significant outbreaks and incidents detailing the lessons learnt. More minor episodes (e.g. sporadic case of typhoid) can be discussed informally

(e.g. at weekly departmental surveillance and information meetings).
• Discussion and monitoring of formal and informal complaints from the public or health professionals.
• It is important in all cases to ensure that someone is responsible for ensuring that identified deficiencies in the service are rectified. Methods of rectifying poor performance are given above.

It is clear that the quality of CDC/HP work and the ability to carry out clinical governance and audit are both dependent upon the level of resources available to the CDC/HP department and the overall culture of the organisation. Nonetheless, the individual practitioner can use his/her leadership, management and professional skills to maximise the resources available and to prioritise their use: clinical governance is a tool that can be used to further those objectives.

4.18 Global health

Global health is the application of public health practice to health issues that transcend national boundaries. Examples of global health issues are summarised in Box 4.18.1.

Box 4.18.1 Examples of global health issues

• Malnutrition and underweight in children
• Low birth weight
• High neonatal mortality
• High pregnancy-related mortality
• Infectious diseases in children including measles, diarrhoea and pneumonia
• Pandemic influenza, West Nile virus, HIV infection, TB, malaria
• Sexually transmitted infections in young women
• Increases in diabetes and cardiovascular disease.
• Violence against women

If health is measured using life-expectancy at birth or child mortality then it is clear that health has improved substantially in many countries in the past 20 years. However, quality and length of life is still low in some countries and in others health is actually deteriorating because of HIV infection and the effects of armed conflict. Between and within countries there are large disparities in access to health services, new technologies for health and the essential prerequisites for health such as income and education.

As a result of globalisation there are large population movements and diseases, and risk factors do not respect national boundaries. Some low and middle income countries are now experiencing the risk factors for non-communicable disease that are familiar in developed countries and are witnessing rising levels of cancer, cardiovascular disease, diabetes and mental health problems.

Global health has been given prominence by the activities of former politicians and celebrities from the world of business and entertainment and is now taught in most university public health programmes. There are several reasons why global health is important. Nations share the threats of infectious diseases and the determinants of disease such as tobacco consumption and modern sedentary lifestyles that cross their boundaries. Economic development of nations is not possible without a healthy population and workforce. Finally, health inequalities between nations present an ethical and moral challenge and may even threaten security.

Global health has developed a number of key concepts and themes which are summarised in Table 4.18.1. In 2000, United Nations member states agreed eight Millennium Development Goals (MDG) to drive progress in tackling poverty, hunger, disease, illiteracy,

Table 4.18.1 Key concepts and themes in global health

Wider determinants of health	Education
	Income and development
	Social capital
	Gender
Measures of health status and the burden of disease	Life expectancy
	Child mortality
	Disability adjusted life years (DALYs)
Effect of culture on health	Health beliefs and practices
	Changing health behaviour
Demographic and lifestyle transitions	Change from high mortality and high fertility to low mortality and low fertility
	Change from a predominance of communicable to non-communicable disease
Health as 'human rights'	
Organisation of health systems	Financing and organising healthcare
	Ensuring quality of care and access
	Integrated outreach, primary healthcare and hospital services
Role of the environment and nutrition	
Maternal and reproductive health	Maternal mortality and morbidity
	Sex-selection abortion
	Female genital cutting
	Sexually transmitted infections
	Violence and sexual abuse

(*Continued on p. 358*)

Table 4.18.1 (*Continued*)

Child health	Neonatal mortality
	Under-5s mortality
Infectious diseases	HIV
	TB
	Malaria
	Diarrhoeal disease
Non-communicable diseases	Cardiovascular disease
	Diabetes
	Cancer
	Mental health
	Tobacco use
	Alcohol
	Drug misuse
Unintentional injury	Emergency medical services
Natural disasters and humanitarian emergencies	
Partnership working	See Table 4.18.2
New technologies	

environmental degradation and discrimination against women by 2015. Three MDGs relate directly to health (MDG 4–6) but all are interdependent. For example, health enables 'children to learn and adults to earn' and health depends on and influences poverty reduction, hunger and environmental degradation. Each MDG has one or more targets (Box 4.18.2). Progress towards the achievement of these goals is regularly monitored and has become an important management and development tool.

Box 4.18.2 The eight Millennium Development Goals

1 To eradicate extreme poverty and hunger.
2 To achieve universal primary education.
3 To promote gender equality and empower women.
4 To reduce child mortality.
  • Target 4a. Reduce by two-thirds, between 1990 and 2015, the under-5s mortality rate.
5 To improve maternal health.
  • Target 5a. Reduce by three-quarters, between 1990 and 2015, the maternal mortality ratio.
  • Target 5b. Achieve, by 2015, universal access to reproductive health.
6 To combat HIV/AIDS, malaria and other diseases.
  • Target 6a. Have halted by 2015 and begun to reverse the spread of HIV/AIDS.
  • Target 6b. Achieve, by 2010, universal access to treatment for HIV/AIDS for all those who need it.
  • Target 6c. Have halted by 2015 and begun to reverse the incidence of malaria and other major diseases.
7 To ensure environmental sustainability.
8 To develop a global partnership for development.

Table 4.18.2 Selected organisations involved in global health

World Health Organization	Specialised UN agency responsible for providing leadership on matters related to global health	http://www.who.int/en/
Joint United Nations Programme on HIV/AIDS (UNAIDS)	Created in 1995, UNAIDS works on the ground in more than 80 countries providing leadership, advocacy, strategic information and mobilising resources	http://www.unaids.org/en/default.asp
Roll Back Malaria (RBM) Partnership	Launched in 1998 by WHO and other partners, provides a co-ordinated global approach to fighting malaria	http://www.rbm.who.int/
World Bank	Source of financial and technical assistance to developing countries to fight poverty by providing financial and infrastructure support	http://www.worldbank.org/
European Centre for Disease Prevention and Control (ECDC)	An EU agency with mission to identify, assess and communicate current and emerging threats to human health posed by infectious diseases. Works mainly within the EU, but supports the EU global health policies	http://www.ecdc.europa.eu
CARE	Non-sectarian federation of relief and development organisations to fight poverty	http://www.care-international.org/
Framework Convention Alliance for Tobacco Control	Works to implement the WHO Framework Convention on Tobacco Control (FCTC)	http://www.fctc.org/
Médecins Sans Frontières (MSF)	Founded in 1971 by a group of French doctors to deliver emergency aid to people affected by armed conflict, epidemics and natural or manmade disasters	http://www.msf.org/
Aga Khan Foundation	Non-denominational development agency established in 1967 with a mission to develop creative solutions to social development problems in the poorest parts of Asia and East Africa	http://www.akdn.org/AKF
Drugs for Neglected Diseases initiative (DNDi)	Not-for-profit partnership working to research and develop new and improved treatments for neglected diseases	http://www.dndi.org/
GAVI Alliance	Unique partnership of public and private sector focused on increasing access to immunisation in poor countries	http://www.gavialliance.org/
Global Fund to Fight AIDS, Tuberculosis and Malaria (Global Fund)	Aims to increase resources to fight these diseases through innovative health financing	http://www.theglobalfund.org/en/
International Committee of the Red Cross (ICRC)	Neutral organisation that ensures humanitarian protection and assistance for victims of war and armed violence	http://www.icrc.org/eng

(*Continued on p. 360*)

Table 4.18.2 Selected organisations involved in global health

Oxfam International	Confederation of 13 independent NGOs dedicated to fighting poverty and related injustice around the world	http://www.oxfam.org/
Rotary International (RI)	Worldwide organisation of business, professional and community leaders to provide service and promote high ethical standards	http://www.rotary.org/en/ EndPolio/Pages/ridefault. aspx
World Medical Association (WMA)	International organisation representing physicians to work for the highest possible standard of ethical behaviour and care	http://www.wma.net/en/ 10home/index.html
Stop TB Partnership	A global movement to accelerate social and political action to stop the spread of TB around the world	http://www.stoptb.org/
Global Health Council	Membership alliance of healthcare professionals and organisations dedicated to saving lives by improving health throughout the world	http://www.globalhealth. org/
Bill and Melinda Gates Foundation Global Health Program	Harnesses advances in science and technology to save lives in poor countries	http://www.gatesfoundation .org/global-health/Pages/ overview.aspx

A recent communication from the European Commission, The EU Role in Global Health (available at http://ec.europa.eu/development/icenter/repository/COMM_PDF_COM_2010_0128_EN.PDF), has addressed the incomplete achievement of the Millennium Development Goals, and emphasised the legitimacy of an EU leadership role in this area.

In addition to government agencies and university institutes, hundreds of other organisations are involved in global health. A selection of these organisations is listed in Table 4.18.2.

Section 5
Communicable disease control in Europe

5.1 WHO and International Health Regulations

World Health Organization

The World Health Organization (WHO) is a United Nations organisation with a strong mandate in global public health. It is organised in a central headquarter in Geneva, and six regional offices. The Regional Office for Europe, located in Copenhagen, serves 53 countries in Europe and Central Asia, including all the EU countries.

Core functions for WHO include provision of technical support and capacity building, knowledge dissemination, health monitoring, shaping research agendas and establishment, promotion and monitoring of norms. The organisation works closely with international and national partners for joint actions, and relies on voluntary contributions for more than 70% of its budget.

In the area of communicable diseases, WHO mainly works on global health control programmes such as HIV/AIDS, tuberculosis and malaria. Following the successful global eradication of smallpox in 1979, WHO is also working to eradicate polio, eliminate measles and rubella through promotion of the expanded programme on immunisation, and provide global leadership on influenza surveillance and control.

WHO provides a global coordination of outbreak control through the Global Outbreak Alert and Response Network (GOARN), which is a technical collaboration of institutions and networks with the capacity to combat international spread of outbreaks and to ensure that technical assistance is effectively deployed to affected outbreak areas.

International Health Regulations

In today's globalised world, many infectious diseases have the potential to spread from one part of the world to another in a very short time. Recent examples are the SARS outbreak in 2003 and the 2009 H1N1 pandemic. To respond effectively to infectious disease outbreaks and other public health risks (e.g. chemical and nuclear accidents) with the potential to affect many countries, the new International Health Regulations (IHR) (http://www.who.int/topics/international_health_regulations/en/) have been set up as an international legal instrument that is binding to 194 countries, including all the WHO Member States.

The new IHR, which entered into force in June 2007, aim to prevent the spread of disease and public health risks while at the same time limiting unnecessary interference with international travel and trade. The IHR provide a framework for the international co-ordination of information sharing, assessment and public health response to events that may constitute a 'public health emergency of international concern' (PHEIC).

Under the IHR, designated National IHR Focal Points in each country are obliged to report potential PHEIC to WHO within 24 hours of assessment and continuously provide the organisation with updated information. The WHO then forward information, in confidence, to other state's parties that may need this information for public health actions. Within the EU, the National IHR Focal Points are normally identical with the EWRS Focal Points (see Chapter 5.2), and the two systems are to a large degree harmonised.

The Director General of WHO also has the right to issue temporary recommendations, including health measures to be implemented in response to a PHEIC. The

Communicable Disease Control and Health Protection Handbook, Third Edition. Jeremy Hawker, Norman Begg, Iain Blair, Ralf Reintjes, Julius Weinberg and Karl Ekdahl.
© 2012 Jeremy Hawker, Norman Begg, Iain Blair, Ralf Reintjes, Julius Weinberg and Karl Ekdahl.
Published 2012 by Blackwell Publishing Ltd.

recommendations may include measures related to individuals (mainly travellers) and transportation of goods. The recommendations on individuals, which shall respect travellers' dignity, human rights, and fundamental freedom, may include the following:
• review travel history in affected areas;
• review proof of medical examination and any relevant laboratory analysis;
• require medical examinations;
• review proof of vaccination or other prophylaxis;
• require vaccination or other prophylaxis;
• place suspect persons under public health observation;
• implement quarantine or other health measures for suspect persons;
• implement isolation and treatment where necessary of affected persons;
• implement tracing of contacts of suspect or affected persons;
• refuse entry of suspect and affected persons;
• refuse entry of unaffected persons to affected areas; and
• implement exit screening and/or restrictions on persons from affected areas.

The IHR also requires the countries to have the capacity to detect, assess, notify and respond to PHEIC and other public health risks. At the request of the affected country, the WHO shall provide technical guidance and assistance when necessary. To have IHR fully implemented thus requires substantial capacity building in many countries.

Point of entry

Also regulated under the IHR is the responsibility for countries to designate specific airports, ports and ground crossings with capacity at all times:
• to provide access to appropriate medical services, staff, equipment and premises for prompt assessment and care of ill travellers;
• to provide access to equipment and personnel for the transport of ill travellers to an appropriate medical facility;
• to provide trained personnel for the inspection of conveyances;

• to ensure a safe environment for travellers using point of entry facilities, including potable water supplies, eating establishments, flight catering facilities, public washrooms, appropriate solid and liquid waste disposal services and other potential risk areas; and
• to provide as far as practicable a programme and trained personnel for the control of vectors and reservoirs in and near points of entry.

For responding to events that may constitute a PHEIC the entry points should also have capacity to:
• provide appropriate public health emergency response by establishing and maintaining a public health emergency contingency plan, including the nomination of a co-ordinator and contact points for relevant point of entry, public health and other agencies and services;
• provide assessment of and care for affected travellers or animals by establishing arrangements with local medical and veterinary facilities for their isolation, treatment and other support services that may be required;
• provide appropriate space, separate from other travellers, to interview suspect or affected persons;
• provide for the assessment and, if required, quarantine of suspect travellers, preferably in facilities away from the point of entry;
• apply recommended measures to disinsect, derat, disinfect, decontaminate or otherwise to treat baggage, cargo, containers, conveyances, goods or postal parcels including, when appropriate, at locations specially designated and equipped for this purpose;
• apply entry or exit controls for arriving and departing travellers; and
• provide access to specially designated equipment, and to trained personnel with appropriate personal protection, for the transfer of travellers who may carry infection or contamination.

Other requirements under IHR

The IHR also include a number of other requirements all aimed at diminishing the risk of transmission of communicable diseases and other public health risks across borders.

Technical requirements pertaining to conveyances and conveyance operators

Conveyance operators shall facilitate:
- inspections of cargo, containers and conveyance;
- medical examinations of persons on board;
- application of other IHR health measures; and
- provision of relevant public health information requested by the country.

Conveyance operators shall provide valid sanitation and health certificates to the national authorities.

Specific measures for vector-borne diseases

Disinfection and other vector control measures shall be recommended for conveyances arriving from certain risk areas. WHO shall on a regular basis publish lists of such areas, and also issue recommendations how such measures should be carried out. To prevent autochthonous spread of infections via imported vectors, countries shall establish vector control programmes for the near vicinity (minimum 400 metres) from point of entry facilities involving passengers or goods from risk areas.

Requirements concerning vaccination or prophylaxis for certain diseases

In addition to vaccinations normally recommended for travel, the IHR can specifically list diseases for which proof of vaccination or prophylaxis may be required for entry to a country. Countries are obliged to offer vaccines or prophylaxis of suitable quality for these diseases and issue international certificate of vaccination or prophylaxis.

Currently, this list includes yellow fever. Yellow fever vaccination may also be required for leaving areas with yellow fever transmis-

sion (as determined by WHO). Countries have the right to quarantine persons arriving from areas with yellow fever up until the day the vaccination certificate becomes valid (10 days post-vaccination) or the full incubation period (6 days), whichever occurs first. India, which is particularly concerned by the possible introduction of yellow fever on its territory, has made a specific reservation regarding yellow fever, including the right to continue all health measures stipulated in previous IHR from 1969.

5.2 Collaboration within the European Union

In 2010, the population of the 27 EU Member States surpassed half a billion people. An unwanted side effect of the free movement of people, goods, services and money within the EU is free movement of microbes. This requires effective, co-ordinated measures for the control of communicable diseases at the EU level. Although mainly the responsibility of the Member States, public health has been covered by EU actions since the Maastricht Treaty of 1992. The three EEA/EFTA countries (Norway, Iceland and Liechtenstein) contribute to the EU public health budget and are included in all EU activities in this field.

The European Commission is responsible for strategy and policy making at EU level in the area of health. It has a part in the decision-making process, notably by introducing new legislation and overseeing the correct implementation of the Treaties and European Law.

The main instrument of the Commission for implementing EU health strategies is the Health Programme through which actions and programmes can be funded. The programme is administered by the Executive Agency for Health and Consumers (http://ec.europa.eu/eahc/). Communicable disease control is under the responsibility of the Directorate-General for Health and

Consumers (DG SANCO) (http://ec.europa.eu/dgs/health_consumer/index_en.htm). Important policy areas include antimicrobial resistance, patient safety, vaccine issues, HIV/AIDS and influenza. DG SANCO also coordinates all issues related to risk management at the EU level.

The framework for EU collaboration in the area of communicable disease is formalised in Decision 2119/98/EC of the European Parliament and of the Council (1998). This establishes the Community Network for the Epidemiological Surveillance and Control of Communicable Diseases with separate pillars for early warning and response and epidemiological surveillance.

Community Network for the Epidemiological Surveillance and Control of Communicable Diseases

The Early Warning and Response System (EWRS) is an important risk management tool, which enables the European Commission and the public health authorities in the Member States to exchange information and co-ordinate measures against major outbreaks and other health threats of importance to more than one country. The EWRS communications are also accessible to the European Centre for Disease Prevention and Control (ECDC) and (most of them) also to the WHO. The system is extensively used during major public health events.

The other pillar of the Community Network concerns EU-level epidemiological surveillance. Amongst the components are disease-specific surveillance networks (DSNs), agreeing a common list of diseases under surveillance, case definitions and laboratory methods. Before 2005, EU-level surveillance was carried out by some 20 DSNs, each with a hub in a Member State. These brought epidemiologists and microbiologists from the countries together to agree surveillance methods for their disease of interest. Each DSN had its own databases and operating protocols. The quality was high, but co-ordination between the DSNs was more or less non-existant.

Supporting the other Community Network activities, a 2-year training programme in intervention epidemiology, EPIET (www.epiet.org) was set up in 1995 and in the same year the scientific journal *Eurosurveillance* (www.eurosurveillance.org) was established to disseminate information from the DSNs and report on communicable disease events of European interest.

European Centre for Disease Prevention and Control

During the 2003 SARS epidemic it became clear that the network approach was insufficient to provide the countries and the Commission with necessary scientific and technical support in a rapidly expanding EU. After a rapid legislative process, the new ECDC (www.ecdc.europa.eu) was established in Stockholm and became formally operational in May 2005. Five years later, by 2010, the ECDC has reached its planned size with some 300 staff members and an annual budget of around €60 million.

ECDC is an independent expert agency of the EU; its role is to provide scientific and technical advice and support (risk assessment). It has only a supporting role when it comes to public health action (risk management) because this is the responsibility of the countries and the Commission. With its limited staff and budget, the strength of ECDC is its ability to co-ordinate and draw from the extensive resources in the countries. The main public health functions of ECDC include the following:

• *Epidemiological surveillance and networking of laboratories:* the ECDC has integrated all the previous DSNs, along with the previously decentralised surveillance databases, into one European Surveillance System (TESSy). The ECDC does not have any laboratories and is developing a network of European reference laboratories.

• *Preparedness and response*: on a 24/7 basis, the ECDC Emergency Operation Centre (EOC) detects and assesses threats, and provides support for response to Member States and the Commission. The technical operation of the EWRS is undertaken by the Centre.

• *Scientific advice*: public health decisions have to be based on independent scientific evidence. Scientific issues arising in the area of communicable diseases vary widely, ranging from questions of clinical medicine and epidemiology through to standardisation of laboratory procedures. ECDC brings together scientific expertise in specific fields through its various EU-wide networks and via ad hoc scientific panels and expert groups.

• *Training*: the EPIET programme has been fully integrated in ECDC since 2007. A new European Public Health Microbiology Training Programme (EUPHEM) was initiated in 2009. These two large programmes are complemented by shorter training courses.

• *Health communication*: ECDC provides independent information to experts, policy makers and the general public, and promotes coherence in risk communication messages at EU level. ECDC also cooperates with the countries on public health campaigns (e.g. by coordinating the annual European Antibiotic Awareness Day, 18 November). The journal *Eurosurveillance* has been published by the ECDC since 2007 with full editorial independence. It is published electronically every Thursday and, with a very short publishing time (12–24 hours for rapid communications), it can provides very timely information on ongoing outbreaks.

• *Country support and capacity building*: ECDC provides technical support and capacity building on all issues within its mandate, including preparedness. This is done not only through training activities, but also through country visits by invitation, in which ECDC experts as well as experts from other countries review present systems and suggest improvements. ECDC mainly works with the EU and EEA/EFTA countries, but increasingly also has a role in integrating the candidate and potential countries and otherwise work on the global public health arena through various Commission mechanisms.

There are six disease programmes within the ECDC which integrate the functions of the previous DSPs:

• respiratory tract infections;
• antimicrobial resistance and healthcare-associated infections;
• vaccine preventable diseases;
• HIV/STI and blood-borne viruses;
• food and water-borne diseases; and
• emerging and vector-borne diseases.

In addition, specific projects cover climate change and infectious diseases and the burden of infectious diseases.

The ECDC works in close collaboration and partnership with other actors in the field, notably the national institutes of public health in Europe and beyond, the WHO and other EU agencies in related fields, including the European Food Safety Agency (EFSA) in Parma (www.efsa.europa.eu), the European Medicines Agency (EMA) in London (www.ema.europa.eu), the European Monitoring Centre for Drugs and Drug Addiction (EMCDDA) in Lisbon (www.emcdda.europa. eu) and the European Environment Agency (EEA) in Copenhagen (www.eea.europa.eu).

5.3 Detailed national example: organisational arrangements for health protection, England, 2010

Health protection describes the subset of public health activities aimed at protecting individuals, groups and populations from infectious diseases and environmental hazards such as chemical contamination and radiation. In England, since 2003, the Health Protection Agency (HPA) has provided support and leadership to the National Health Service (NHS) and other agencies for health

Table 5.3.1 The organisations of the Health Protection Agency (HPA), 2010

Health Protection Services Division 1. Local and regional services	Comprises regional offices, 26 Health Protection Units (HPUs) and the Emergency Response Department. Responds directly to cases and incidents and strengthens the front line by being a source of specialist advice and operational support and by contributing to policy making and implementation in partnership with NHS, Local Authorities and other agencies.
2. Epidemiology Service	Prevention of infectious disease by surveillance, supporting the investigation of national and uncommon outbreaks, advising government on the risks posed by various infections and responding to international health alerts.
Microbiology Services Division	Prevention of infectious disease through the provision of specialist and reference microbiology services from national reference laboratories. Eight Regional Microbiology Laboratories and local collaborating hospital microbiology laboratories.
	Carries out research into infectious diseases and develops and tests healthcare products and interventions including manufacture of vaccines. Role in planning and response for health emergencies, including possible acts of deliberate release.
Centre for Radiation, Chemical and Environmental Hazards	Radiation Protection staff carry out work on ionising and non-ionising radiation, research methods of protection, provide laboratory and technical services and provide training and expert advice. Chemical Hazards and Poisons staff provide advice on toxicology and the human health effects of chemicals.
National Institute for Biological Standards and Control	Ensures quality of biological medicines, custodian of WHO standards and reference material, ensures products comply with specifications and conducts leading edge scientific research.

protection. The HPA advises government on health protection policies and programmes, it provides authoritative information and advice to professionals and the public and it responds to emerging threats to public health and health emergencies including outbreaks and deliberate release incidents. The HPA also has a key role in health emergency planning. The HPA has national, regional and local tiers (Table 5.3.1). From 2010, the HPA will undergo major re-organisation (which is under consultation at the time of writing), probably including its incorporation into a new service, Public Health England, which will be part of the Department of Health, although it is expected that its functions will be preserved.

Health Protection Units

The local tier of the HPA in England comprises 26 Health Protection Units (HPUs), each covering a population of about 2 million people.

Each unit is staffed by Consultants in Communicable Disease Control (CCDCs; now sometimes called Consultants in Health Protection), health protection nurses and other support staff. The HPU (Box 5.3.1) undertakes local surveillance, investigation and management of incidents and outbreaks and the delivery of national action plans in collaboration with Primary Care Trusts (PCTs), Hospital Trusts and Local Authorities.

The NHS and Department of Health

The UK NHS was set up 56 years ago and is now the largest organisation in Europe. The overall aim of the government's Department of Health is to improve the health and wellbeing of the population by supporting activity to protect, promote and improve health and securing the provision of high quality health and social care services.

Box 5.3.1 Core activities of local health protection teams

- The surveillance of infectious diseases, and tracking health protection incidents and exposures, to inform local action.
- Alerting partners to emerging infectious and environmental threats to health.
- The timely investigation of incidents, outbreaks and trends and clusters of disease.
- The provision of evidence-based specialist health protection advice for action across the full range of health protection hazards.
- Preparing for and taking action to manage and control health protection incidents and emergencies.
- Working with stakeholders to identify training and planning needs and providing specialist input to the design and delivery of training.
- Working with stakeholders to the develop strategies and plans to protect health.
- Support NHS and local authority partners in their statutory responsibilities.
- Leading or contributing to prevention and control programmes and other actions to protect health.

Primary Care Trusts

At the time of writing, PCTs are local health organisations that are responsible for health services and improving health in their areas. PCTs carry out most of the functions that were previously the responsibility of health authorities including assessing health needs and ensuring that a full range of services is provided (Table 5.3.2). PCTs are also responsible for health protection and health emergency planning but receive assistance from the HPA to do this. PCTs are responsible for the delivery of immunisation services, HIV prevention services and infection control services in their community facilities. Some PCTs provide genitourinary medicine (GUM) services and tuberculosis services while in other areas they commission these services from acute trusts. From 2010, as a result of NHS re-organisation it is anticipated that PCTs will disappear, but their key functions will be transferred to other bodies such as local consortia of GPs (particularly for commissioning services) and local government authorities (particularly for health improvement).

Local government authorities

Local government in England and Wales is based on elected councils, which are accountable to the residents that they serve. In most areas there are two levels: a county council and a district council, although some areas have single 'unitary' authorities. County councils provide most public services, including schools, social services, waste disposal, civil defence, highways, consumer protection and planning and public transportation. Each county has several district councils that provide local services, including environmental health, housing, planning, refuse collection, cemeteries and crematoria, markets and fairs, licensing activities and leisure and recreation. In most large towns and cities a single level unitary authority will be responsible for all local services. Police and fire services are organised at county level but under separate organisational structures. Councils consist of elected members or councillors and exercise their powers through committees, subcommittees or delegation to salaried officers. Officers acting on behalf of a council must ensure that the powers and responsibilities they exercise have been lawfully delegated to them by the elected members. Often legislation requires that the council exercises its power through a specific officer, usually referred to as the proper officer. For some public health legislation the proper officer would be the CCDC.

Table 5.3.2 Local health services, England, 2010

Primary care trusts	Manage front-line health services including GPs, dentists, opticians, NHS walk-in centres, NHS Direct and pharmacies. Control 80% of the NHS budget.
Primary care services	Includes GPs, dentists, opticians and pharmacists, who often work as independent contractors. GPs care for patients with infection including diagnosis and treatment. They notify cases of infection to the CCDC/HPU. They advise on hygiene, other infection control measures and travel health and deliver immunisation programmes.
NHS community trusts	Provide non-acute health services and comprise community-based healthcare workers, clinics, community hospitals and nursing homes. Community nurses and other community-based healthcare workers usually work as members of a primary health care team; they manage infection problems and require access to infection control advice. Community trusts vary but they should have an infection control doctor (ICD), now called Director of Infection Prevention and Control, and one or more community infection control nurses (CICNs).
NHS Walk-in Centres	Prompt access to health advice and treatment.
NHS Direct	24-hour phone line, staffed by nurses, healthcare advice to the general public.
Care Trusts	NHS and Local Authorities work together to provide both health and social care.
Mental Health Trusts	There are 58 mental health trusts in England providing specialist health and social care services for people with mental health problems.
Acute Trusts	Manage hospitals to ensure they provide high quality healthcare and that they spend their money efficiently. Plan developments and improvements. May be regional or national centres for more specialised care. May provide services in the community. Provide NHS microbiology services and clinical infectious disease services.
Foundation Trusts	NHS hospital run by local managers, staff and members of the public and provided with financial and operational freedom in an attempt to de-centralise public services. Subject to NHS inspection.
Strategic health authorities	Strategic health authorities were created by the government in 2002 to manage the local NHS on behalf of the Secretary of State. From 2010 as a result of the proposed NHS re-organisation, it is anticipated they will disappear and their functions will transferred to other bodies (e.g. the proposed NHS Commissioning Board).
Ambulance Trusts	There are 12 ambulance services in England, providing emergency access to healthcare.
Special health authorities	Provide national level specialist services. The National Blood Authority is an example.

Environmental Health Departments and Environmental Health Officers

The responsibilities of Environmental Health Departments include food safety, air quality, noise, waste, health and safety, water quality, port health controls at air and sea ports, refuse collection and pest control. Environmental Health Officers (EHOs) investigate outbreaks of food and water-borne infections, advise on and enforce food safety legislation, inspect food premises and investigate complaints and provide food hygiene training. EHOs liaise with a wide range of other professionals including the CCDC, GPs, teachers, microbiologists and veterinarians. Other agencies with a role in infectious disease control are summarised in Tables 5.3.3 and 5.3.4. From 2010, as a result of the proposed UK government

Table 5.3.3 Other agencies with a role in infectious disease control

Department for the Environment, Food and Rural Affairs (DEFRA)	Promotes sustainable development and a better environment, protects public health in relation to food-borne disease and zoonoses.
Drinking Water Inspectorate (DWI)	Ensures safety of public water supplies and regulates the performance of water companies.
Animal Health	Formed in 2007 by merger of State Veterinary Service and other bodies to manage the economic and public health risks arising from animal diseases.
Environment Agency (EA)	Responsible for assessing, monitoring and reporting on waste disposal and environmental impact of environment on human health.
Health and Safety Executive (HSE)	Improves health and safety at work, reduces risks to workers and the public from work activities, controls and investigates Legionnaires' disease, enforces Control of Substances Hazardous to Health Regulations, controls infectious disease risks in the workplace.
Food Standards Agency (FSA)	Protects the public from risks from consumption of food and advises on nutrition.
Occupational Health Services	Advise managers and employees about the effect of work on health and of health on work, minimises infectious hazards at work including advising on immunisation of staff.

Table 5.3.4 Agencies and individuals involved in local health protection

Health Protection Agency	Consultant for Communicable Disease Control
	Consultant/Specialist in Health Protection
	Health protection nurse
	Regional HPA laboratory
	Regional epidemiologist
	Health emergency planning adviser
Primary Care Trust	Director of Public Health
	Director for Infection Prevention and Control
	Community infection control nurse
	Health visitors, district nurses, school health nurses
Hospitals	Director for Infection Prevention and Control
	Infection control doctor
	Medical microbiologist
	Infection control nurse
	Infectious disease specialist
	TB specialist, TB nurse advisers
	Genitourinary medicine specialist, GUM health adviser
Local Authority departments (environmental health, education, social services)	Environmental Health Officers
	Trading Standards Officers
	Teachers, social workers, home carers
	Residential home managers, safety managers
Primary care	GPs, practice nurses and other practice staff, community pharmacists, general dental practitioners
Private nursing homes, residential homes	Managers, nursing staff, carers
Occupational health departments	Occupational health doctors and nurses
Day nurseries	Managers, nursery nurses
General public	Citizens, consumers, newspapers, radio, TV
Water companies	Quality managers

re-organisation, it is anticipated that some of these may disappear in name with their functions transferred to other bodies.

5.4 Austria

Austria (population 8,210,000) is a federal republic with nine federal states (*Bundesländer*), subdivided into 99 districts (*Bezirke*) and 15 autonomous cities (*Statutarstädte*).

The prevention, control and surveillance of infectious diseases are regulated by federal law. The responsibility for the public health services, including control of communicable diseases is shared between the Ministry of Health at the federal level, and the states and local health departments within the states. The Ministry of Health has a key role, with responsibility for implementation of the legislation, national surveillance and international contacts (EU and WHO).

In each federal state, the infectious disease control, including surveillance, is the responsibility of a State Department for Health, led by the State Health Director. At the level of districts and autonomous cities there are District/City Health Offices. Specific public health functions are carried out by antenatal clinics, vaccination centres, AIDS help centres, etc.).

The Austrian Agency for Health and Food Safety (AGES) is a state-owned enterprise that carries out expert tasks in the area of food safety and communicable disease control on behalf of the Austrian Government. The agency has activities in the area of epidemiology, microbiology (reference laboratory functions), threat detection, outbreak control and supports the national surveillance system for infectious diseases.

National competent authorities for communicable disease control

Ministry of Health (Bundesministerium für Gesundheit; BMG): www.bmg.gv.at

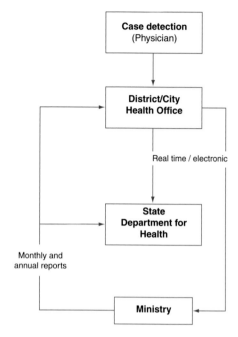

Fig. 5.4.1 Flow chart of statutory notification: Austria.

Austrian Agency for Health and Food Safety (Österreichische Agentur für Gesundheit und Ernährungssicherheit GmbH; AGES): www.ages.at

Surveillance of communicable diseases

Surveillance of communicable diseases is regulated by federal law, and the Ministry of Health is responsible for introducing changes in the statutory notification system (Figure 5.4.1). Some 51 diseases are notifiable by physicians and laboratories. No financial incentives are given.

The reporting is hierarchical with first-level reporting to the District Health Offices which report into an electronic reporting system, which can be accessed at any time by the health authorities on state and national level according the data protection rules. Data dissemination is carried out by the Ministry of Health, and annual and monthly reports are available on the Internet (http://www.bmg.gv.at/cms/site/thema.html?channel=CH0745). There is a separate reporting system for AIDS.

Outbreak investigation and control

In the case of an outbreak affecting more than one state, the Ministry of Health has to be informed. District and state health administrations have the legal responsibility for detection and investigation of outbreaks and for public health action on outbreaks in co-operation with regional food and veterinary administration and AGES.

Childhood vaccination schedule

Updated data on the Austrian childhood vaccination schedule are available from EU-VAC.NET (www.euvac.net). The national programme includes DTaP, dTaP, dT-IPV, HepB, Hib, HPV, IPV, MMR, PCV7, RV and Var (see List of abbreviations).

Updated data on vaccine coverage are available from the WHO Regional Office for Europe (http://data.euro.who.int/cisid/). Recent vaccine coverage rates: DTP4 (72.5%), HepB3 (83.3%), Hib3 (83.3%), MCV2 (64%) and Polio3 (83%).

5.5 Belgium

Belgium (population 10,414,000) is a federal state with three levels of government: (i) federal; (ii) regional (Brussels: Capital Region, Flanders and Wallonia); and (iii) linguistic communities (Flemish Community, French Community and German Community). Each community and each region has its own administration of public health and different responsibilities are shared in a complex way.

Surveillance and control of communicable diseases is mainly the responsibility of the three Communities, and the Communities have infectious disease control units in the provinces. The German-speaking Community is located entirely within the Province of Liège in Wallonia. The Flemish and French Communities share the responsibilities for communicable disease control in Brussels, in a separate commission with its own infectious disease control unit.

Emergency planning, crisis management and health security issues (e.g. bioterrorism) are the responsibility of the federal government (Federal Public Service, Health, Food Chain Safety and Environment). At the federal level, the Scientific Institute of Public Health is, on behalf of Communities, responsible for the co-ordinated surveillance of communicable diseases, including HIV/STI surveillance, influenza sentinel surveillance and surveillance based on data from reference laboratories.

National competent authorities for communicable disease control

Scientific Institute of Public Health (Institut Scientifique de la Santé Publique/Wetenschappelijk Instituut Volksgezondheid): www.wiv-isp.be

Federal Public Service, Health, Food Chain Safety and Environment: http://www.health.belgium.be/eportal/?fodnlang=en

Flemish Agency for Care and Health (Vlaams Agentschap Zorg en Gezondheid): http://www.zorg-en-gezondheid.be/EN/

Ministry of the French Community, Directorate General of Health (Le Ministère de la Communauté française, Direction générale de la Santé): http://www.cfwb.be/index.php?id=225

Ministry of the German-Speaking Community (Das Ministerium der Deutschsprachige Gemeinschaft): http://www.dglive.be/en/Desktopdefault.aspx/tabid-1263/2264_read-27181/

Flemish Communities

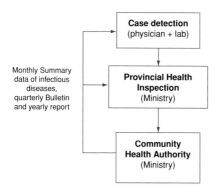

French Community (including data from the German Community):

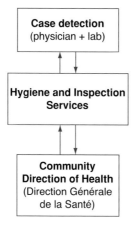

Fig. 5.5.1 Flow chart of statutory notification: Belgium.

Surveillance of communicable diseases

The Ministry of Health of each Community is responsible for introducing changes in the statutory notification system (Figure 5.5.1). About 35 diseases are notifiable in the Communities. The responsibility for case management is held by the treating physician. No financial incentives are given for notifying physicians or laboratories in Belgium. The local reporting is to the health inspector of the provincial infectious disease unit.

Surveillance data are disseminated via the *Flemish Infectious Disease Bulletin* (quarterly, print and online in Flemish with summaries in English) (http://www.infectieziekte bulletin.be), published by the Department of Infectious Diseases Control, Flanders and via the monthly *Bulletin d'information de la section d'Epidémiologie/Bulletin van de Afdeling Epidemiologie,* published by the Federal Scientific Institute of Public Health.

Outbreak investigation and control

The Health Inspectors of the Communities have the legal responsibility for detection, investigation and public health action within their Community in co-operation with other local/regional authorities (environmental health, veterinarians, etc.). The Federal Public Service, Health, Food Chain Safety and Environment is involved whenever there is a health security issue with international dimension (e.g. pandemic, bioterrorism) and provides the IHR focal point.

Childhood vaccination schedule

Updated data on the Belgian childhood vaccination schedule are available from EU-VAC.NET (www.euvac.net). The programme includes DTaP, DTpa, HepB, Hib, HPV, IPV, MenC, MMR, PCV7 and RTV (see List of abbreviations).

Updated data on vaccine coverage are available from the WHO Regional Office for Europe (http://data.euro.who.int/cisid/). Recent vaccine coverage rates: DTP4 (92%), HepB3 (97%), HiB3 (97%), MCV2 (83%) and Polio3 (99%).

5.6 Bulgaria

Bulgaria is a republic (population 7,149,000) divided into 28 provinces (*oblasts*) named after its main city, and subdivided into 263 municipalities.

The Bulgarian public health system is supervised by the Ministry of Health. The Chief State Health Inspector (within the Ministry of Health) is responsible for preparing guidelines and issues related to preparedness and response. At provincial level, 28 Regional Inspectorates for Protection and Control of Public Health (RIPCPHs) have important roles in communicable disease surveillance and control. Currently (autumn 2010) the Bulgarian Parliament is in the process of changing the Bulgarian Health Law in order to unite the RIPCPH and Regional Health Centres (RHC) in each province. The new structure will be named Regional Health Inspectorates.

The National Centre for Infectious and Parasitic Diseases acts under the Ministry as the main national research and reference centre on infectious diseases. It provides the evidence-base for the control of communicable diseases, it runs the national microbiological reference laboratories, analyses the epidemiological surveillance data on communicable diseases and antimicrobial resistance, issues guidelines, supports the national immunisation programme and provides graduate and postgraduate training in the field.

As the main institution for health statistics, the National Centre of Health Informatics has an important role in the compilation of national surveillance data on communicable diseases but is not involved in the data analysis.

National competent authorities for communicable disease control

The main institutions in the field of public health and communicable diseases are as follow:

Bulgaria Ministry of Health, Directorate of Public Health: http://www.mh.government.bg

Bulgaria National Center of Infectious and Parasitic Diseases (NCIPD): http://www.ncipd.org

National Center of Health Informatics: http://www.nchi.government.bg

Surveillance of communicable diseases

The surveillance of communicable diseases in Bulgaria is regulated by the Law on Health from 2005. All physicians and microbiological laboratories are obliged to report 60 mandatory notifiable diseases (suspected and confirmed cases) within 24 hours to the district RIPCPH. The RICPH are passing on aggregated information (number of cases and place of origin) to the NCHI on a daily basis. These reports are followed up on a monthly basis with aggregated information on confirmed cases, outcome and place of origin. At the national level, NCHI reports aggregated information to the Ministry of Health and the NCIPD on, daily, weekly and monthly basis.

Data analysis is performed both at district (RIPCPH) and national level (NCIPD). The surveillance system is supported by a network of microbiology laboratories and the reference laboratories at the NCIPD, and the NCIPD provides necessary support (Figure 5.6.1). A weekly bulletin on the epidemiological situation is issued by NCIPD (in Bulgarian): http://www.ncipd.org/index.php?news=disease.

Specific diseases, such as tuberculosis, influenza, acute respiratory tract infections, STIs and healthcare-associated infections are reported through parallel vertical systems.

Outbreak investigation and control

The RIPCPHs are responsible for outbreak investigations and control measures with support from national level when necessary. RICPHs are obliged to immediately inform the Ministry of Health of any communicable disease outbreak.

Childhood vaccination schedule

Updated data on the Bulgarian childhood vaccination schedule are available from EU-VAC.NET (www.euvac.net). The national

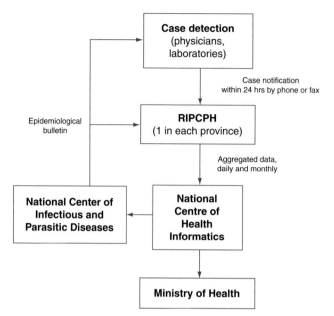

Fig. 5.6.1 Flow chart of statutory notifications: Bulgaria.

programme includes BCG, DTaP, dT, HepB, Hib, IPV, MMR, PCV (see List of abbreviations).

Updated data on vaccine coverage are available from the WHO Regional Office for Europe (http://data.euro.who.int/cisid/). Recent vaccine coverage rates: BCG (97.8%), DTP4 (93.2%), HepB3 (95.6%), MCV2 (93.8%) and Polio3 (94.3%).

5.7 Cyprus

Cyprus (population 796,000 in government controlled areas) is a republic, administratively divided in six districts. Since 1974, when Turkey invaded the northern part of the country, the northern third of the country is not under effective control of the Government of the Republic of Cyprus. The northern part of the island is thus not included in the public health and surveillance systems of the Republic of Cyprus.

The responsibility for communicable disease control in the country lies with the Department of Medical and Public Health Ser-

vices of the Ministry of Health, specifically within its Unit for Surveillance and Control of Communicable Diseases. The Director of Medical and Public Health Services (or a person authorised by him/her) is responsible for issuing guidelines, surveillance, threat detection, preparedness, outbreak control and communication, as well as contacts with the EU on communicable diseases.

National competent authority for communicable disease control

Ministry of Health, Directorate Medical and Public Health Services: http://www.moh.gov.cy/moh/moh.nsf/index_en/index_en

Surveillance of communicable diseases

The surveillance of communicable diseases is regulated in the Quarantine Law. A total of 60 communicable diseases are notifiable; 12 to be notified within 24 hours. All physicians are obliged to report these diseases to the

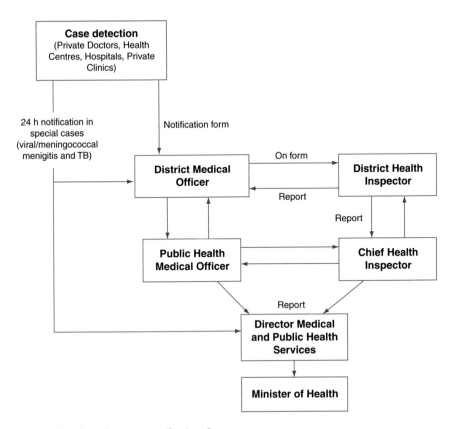

Fig. 5.7.1 Flow chart of statutory notification: Cyprus.

District Medical Officers who forward the information to the Medical and Public Health Services. For diseases notifiable within 24 hours, simultaneous reporting is to the District Medical Officer and to the Medical and Public Health Services (Figure 5.7.1).

Surveillance data are disseminated via the *Newsletter of the Network for Surveillance and Control of Communicable Diseases in Cyprus* (biannual, print and online in Greek), published by the Medical and Public Health Services.

Outbreak investigation and control

Control measures including contact tracing and outbreak investigation is generally the responsibility of the District Medical Officer and his/her team, supported when necessary by the Medical and Public Health Services.

Childhood vaccination schedule

Updated data on the Cypriot childhood vaccination schedule are available from EUVAC. NET (www.euvac.net). The national programme includes BCG, DTaP, HepB, Hib, IPV, MenC, MMR, PCV7 and Var (see List of abbreviations).

Updated data on vaccine coverage are available from the WHO Regional Office for Europe (http://data.euro.who.int/cisid/). Recent vaccine coverage rates: BCG (9%), HepB3 (96%), HiB3 (96%), MCV2 (88%) and Polio3 (99%).

5.8 Czech Republic

The Czech Republic (population 10,211,000) is divided in 13 administrative regions. All public health services (central governmental and regional) are centralised under the Ministry of Health. The Ministry of Health is responsible for issuing guidelines, threat detection, preparedness, outbreak control and communication.

The National Institute of Public Health (SZÚ) is a scientific institute directly managed by the Ministry of Health. The Institute works with both communicable and chronic diseases. A main task is communicable disease control; epidemiology, microbiology and hygiene. The NIPH provides scientific advice and is responsible for surveillance of infectious diseases. Furthermore, it provides methodological support and operates most of the national reference laboratories in the country.

Regional public health offices are responsible for the basic public health services, including surveillance and implementation of the general immunisation programmes.

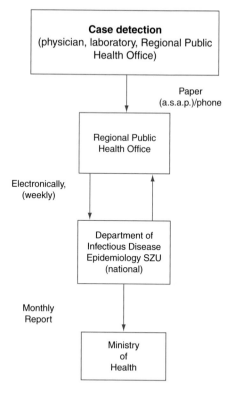

Fig. 5.8.1 Flow chart of statutory notifications: Czech Republic.

National competent authorities for communicable disease control

Ministry of Health (Ministerstvo Zdravotnictví): http://www.mzcr.cz

National Institute of Public Health (Státní Zdravotní Ústav – SZÚ): http://www.szu.cz

Surveillance of communicable diseases

Communicable diseases are by law notifiable by physicians, laboratories and detached Regional Public Health Offices (Figure 5.8.1). The notifications are sent to the Regional Public Health Offices, which forward the information, usually within a week, to the NIPH who coordinates the national reporting system

(EPIDAT). The responsibility for case management is held by the notifier.

Surveillance data are disseminated via the *Zprávy Epidemiologie a Mikrobiologie* (*Bulletin of Epidemiology and Microbiology*) (monthly, print and online in Czech and English) published by the SZÚ, and as tabular data (in Czech): http://www.szu.cz/publikace/data/infekce-v-cr.

Outbreak investigation and control

Directors of all healthcare facilities are required by law to notify unusually high occurrence or severity. Control measures including contact tracing and outbreak investigation is generally the responsibility of the Public Health Service, primarily on regional level with support from national level (national outbreak management team) when necessary.

Childhood vaccination schedule

Updated data on the Czech childhood vaccination schedule are available from EUVAC. NET (www.euvac.net). The national programme includes BCG, DTaP, HepB, Hib, IPV and MMR (see List of abbreviations).

Updated data on vaccine coverage are available from the WHO Regional Office for Europe (http://data.euro.who.int/cisid/). Recent vaccine coverage rates: BCG (99.0%), DTP4 (99.5%), HepB3 (99.3%), HiB3 (99.4%), MCV2 (97.9%) and Polio3 (99.0%).

5.9 Denmark

Denmark (population 5,500,000) is a constitutional monarchy, administratively divided in five regions. Healthcare is predominantly managed at the regional level. At the national level, the Ministry of Interior and Health oversees the two main national public health authorities.

The National Board of Health is the supreme healthcare authority in Denmark, and has an important role in overseeing all communicable disease control activities, issuing guidelines, providing scientific advice, reviewing the national immunisation programme and co-ordinating local efforts to control outbreaks. The National Board of Health is also responsible for preparedness, risk management and communication.

The Statens Serum Institut (SSI) is a public enterprise under the Ministry of Interior and Health. It is the main national expert agency working with communicable disease control and is the main adviser to the National Board of Health. Main tasks of the SSI are research, scientific advice, national surveillance of infectious diseases, microbiological diagnostics (including reference laboratories), technical assistance in outbreak management, vaccine production and procurement and preparedness against bioterrorism.

The Medical Officers of Health (embedslæger) have offices in the five regions, and are responsible for a number of tasks in relation to prevention and control of infectious diseases. They are a part of the National Board of Health, and the main implementers of the day-to-day local communicable disease control activities.

National competent authorities for communicable disease control

Ministry for Health and Prevention (Indenrigs og Sundhedsministeriet): www.ism.dk

National Board of Health (Sundhedsstyrelsen): www.sst.dk

Statens Serum Institut (SSI): www.ssi.dk

Surveillance of communicable diseases

The surveillance of communicable diseases is regulated by law. Forty diseases are notifiable on person identifiable basis, and four diseases are notifiable on an anonymous basis. Laboratories report identification of nine specific microbial agents as well as all gastrointestinal bacteria to the SSI (Figure 5.9.1). In addition, the number of positive and negative HIV test results are reported. All physicians and laboratories are obliged to notify cases of notifiable diseases in parallel to the Regional Medical Officers of Health and to the SSI. Surveillance data are disseminated via *Epi-Nyt* (*Epi-News*) and ssi.dk (weekly, online in Danish and English) published by the SSI (www.ssi.dk).

Outbreak investigation and control

Physicians are required by law to report any abnormal event or outbreak of any disease immediately by phone to the Medical

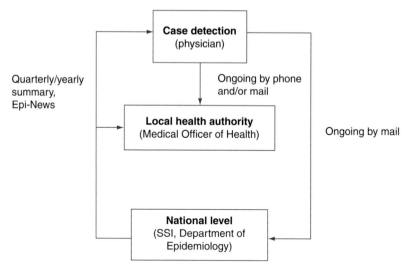

Fig. 5.9.1 Flow chart of statutory notifications: Denmark.

Officers of Health. They also have to notify to the national level (SSI) by mail using a written form. Local and national reference laboratories also detect and report outbreaks. The Medical Officers of Health have responsibility for outbreak control at regional and local level, including contact-tracing. The SSI has national responsibility as a reference centre for surveillance and is involved in outbreak investigation and control on request. There is a permanent committee for the management of food-borne outbreaks, including the Danish Veterinary and Food Administration, the National Food Institute DTU and SSI.

Childhood vaccination schedule

Updated data on the Danish childhood vaccination schedule are available from EUVAC. NET (www.euvac.net). The national programme includes DTaP, dTaP, HepB, Hib, HPV, IPV, MMR and PCV7 (see List of abbreviations).

Updated data on vaccine coverage are available from the WHO Regional Office for Europe (http://data.euro.who.int/cisid/). Recent vaccine coverage rates: DTP4 (87%), HiB3 (89%), MCV2 (85%) and Polio3 (89%).

5.10 Estonia

Estonia (population 1,340,000) is a republic, administratively divided in 15 counties. The main bodies responsible for communicable disease control are the Ministry of Social Affairs and its agencies. The Ministry has a supervising role and responsibility for public health policy and strategies and introduction of new legislation, while surveillance and control activities are carried out by the Health Board under the Ministry. The Health Board was created on 1 January 2010, joining together the Health Protection Inspectorate, the Health Care Board and the Chemicals Notification Centre.

The former Health Protection Inspectorate (now part of the Health Board) is the main public health institution working with communicable diseases. It is responsible for surveillance of infectious diseases, outbreak management, preventive measures, supervision and monitoring of the national immunisation programme, and organises public health microbiology, as well as responsible for early warning and response. Four regional Health Board Services are part of the organisation.

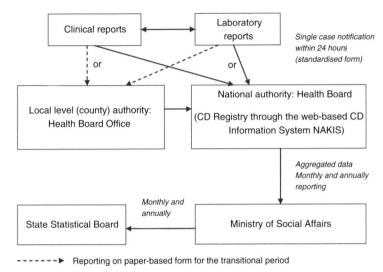

Fig. 5.10.1 Flow chart of statutory notifications: Estonia.

Surveillance and control of tuberculosis and HIV are carried out by the National Institute for Health Development.

In each of the 15 counties, local communicable disease control is carried out by the County Health Board Offices.

National competent authorities for communicable disease control

Ministry of Social Affairs (Sotsiaalministeerium; SM): www.sm.ee

Health Board (Terviseamet; TA): www.terviseamet.ee

National Institute for Health Development (Tervise Arengu Instituut) HIV/AIDS and TB surveillance: http://www.tai.ee/?lang=en

Surveillance of communicable diseases

The surveillance of communicable diseases is regulated by law (Communicable Diseases Prevention and Control Act). A total of 62 communicable diseases are notifiable to the County Health Board Offices or to the web-based CD Information System (NAKIS). All physicians and laboratories are obliged to no-

tify cases that fulfil the criteria for notifiable diseases. No financial incentives are given for notifying. The responsibility for case management is held by the physicians (including contact tracing), supported by the County Health Board Office (Figure 5.10.1).

Surveillance data are disseminated via *EstEpi Report* (*Estonian Communicable Disease Bulletin*) (monthly, print and online in Estonian and English), published by the Health Board (www.terviseamet.ee).

Outbreak investigation and control

A variety of information sources are used to detect possible outbreaks. The information is forwarded to County Health Board Offices, responsible for investigation and public health action at local level. The County Health Board Offices report to the Health Board, responsible for outbreak detection and management at national level.

Childhood vaccination schedule

Updated data on the Estonian childhood vaccination schedule are available from

EUVAC.NET (www.euvac.net). The national programme includes BCG, DTaP, dT, HepB, Hib, IPV and MMR (see List of abbreviations).

Updated data on vaccine coverage are available from the WHO Regional Office for Europe (http://data.euro.who.int/cisid/). Recent vaccine coverage rates: BCG (97.2%), DTP4 (93%), HepB3 (95.3%), HiB3 (95%), MCV2 (96%) and Polio3 (95.3%).

5.11 Finland

Finland (population 5,250,000) is a republic, divided into six administrative provinces. The main bodies responsible for communicable disease control are the Ministry of Social Affairs and Health and the National Institute for Health and Welfare. The Ministry has a supervising role with responsibility for public health policy and strategies, proposing legislation and monitoring its implementation.

The newly formed (merger of two previous institutions in January 2009) National Institute for Health and Welfare (THL), acting under the Ministry of Social Affairs and Health, is the main scientific institute working with communicable disease control. With a strong research base, the institute is responsible for epidemiological surveillance and response, threat detection, the Finnish vaccination programme, scientific advice and communication.

At the local level, Municipal Health Authorities are in primary charge of control measures.

National competent authorities for communicable disease control

Ministry of Social Affairs and Health (Department for Promotion of Welfare and Health): www.stm.fi

National Institute for Health and Welfare (Terveyden Ja Hyvinvoinnin Laitos; THL): http://www.thl.fi/en_US/web/en

Surveillance of communicable diseases

The surveillance of communicable diseases is regulated by the Law and Act of Communicable Diseases. A total of 79 diseases are notifiable. They are classified into three categories. For some diseases both the physician and the laboratory must report the case, for others only laboratory reports are collected (more than half of all infections). The information is entered into the National Infectious Disease Register (NDR) and duplicate notifications are merged. Data from individual cases are linked by the unique personal identifying number. There are no financial incentives for notifying physicians.

Laboratory notifications are sent directly to the national level at National Institute for Health and Welfare. In addition, laboratories send microbes to a national strain collection. Physician notifications are sent through the regional level to the national level. The notifying physicians are responsible for detection and notification of cases and for necessary action to stop spread. They are assisted by infectious disease specialists and microbiologists (Figure 5.11.1).

All registry data are compiled and arranged at National Institute for Health and Welfare and accessible through encrypted www-communication to health authorities in charge at district and municipal levels. A weekly updated www-version is available for the public and includes comments and epidemiological observations (http://www3.ktl.fi/stat/). The data format allow compilations of tables, trend analysis, etc. by the user.

Outbreak investigation and control

Control measures including contact tracing and outbreak investigation are generally the responsibility of the Public Health Service, primarily on local level with support from national level. In outbreak situations, local health authorities are primarily responsible

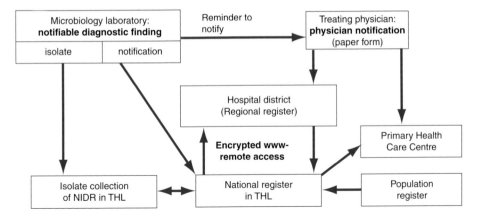

Fig. 5.11.1 Flow chart of statutory notifications: Finland.

for situation analysis and action. In cases where several municipalities are involved, the hospital district specialist and/or the provincial veterinary and food authorities act as co-ordinator and consultant. The National Institute for Health and Welfare is involved in wider outbreaks and provides co-ordination and expert help.

Childhood vaccination schedule

Updated data on the Finnish childhood vaccination schedule are available from EU-VAC.NET (www.euvac.net). The national programme (for all children) includes DTaP, Hib, influenza, IPV, MMR, PCV and RTV (see List of abbreviations).

Updated data on vaccine coverage are available from the WHO Regional Office for Europe (http://data.euro.who.int/cisid/). Recent vaccine coverage rates: BCG (98.5%), DTP4 (97%), HiB3 (98.5%) and Polio3 (99%).

5.12 France

France (population 64,057,000) is a republic, divided into 22 metropolitan and 4 overseas administrative regions, and subdivided in 96

metropolitan departments and 4 overseas departments (same as the overseas regions).

The main bodies responsible for communicable disease control are the Ministry of Health and Sports with its General Directorate of Health (DGS) and the National Institute for Public Health Surveillance (InVS). The DGS has a supervising role with responsibility for public health policy and strategies, proposing legislation and monitoring its implementation. The DGS is further responsible for issuing guidelines, preparedness and response, health emergencies including bioterror threats, risk communication and EU contacts on risk management issues.

The InVS has national responsibility for threat detection, surveillance of infectious diseases, risk analysis and acts as an advisor to the DGS recommending measures against detected threats as well as contributes to the management of health crises. The responsibility of the institute includes the overseas departments.

The National Institute for Prevention and Health Education (INPES) is the reference institute for health education, prevention and promotion.

In each region a Regional Health Agency (ARS) is responsible for carrying out public health actions at local level. The InVS have regional offices (Cellule Régionale d'Epidémiologie; CIRE) within ARS to develop local surveillance and investigation activities and support response to public health threat, including those of infectious origin at the regional level.

National competent authorities for communicable disease control

Ministry of Health and Sports, General Directorate of Health (Ministère de la Santé et des Sports, Direction Générale de la Santé; DGS): www.sante-sports.gouv.fr

National Institute for Public Health Surveillance (Institut de Veille Sanitaire; InVS): www.invs.sante.fr

National Institute for Prevention and Health Education (Institut National de Prévention et d'Education pour la Santé; IN-PES): public communication: www.inpes.fr

Surveillance of communicable diseases

The surveillance of communicable diseases is regulated by law. The Ministry of Health and Sports has the responsibility for modifications in the notification system based on proposals made by the InVS.

For 26 diseases, notification is mandatory. All physicians, biologists and hospitals are obliged by law to notify all cases that fulfil the criteria for mandatory notification (Figure 5.12.1). No financial incentive is given to notifiers. Individual cases are anonymously notified to the ARS that forwards the notifications to the InVS (usually within 1–2 days). The responsibility for case management is held by the notifier.

According to the disease, a case detection may lead to two levels of action. All the diseases – except for HIV/AIDS, acute hepatitis B and tetanus – have to be reported in emergency and then notified for immediate action.

InVS is responsible for managing surveillance activities at national level while DGS is responsible for policy and decision. InVS performs trend analysis, outbreak detection

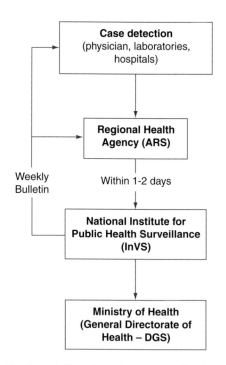

Fig. 5.12.1 Flow chart of statutory notifications: France.

based on the surveillance and epidemic intelligence and carry out outbreak investigation.

Surveillance data are disseminated via annual surveillance reports at the national and regional level and the *Bulletin Épidemiologique Hebdomadaire* (*Weekly Epidemiological Bulletin*) (print and online in French) (http://www.invs.sante.fr/beh/index.html), published by the InVS.

Outbreak investigation and control

All health professionals are obliged to inform the ARS of any abnormal health event or outbreak of any disease. The ARS is responsible for investigation and control with the assistance from the regional (CIRE of the InVS) or national level (InVS) when necessary. Control of the outbreak is the responsibility of the ARS and the DGS, and the Ministry of Agriculture may be involved in food-borne outbreaks.

Childhood vaccination schedule

Updated data on the French childhood vaccination schedule are available from EUVAC. NET (www.euvac.net). The national programme includes aP, BCG, DT, dT, HepB, Hib, HPV, IPV, MMR, PCV7 and Var (see List of abbreviations).

Updated data on vaccine coverage are available from the WHO Regional Office for Europe (http://data.euro.who.int/cisid/). Recent vaccine coverage rates: BCG (78.2%), DTP4 (88%), HepB3 (41.9%), HiB3 (96.7%) and Polio3 (98%).

5.13 Germany

Germany (population 82,330,000) is a federal republic, administratively divided in 16 states (*Bundesländer*), and subdivided in 439 districts (*Kreise*) and cities (*kreisfreie Städte*). The decision-making power is shared between the federal and the state governments, and the responsibility for health is at state level. The main national authorities responsible for communicable disease control are the Federal Ministry of Health (BMG) and the Robert Koch Institute (RKI).

The BMG has a supervising role with responsibility for public health policy and strategies, drafting legislation and monitoring its implementation, as well as for preparedness, health protection, disease prevention, risk communication and EU contacts on risk management issues.

The RKI is the central federal expert institution responsible for communicable disease prevention and control. The RKI work is research-based, and includes compiling scientific findings as a basis for political decisions, infectious disease surveillance (including surveys and sentinel studies), and threat detection (national and international), as well as identification and prevention of bioterror attacks. To achieve its objectives, the RKI cooperates closely with the federal ministries, with the state governments, local

authorities and European and international institutions.

Federal Centre for Health Education (BZgA) is responsible for the implementation of health educational programmes of national importance.

At state level, communicable disease control is carried out by the state health department (*Landesgesundheitsamt*), and at district level by the local health department (*Gesundheitsamt*).

National competent authorities for communicable disease control

Federal Ministry for Health (Bundesministerium für Gesundheit; BMG): www.bmg. bund.de

Robert Koch Institute (RKI): www.rki.de

Federal Centre for Health Education (Bundeszentrale für gesundheitliche Aufklärung; BZgA): www.bzga.de

Surveillance of communicable diseases

The surveillance of communicable diseases is regulated by law, with a new law in force in 2001. Some 47 diseases/infections are notified with identifiers of the patient. Six other diseases/infections are notified without personal identifiers. All physicians and medical microbiology laboratories are obliged to report notifiable disease, and no financial incentives are given for notifying physicians.

For most notifiable diseases, notifications from physicians and laboratories go to local health departments. From there they are forwarded via the state health departments to the RKI at federal level. The notifications usually reach the state level within 1 week and the RKI within 2 weeks (Figure 5.13.1).

Surveillance data are disseminated via annual surveillance reports and the *Epidemiologisches Bulletin* (*Epidemiological Bulletin*) (weekly online in German) (http://www.rki.

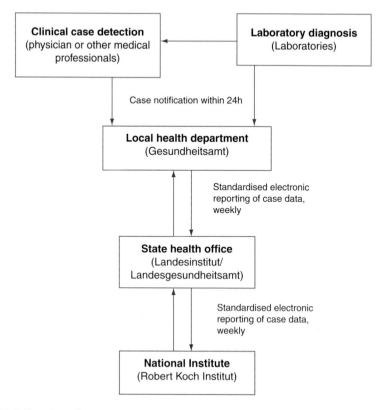

Fig. 5.13.1 Flow chart of statutory notifications: Germany.

de/DE/Content/Infekt/EpidBull/epid__bull__ node.html), published by the RKI. The data can also be accessed and used via an Internet application, SurvStat@RKI (http://www3.rki. de/SurvStat).

Outbreak investigation and control

Outbreak investigation and management, including contact tracing, is generally the responsibility of the local health department with support from the state health department and RKI when necessary.

Childhood vaccination schedule

Updated data on the German childhood vaccination schedule are available from EUVAC.

NET (www.euvac.net). The national programme includes DTaP, dTaP, HepB, Hib, HPV, IPV, MenC, MMR, PCV7 and Var (see List of abbreviations).

Updated data on vaccine coverage are available from the WHO Regional Office for Europe (http://data.euro.who.int/cisid/). Recent vaccine coverage rates: DTP4 (96.4%), HepB3 (90.4%), HiB3 (94.1%), MCV2 (91.4%) and Polio3 (95.7%).

5.14 Greece

Greece (population 10,737,000) is a parliamentary republic, administratively divided into 13 peripheries and subdivided into 51 prefectures. The main national authorities

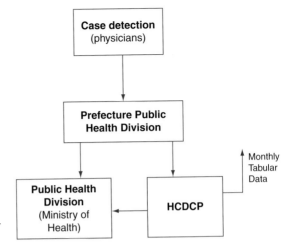

Fig. 5.14.1 Flow chart of statutory notifications: Greece.

responsible for communicable disease control are the Ministry of Health and Social Solidarity with its Directorate of Public Health and the Hellenic Centre for Disease Control and Prevention (HCDCP).

The Ministry of Health and Social Solidarity has a supervising role with responsibility for public health policy and strategies, proposing legislation and monitoring its implementation. The Directorate of Public Health is further responsible for preparedness, risk communication and EU contacts on risk management issues.

The HCDCP is an independent expert institution working under the supervision of the Ministry, collaborating closely with other public health authorities. The HCDCP provides scientific advice, preparing guidelines, organising educational campaigns and is responsible for the national surveillance of communicable diseases. It also intervenes in cases of outbreaks of national significance (in collaboration with local public health authorities), provides information to the general public (including travel advice), provides risk assessment for communicable diseases and works on bioterror preparedness. Finally, HCDCP together with the National School of Public Health coordinates the function of the National and District Public Health laboratories.

National competent authorities for communicable disease control

Ministry of Health and Social Solidarity, Directorate of Public Health: www.yyka.gov.gr

Hellenic Centre for Disease Control and Prevention (HCDCP): http://www.keelpno.gr/en/

Surveillance of communicable diseases

The surveillance of communicable diseases is regulated by law. A total of 48 diseases, divided into three categories (depending on urgency of notification), are notifiable. No financial incentive is given to physicians to notify. The responsibility for case management is held by the notifier. Physicians notify cases to the Prefecture Public Health Division, being responsible for case investigation (Figure 5.14.1). Monthly aggregate data are sent to the Ministry of Health and to the HCDCP. The HCDCP is responsible for the analysis of the data. Tabulated surveillance data are accessible on the HCDCP website. Separate surveillance and other action programmes are established within the HCDCP to assess and intervene in surveillance issues with migrants, HIV and STIs, viral hepatitis and nosocomial infections.

Outbreak investigation and control

Control measures including contact tracing and outbreak investigation is generally the responsibility of the Public Health Service, primarily on local level with support from the HCDCP when necessary.

Childhood vaccination schedule

Updated data on the Greek childhood vaccination schedule are available from EU-VAC.NET (www.euvac.net). The national programme includes BCG, DTaP, dT, HepB, Hib, IPV, MenC, MMR, PCV7 and Var (see List of abbreviations).

Updated data on vaccine coverage are available from the WHO Regional Office for Europe (http://data.euro.who.int/cisid/). Recent vaccine coverage rates: BCG (90.6%), DTP4 (82.4%), HepB3 (95.3%), HiB3 (83%), MCV2 (77.1%) and Polio3 (99.1%).

5.15 Hungary

Hungary (population 10,013,000) is a parliamentary republic, administratively divided into 19 counties and the capital city (Budapest). These are further subdivided into 174 subregions, with Budapest comprising its own subregions. Since 1999 the counties and Budapest have been grouped into seven planning and statistical regions.

Directly under the Ministry of National Resources, the Chief Medical Officer of Hungary leads the Hungarian National Public Health and Medical Officers' Service (NPH-MOS), which operates as a public administration agency. The NPHMOS is organised at na-

tional, regional and local levels and is responsible for controlling, co-ordinating and supervising all public health activities. The NPH-MOS includes the Office of the Chief Medical Officer (OCMO), a number of national scientific institutes as well as regional and subregional institutions.

The National Centre for Epidemiology (NCE) is part of NPHMOS, but acts as a scientifically independent expert institution with main responsibilities including surveillance, threat detection, prevention and control of infectious diseases, vaccine safety, laboratory and reference laboratory functions, training of the health officers and postgraduate training. The NCE also provides expertise for epidemiological preparedness and emergency situations (including bioterror events) of national importance, and is the leading institution against nosocomial infections. NCE is responsible for the development of the national immunisation programme.

The Koranyi National Institute of Tuberculosis and Pulmonology is responsible for surveillance and control of tuberculosis.

The implementation of communicable disease surveillance and control at county and municipality level is carried out by the regional and subregional institutions of the NPHMOS.

National competent authorities for communicable disease control

Ministry of National Resources (Nemzeti Erőforrás Minisztérium): www.nefmi.gov.hu

Hungarian National Public Health and Medical Officer Service (Állami Népegészségügyi és Tisztiorvosi Szolgálat): http://www.antsz.hu/portal/portal/bemutatkozasangol.html

National Centre for Epidemiology (Országos Epidemiológiai Központ): www.oek.hu

Koranyi National Institute of Tuberculosis and Pulmonology: www.koranyi.hu

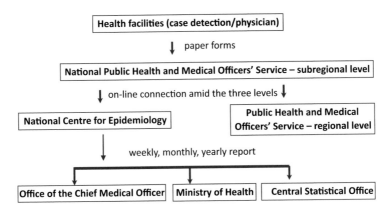

Fig. 5.15.1 Flow chart of statutory notifications: Hungary.

Surveillance of communicable diseases

The surveillance of communicable diseases is regulated by legislation from 1997. The basis for the national surveillance system (except TB) is the NPHMOS. Communicable diseases, even the suspicion of the disease, are reported on paper forms by mail by health service providers to the subregional level of the NPHMOS where data are entered immediately into the electronic database of NPHMOS. Access to the database is provided online for the subregional, regional and national level of NPHMOS, according to rights of access authorisation based on the hierarchical institutional tasks (Figure 5.15.1).

The mandatory notification is required for 72 diseases with personal identifying data and for 13 diseases without identifying data.

The NCE issues an epidemiological bulletin (*Az Országos Epidemiológiai Központ epidemiológiai információs hetilapja; Epinfo*) (weekly electronic in Hungarian) (http://www.oek.hu/oek.web?to=,839&nid=41&pid=1&lang=hun).

Outbreak investigation and control

Control measures including contact tracing and outbreak investigations are generally the responsibility of the subregional and regional institutes of the NPHMOS, with the support of the NCE.

Childhood vaccination schedule

Updated data on the Hungarian childhood vaccination schedule are available from EUVAC.NET (www.euvac.net). The national programme includes BCG, DTaP, HepB, Hib, IPV, MMR and PCV71 (see List of abbreviations).

Updated data on vaccine coverage are available from the WHO Regional Office for Europe (http://data.euro.who.int/cisid/). Recent vaccine coverage rates: BCG (90.6%), DTP4 (99.8%), HepB3 (99.9%), HiB3 (99.9%), MCV2 (99.3%) and Polio3 (99.8%).

5.16 Iceland

Iceland (population 318,000) is a republic divided into 8 regions, and subdivided into 78 municipalities. The Ministry of Health and Social Security is responsible for health services including public health, policy issues, strategic planning. The main national health authority is the Directorate of Health. Within the Directorate is a specific Unit for Infectious Disease Control, headed by the

Chief Epidemiologist. The Chief Epidemiologist has a broad mandate including organising and co-ordinating communicable disease prevention and control in the country, surveillance of communicable diseases, monitoring use of and resistance to antimicrobial agents, supervision of preventive measures, including the national immunisation programme, health information, providing advice and guidelines, and measures in the case of outbreaks and other health threats due to communicable diseases.

Under the Chief Epidemiologist, regional epidemiologists in selected healthcare centres have local responsibility for preventive measures and control measures against infectious diseases.

National competent authorities for communicable disease control

Ministry of Health (Heilbrigðisráðuneytið): eng.heilbrigdisraduneyti.is

Directorate of Health (Landlæknisembættið): www.landlaeknir.is

Surveillance of communicable diseases

The national surveillance is regulated in the Act on Health Security and Communicable Diseases of 1997. Physicians and laboratories are obliged to report 46 statutory notifiable infectious diseases and serious public health events, with full identity to the Chief Epidemiologist. Data dissemination is done through the website of the Directorate of Health, with statistical information and a quarterly bulletin available in English: http://www.landlaeknir.is/Utgafa/EPI—ICE .

There is no alert system in place in the country.

Childhood vaccination schedule

Updated data on the national childhood vaccination schedule are available from EU-VAC.NET (www.euvac.net). The national programme includes DTaP, Hib, IPV, MenC and MMR (see List of abbreviations).

Updated data on vaccine coverage are available from the WHO Regional Office for Europe (http://data.euro.who.int/cisid/). Recent vaccine coverage rates: DTP4 (95%), HiB3 (96%), MCV2 (93%) and Polio3 (96.2%).

5.17 Ireland

Ireland (population 4,203,000) is a republic, administratively divided in 26 counties and 5 cities. For health purposes the country is divided into four Health Service Executive Areas. The main bodies responsible for communicable disease control are the Department (Ministry) of Health and Children and the Health Protection Surveillance Centre (HPSC). The Ministry has a supervising role with responsibility for public health policy and strategies, proposing legislation and monitoring its implementation.

The HPSC is the national specialist institution for surveillance of communicable diseases. Other key tasks of the centre are providing independent advice to government departments and other agencies, issuing guidelines, epidemiological investigations, applied research, communication and training in communicable disease control. The HPSC is part of the Health Service Executive (HSE), and works closely with the public health officers in eight departments of public health.

National competent authorities for communicable disease control

Department of Health and Children: www.dohc.ie

Health Protection Surveillance Centre (HPSC): http://www.hpsc.ie/hpsc

Surveillance of communicable diseases

The surveillance of communicable diseases is regulated by law. The Department of Health and Children has the responsibility for modifications. A total of 68 diseases are notifiable, and 2€ per notification is given to physicians as financial incentive to notify. Notifications are made by both medical practitioners and microbiological laboratories. The responsibility for case management is held by the notifier.

The reporting is increasingly being done through the Computerised Infectious Disease Reporting (CIDR) system, which is a shared system between HPSC, the former Health Boards, the Food Safety Authority of Ireland, the Food Safety Promotion Board and the Department of Health and Children (Figure 5.17.1).

Surveillance data are disseminated via *Epi-Insight* (monthly, print and online) (http://www.ndsc.ie/hpsc/EPI-Insight) and via annual surveillance reports published by the HPSC.

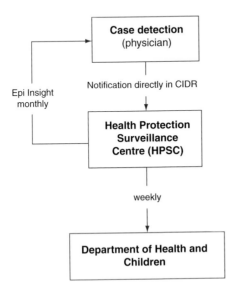

Fig. 5.17.1 Flow chart of statutory notifications: Ireland.

Outbreak investigation and control

Control measures including contact tracing and outbreak investigation is generally the responsibility of the HSE public health service, primarily on local level with support from national level. The HPSC is responsible for investigation and control of national outbreaks, liaising with laboratories and the Food Safety Authority.

Childhood vaccination schedule

Updated data on the Irish childhood vaccination schedule are available from EUVAC.NET (www.euvac.net). The national programme includes BCG, DTaP, HepB, Hib, HPV, IPV, MenC, MMR, PCV7 and Td (see List of abbreviations).

Updated data on vaccine coverage are available from the WHO Regional Office for Europe (http://data.euro.who.int/cisid/). Recent vaccine coverage rates: BCG (93.7%), HiB3 (98.4%) and Polio3 (93.7%).

5.18 Italy

Italy (population 60,045,068) is a republic divided in 19 regions, 2 autonomous provinces and 110 provinces. The regions have large autonomy in terms of healthcare organisation (including public health). The main national authorities responsible for communicable disease control are the Ministry of Health, with its General Directorate of Health Prevention, and the National Health Institute (ISS).

The Ministry of Health is the national authority in the Italian National Health Service (NHS) and has a supervising role with responsibility for public health policy and planning, proposing legislation and regulations and monitoring their implementation. The Directorate General of Health Prevention within the Ministry of Health has the national co-ordinating responsibility for infectious disease control, including issuing guidelines, preventive measures, bioterrorism, antimicrobial resistance, hospital-acquired infections and international co-operation.

The ISS is the leading national scientific institution of the NHS, active on many issues related to human health. It has a broad public health mandate. Activities related to communicable diseases are mainly carried out within the National Centre for Epidemiology, Surveillance and Health Promotion (CNESPS) and the AIDS Centre. Main tasks of ISS include national surveillance, threat detection, rapid response, scientific advice (including on vaccines), training and applied research. Support to the local health authorities in outbreak investigations and public health activities is provided upon request.

The hospital Lazzaro Spallanzani is a national reference institution for the diagnosis and care of severe infectious diseases, including HIV/AIDS, and rare imported infections. A biosafety level 4 laboratory is available at the hospital.

Regional public health agencies have an important role in guiding the activity of the 194 local health units, in charge of delivering primary health care and prevention.

National competent authorities/bodies for communicable disease control

Ministry of Health (Ministero della Salute): www.ministerosalute.it

National Health Institute (Istituto Superiore di Sanità-ISS): www.iss.it

National Institute for Infectious Diseases (Istituto Nazionale per le Malattie Infettive L. Spallanzani): www.inmi.it

Surveillance of communicable diseases

Reporting of communicable diseases is regulated by law, last updated in 1990 by a ministerial decree. All detected infections posing a risk to public health are principally notifi-

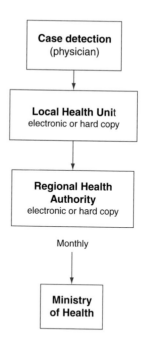

Fig. 5.18.1 Flow chart of statutory notifications: Italy.

able; however, 48 diseases are listed in the national regulation. These are divided into five classes, which differ by flow of information, timeliness of reporting and by the degree of ascertainment requested. Each case of disease has to be reported on an individual notification form. Diagnosing physicians are obliged by law to notify all cases that fulfil the criteria for notifiable diseases.

Cases of notifiable diseases are reported to the public hygiene departments of local health units, which have to check and carry out additional investigations (e.g. in case of outbreaks) (Figure 5.18.1). Data from individual notification forma are entered in a computerised database and a common subset of data is periodically extracted (usually monthly) and forwarded to the regional health authorities who in turns forward the aggregated data set to the Ministry of Health. The system is currently under revision with the aim of building a national web-based database to be updated in real time.

Data on relevant communicable diseases not included in the notification list as well as on 'emerging' issues are obtained by means of 'special' surveillance systems set up by ISS in collaboration with the regional authorities and the Ministry of Health. In these systems, data are collected at ISS and made available to the Ministry.

Data on common notifiable diseases are available on the Ministry of Health website (www.ministerosalute.is).

Outbreak investigation and control

Control measures including contact tracing and outbreak investigation are generally the responsibility of the local health units, with support from regional and national level when deemed necessary. ISS performs field investigations only upon request of the Ministry of Health or the regional authority.

Childhood vaccination schedule

Updated data on the Italian childhood vaccination schedule are available from EU-VAC.NET (www.euvac.net). The national programme includes DTaP, HepB, Hib, HPV, IPV, MenC, MMR, PCV (with regional differences) and Var (see List of abbreviations).

Updated data on vaccine coverage are available from the WHO Regional Office for Europe (http://data.euro.who.int/cisid/). Recent vaccine coverage rates are HepB3 (96.2%), HiB3 (95.6%) and Polio3 (96.1%).

5.19 Latvia

Latvia (population 2,248,000) is a republic administratively divided in 9 cities and 109 municipalities. For public health purposes epidemiologists are situated in the eight largest cities of the country. The Ministry of Health has a leading role with responsibility for public health policy and strategies, health promotion, proposing legislation and monitoring its implementation, as well as overseeing the work of its subordinate institutions.

The Infectology Centre of Latvia (LIC) is a government institution under the Ministry of Health. After a reform in 2009, it has taken over the previous functions of the Public Health Agency in areas of infectious diseases and also integrated the State Agency of Tuberculosis and Lung Diseases and its branches. The LIC is now responsible for threat detection, control, prevention and national surveillance of all communicable diseases, including STI, HIV/AIDS and tuberculosis, as well as overseeing the national immunisation programme. The LIC gives scientific advice, prepares guidelines, provides training and conducts applied research. The LIC also provides care for patients with infectious diseases as well as diagnostic and reference laboratory functions.

The State Emergency Medical Service is responsible for co-ordination of emergency management for public health threats, and acts as WHO liaison point for International Health Regulations.

National competent authorities for communicable disease control

Ministry of Health (Veselības ministrija): www.vm.gov.lv

Infectology Center of Latvia (Valsts aģentūra 'Latvijas Infektoloģijas Centrs'): www.lic.gov.lv

State Emergency Medical Service (Neatliekamās medicīniskās palīdzības dienests; NMPD): www.nmpd.gov.lv

Surveillance of communicable diseases

The surveillance of communicable diseases is regulated by the Epidemiological Safety Law. All physicians are obliged to report 72 notifiable diseases and conditions and laboratories are obliged to report 49 pathogens.

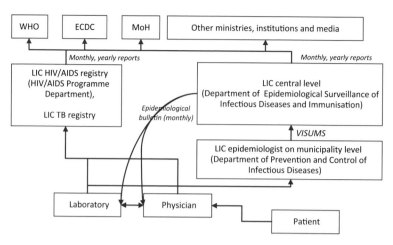

Fig. 5.19.1 Flow chart of statutory notifications: Latvia.

Notifications (except HIV/AIDS and tuberculosis) are made by the epidemiologists of LIC working at the local level (Figure 5.19.1). They organise epidemiological investigations and control measures as well as forward the reports to the central level. Surveillance data are disseminated via the *Epidemiological Bulletin* (in Latvian).

Case notification from physician or laboratory is being done through phone or paper, within 12–72 hours depending on disease (condition).

VISUMS, LIC computerised infectious diseases surveillance and monitoring system.

Outbreak investigation and control

The epidemiologists of the LIC working at the municipality level are responsible for control of outbreaks.

Childhood vaccination schedule

Updated data on the Latvian childhood vaccination schedule are available from EU-VAC.NET (www.euvac.net). The national programme includes BCG, DTaP, dT, HepB, Hib,
IPV, MMR, PCV7 and Var (see List of abbreviations).

Updated data on vaccine coverage are available from the WHO Regional Office for Europe (http://data.euro.who.int/cisid/). Recent vaccine coverage rates: BCG (98.8%), DTP4 (90.2%), HepB3 (93.6%), HiB3 (95%), MCV2 (96.5%) and Polio3 (95.9%).

5.20 Lithuania

Lithuania (population 3,545,000) is a republic, administratively divided into 10 counties, further subdivided into 60 municipalities.

The Ministry of Health is responsible for general supervision of the healthcare system. The Centre for Communicable Diseases and AIDS (ULAC) is a governmental institution under the Ministry of Health, established in 2009 in a merger of two previous institutions: the Centre for Communicable Diseases Prevention and Control and the Lithuanian AIDS Centre. ULAC organises and implements prevention and management of communicable diseases, including national surveillance and the national immunisation programme.

Public health centres are established in every county. These institutions are under the supervision of the State Public Health Service. Public health centres receive information from personal healthcare settings about cases of communicable diseases, they investigate outbreaks and are responsible for prevention and control of communicable diseases at local and regional level.

The Health Emergency Situation Centre is responsible for emergency preparedness and response. This institution is a 24/7 focal point in Lithuania and is responsible for information and co-ordination after work, during weekends and holidays.

The Lithuanian Institute of Hygiene dates back to 1808, and is responsible for prevention of nosocomial infections and rational use of antimicrobial agents, including surveillance in these areas.

National competent authorities for communicable disease control

The main institutions in the field of public health and communicable diseases are as follows:

Ministry of Health (Sveikatos apsaugos ministerijos; SAM): www.sam.lt

State Public Health Service (Valstybinę visuomenės sveikatos priežiūros tarnybą; VVSPT): www.vvspt.lt

Centre for Communicable Diseases and AIDS (Užkrečiamųjų ligų ir AIDS centro; ULAC): www.ulac.lt

National Public Health Surveillance Laboratory (Nacionalinė visuomenės sveikatos priežiūros laboratorija; NVSPL): www.nvspl.lt

Lithuania Health Emergency Situations Centre (Ekstremaliųjų sveikatai situacijų Centras; ESSC): www.essc.sam.lt

Lithuania Institute of Hygiene (Higienos Institutas; HI), provides scientific advice, communication and surveillance of hospital infections and antimicrobial resistance: www.hi.lt

Surveillance of communicable diseases

There are 84 communicable diseases notifiable by law, through a hierarchical system. Physicians report case data (within 12 hours) to public health institutions, who report aggregated data to the 11 regional public health centres (Figure 5.20.1). Communicable disease report forms are completed by every regional public health centre and sent to the ULAC, monthly and annually. The individual case reporting system is being implemented in Lithuania and will start from 2011. When it is fully implemented, monthly and annual reports from public health centres will no longer be required.

Surveillance data are disseminated via monthly and annual surveillance overviews on the ULAC website.

Outbreak investigation and control

Regional public health centres are responsible for outbreak investigations and control measures. For food-borne outbreaks, food and veterinary services are also involved. The ULAC supports systematic outbreak investigations and informs media and the Ministry of Health.

Childhood vaccination schedule

Updated data on the Lithuanian childhood vaccination schedule are available from EUVAC.NET (www.euvac.net). The national programme includes BCG, DTaP, dT, HepB, Hib, IPV and MMR (see List of abbreviations).

Updated data on vaccine coverage are available from the WHO Regional Office for Europe (http://data.euro.who.int/cisid/). Recent vaccine coverage rates: BCG (99%), DTP4 (90.1%), HepB3 (95%), HiB3 (98%), MCV2 (94%) and Polio3 (98%).

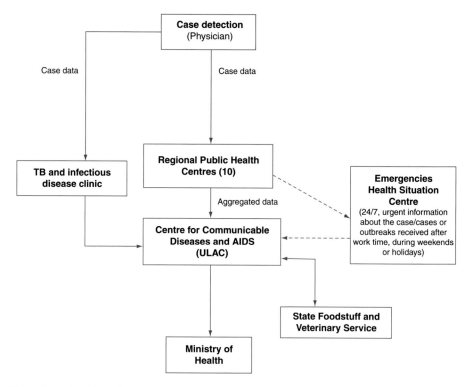

Fig. 5.20.1 Flow chart of statutory notification: Lithuania.

5.21 Luxembourg

Luxembourg is a constitutional monarchy (grand duchy) (population 500,000), administratively divided into 3 districts, which are further divided into 12 cantons. Public health is the responsibility of the Ministry of Health, and interventions are provided by a few public services and by private practitioners and non-profit associations paid for out of the Ministry budget.

The Health Directorate within the Ministry of Health is responsible for communicable disease control, especially policy issues, preparing and implementing guidelines, threat detection, preparedness and response, as well as training and communication. The national surveillance is carried out by the Division of Health Inspection within the Health Directorate, supported by experts in the National Health Laboratory (also responsible for sentinel surveillance of influenza and food poisoning) and the National Service of Infectious Diseases within the Central Hospital of Luxembourg.

National competent authorities for communicable disease control

The main institutions in the field of public health and communicable diseases are as follows:

Ministry of Health (Ministère de la Santé): http://www.ms.public.lu/fr/ministere/index.html

Ministry of Health, Health Directorate (Direction de la Santé): http://www.ms.public.lu/fr/direction/index.html

National Health Laboratory: www.lns.public.lu

Surveillance of communicable diseases

The infectious or communicable diseases subject to compulsory notification are regulated in the Règlement Grand-Ducal of 10 September 2004. The notifiable diseases are grouped into eight classes. A small fee per notified patient is given to physicians as financial incentive to notify. The estimated time to inform the national level is 2 days. Notifications are submitted to the Health Directorate, which publishes surveillance data every month with a yearly summary report (Figure 5.21.1).

Outbreak investigation and control

Control measures including contact tracing and outbreak investigation is the responsibility of the Health Directorate.

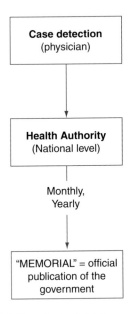

Fig. 5.21.1 Flow chart of statutory notification: Luxembourg.

Childhood vaccination schedule

Updated data on the Luxembourg childhood vaccination schedule are available from EU-VAC.NET (www.euvac.net). The national programme includes DTaP, dTap, HepB, Hib, HPV, IPV, MenC, MMRV, PCV13 and RTV (see List of abbreviations).

Updated data on vaccine coverage are available from the WHO Regional Office for Europe (http://data.euro.who.int/cisid/). Recent vaccine coverage rates: DTP4 (94.6%), HepB3 (94.5%), HiB3 (98.5%) and Polio3 (99.1%).

5.22 Malta

Malta (population 407,000) is a republic administered directly from the capital Valletta, subdivided into 6 districts (mainly for statistical purposes) and 54 local councils. The health system is entirely organised at national level. The Ministry of Health, the Elderly and Community Care has overall responsibility for the health services, including public health.

Within the Ministry the responsibility for communicable disease surveillance and control rests with the Department for Health Promotion and Disease Prevention and its Infectious Disease Prevention and Control Unit (IDCU). The IDCU is responsible for the national surveillance of communicable diseases, data dissemination, epidemiological research, as well as managing outbreaks. The unit also provides advice to health professionals and the general public and contributes to training in communicable disease control.

National competent authority for communicable disease control

Infectious Disease Prevention and Control Unit (IDCU) within the Department of Health Promotion and Disease Prevention of

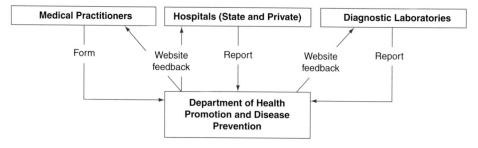

Fig. 5.22.1 Flow chart of statutory notification: Malta.

the Ministry for Social Policy, Health, the Elderly and Community Care: https://ehealth.gov.mt/HealthPortal/public_health/idcu/introduction.aspx

Surveillance of communicable diseases

The communicable diseases control is governed by the Prevention of Disease Ordinance Act and the Public Health Act. Some 67 communicable diseases are notifiable by law for all doctors in both public and private sectors. In addition, reports are filed from the microbiological laboratories (public and private) (Figure 5.22.1). Reports are filed via postal mail, fax and telephone and also via a secure e-mail system. The estimated time for reporting is 2 days. Data are collected and analysed by IDCU.

Reports on notified and confirmed cases are issued on the IDCU website as monthly and annual tables, and annual reports (https://ehealth.gov.mt/HealthPortal/public_health/idcu/library/library_menu.aspx).

Outbreak investigation and control

Reports of outbreaks are collected at the IDCU, which when necessary sets up outbreak control teams to investigate and follow up outbreaks so that timely control measures can be taken.

Childhood vaccination schedule

Updated data on the Maltese childhood vaccination schedule are available from EUVAC.NET (www.euvac.net). The national programme includes BCG, DT, Dt, DTaP, DTwP, HepB, Hib, IPV, MMR and OPV (see List of abbreviations).

Updated data on vaccine coverage are available from the WHO Regional Office for Europe (http://data.euro.who.int/cisid/). Recent vaccine coverage rates: BCG 82.3%), DTP4 (63.4%), HepB3 (86%), HiB3 (73%), MCV2 (85%) and Polio3 (73%).

5.23 The Netherlands

The Netherlands (population 16,609,000) is a constitutional monarchy divided into 12 provinces and subdivided into 431 municipalities. The Ministry of Health Welfare and Sports has the overall responsibility for the provision and infrastructure of public health in the country. Public health is regulated in the revised Dutch Public Health Act of 2008.

Public health is executed by 28 Municipal Health Services (GGDs), each under the responsibility of a group of collaborating municipalities. The Municipal Health Services take care of child health examinations, vaccinations, environmental health, medical disaster relief, health protection and health promotion activities. Local public health includes all aspects of infectious disease control, general hygiene, school health and public health education.

The centralised steering of outbreak control by the Minister is limited in the law to outbreaks of category A diseases and incidents/outbreaks with international impact. The Health Care Inspectorate (IGZ) under the Ministry monitors and assesses public healthcare, primarily on quality and safety.

The National Institute for Public Health and the Environment (RIVM) is a broad public health research institute acting in the fields of health, nutrition and environmental protection. RIVM is an agency of the Ministry of Health and mainly works for the Dutch government. RIVM has an important role in the co-ordination, prevention and control of infectious diseases, through its Centre for Infectious Disease Control (CIb) which hosts laboratories, epidemiology and the national co-ordination and response department. RIVM/CIb is responsible for the national surveillance of infectious diseases. It is designated national focal point for the communication with WHO and the EU, and it provides advice, support and co-ordination of outbreak management between the 28 municipal health services. RIVM/CIb issues guidelines for communicable disease prevention and control and is responsible for the national child immunisation programmes as well as for emergency vaccination campaigns.

National competent authorities for communicable disease control

Ministry of Health, Welfare and Sport (Ministerie van Volksgezondheid, Welzijn en Sport), Directorate-General of Public Health, policy issues and preparedness: http://www.rijksoverheid.nl/ministeries/vws

The Dutch Health Care Inspectorate (Inspectie voor de Gezondheidszorg; IGZ): www.igz.nl

Netherlands National Institute for Public Health and the Environment (Rijksinstituut voor Volksgezondheid en Milieu; RIVM): http://www.rivm.nl/en/

RIVM, Centre for Infectious Disease Control (Centrum Infectieziektebestrijding; CIb), national focal point, research, surveillance, secondary diagnostics, preparedness and response: http://www.rivm.nl/en/infectious-diseases/

Surveillance of communicable diseases

Notification and surveillance of communicable diseases is regulated in the Public Health Act 2008. The Ministry of Health is responsible for changes in statutory notification. The system is based on notifications both from physicians and laboratories to the Municipal Health Services (GGD). The national surveillance system (Osiris) at CIb is updated on a daily basis from the GGDs (Figure 5.23.1).

A total of 42 diseases in three groups are notifiable, either instantly on suspicion or within 24 hours after confirmation. No financial incentive is given to physicians to notify. A laboratory-based surveillance system for antimicrobial resistance (ISIS-AR) is run by RIVM-CIb together with the clinical microbiological laboratories run by the private sector.

Data dissemination is performed instantly through an electronic information system (inf@ct) in the case of an emergency, 2-monthly via a surveillance bulletin (*Infectieziekten Bulletin*) and through updates and reports on the RIVM-CIb website (http://www.rivm.nl/cib/publicaties/bulletin/).

Outbreak investigation and control

Under supervision of the mayor, the Municipal Health Service GGD is responsible for control measures including source and contact tracing and outbreak investigation, with assistance and co-ordination from the RIVM/CIb when necessary. In the case of a category A disease (polio, SARS, smallpox, haemorrhagic fever), or when international implications are expected, RIVM/CIb is in charge and gives out

Governors   **Professional**   **Inspection**

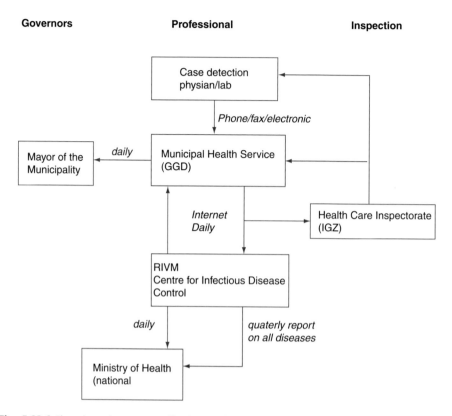

Fig. 5.23.1 Flow chart of statutory notification: Netherlands.

directives to the GGDs under supervision of the Minister. Measures to control an outbreak that violate human rights are exhaustively described in the law and assessed by court immediately after they are imposed.

Childhood vaccination schedule

Updated data on the Dutch childhood vaccination schedule are available from EU-VAC.NET (www.euvac.net). The national programme includes DTaP, dT, HepB, Hib, IPV, MenC, MMR and PCV (see List of abbreviations).

Updated data on vaccine coverage are available from the WHO Regional Office for Europe (http://data.euro.who.int/cisid/). Recent vaccine coverage rates: DTP4 (95.0%), HiB3 (96.7%), MCV2 (93.1%) and Polio3 (96.3%).

5.24 Norway

Norway (population 4,676,000) is a constitutional monarchy, administratively divided into 19 counties (*fylker*) and subdivided in 430 municipalities.

The Ministry of Health and Care Services (HOD) has the overall responsibility for the public health services in Norway. Among the main tasks of the Department of Public Health within the Ministry are protection against communicable diseases and the prevention of HIV/AIDS.

The Directorate of Health is a specialist directorate under the Ministry of Health and Care Services. Headed by the Chief Medical Officer, it has regulatory and implementing functions in the areas of health and care policy, and it monitors the conditions that affect public health. The directorate provides advice and guidance, and has authority to apply and interpret laws and regulations in the health sector.

The Norwegian Institute for Public Health (FHI) is a broad public health institution, acting as a national competence institution. The Division of Infectious Disease Control is responsible for prevention and control of communicable diseases. The activities include national surveillance of infectious diseases and infectious agents, specialised microbiological services, the national immunisation programme and vaccine supply. The division provides advice and recommendations and performs applied research.

National competent authorities for communicable disease control

Ministry of Health and Care Services (Helse og omsorgsdepartmentet HOD): http://www.regjeringen.no/en/dep/hod.html?id=421

Norwegian Directorate of Health (Helsedirektoratet): www.shdir.no

Norwegian Institute of Public Health (Folkehelseinstituttet; FHI): www.fhi.no

Surveillance of communicable diseases

The Norwegian Surveillance System for Communicable Diseases (MSIS) was established nationwide in 1975. Notifications are based on the Communicable Diseases Control Act from 1995 and Health Register Act from 2002. All physicians and medical microbiology laboratories are obliged to report notifiable disease directly to the FHI with copies for some diseases to municipal medical officer (Figure 5.24.1). Some 51 diseases are reported with full patient identification. HIV, gonorrhoea and syphilis are reported anonymously using non-unique identifier linking reports from clinicians and laboratories. There are no financial incentives for notifying physicians.

Searchable surveillance data are directly accessible on the Internet via www.msis.no.

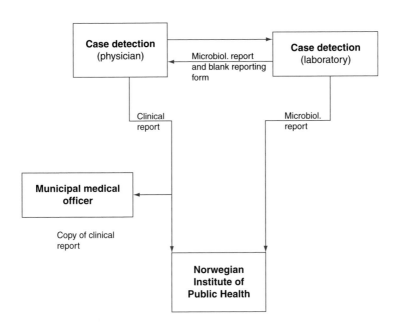

Fig. 5.24.1 Flow chart of statutory notification: Norway.

Outbreak investigation and control

The municipal medical officers have the legal responsibility for detection, investigation and public health actions within their municipality, in co-operation with other local authorities (e.g. food safety authorities). If more than one municipality is involved or otherwise needed NIPH will provide assistance.

Childhood vaccination schedule

Updated data on the Norwegian childhood vaccination schedule are available from EU-VAC.NET (www.euvac.net). The national programme includes BCG, DTaP, dT, HepB, Hib, HPV, IPV, MMR and PCV7 (see List of abbreviations).

Updated data on vaccine coverage are available from the WHO Regional Office for Europe (http://data.euro.who.int/cisid/). Recent vaccine coverage rates: HiB3 (94%), MCV2 (97%) and Polio3 (93%).

5.25 Poland

Poland (population 38,167,000) is a republic, administratively divided into 16 provinces (*voivodeships*) and further subdivided in 379 districts (*powiats*), including 65 cities with *powiat* status.

The Ministry of Health is responsible for national public health policy and implementing the national public health programmes. The Chief Sanitary Inspectorate (GIS) is a central administration body under the Minister of Health, with public health protection as the main mission. The GIS works with communicable disease control, and other issues related to public health, through a system of provincial, county and border sanitary–epidemiological stations. The GIS leads and coordinates the work of the 16 provincial (*voivodeship*) sanitary–epidemiological sta-

tions (WSSE), and the 10 border sanitary–epidemiological stations (GSSE), while district (*powiat*) and city sanitary–epidemiological stations (PSSE) are under the provincial sanitary–epidemiological stations. The GIS is also responsible for preparedness, response, threat detection and communication to the public on the national level.

The National Institute of Public Health – National Institute of Hygiene (NIZP-PZH) has a broad public health mission including infectious disease surveillance, microbiological services, food safety, scientific research and training. NIZP-PZH provides expertise and advice to the government and conducts vaccine research.

Surveillance and laboratory work on antimicrobial resistance is the responsibility of the National Medicines Institute (IL). The Polish National Tuberculosis and Lung Disease Institute (IGICHP) performs surveillance, research and gives scientific advice on all issues related to tuberculosis.

National competent authorities for communicable disease control

Ministry of Health (Ministerstwo Zdrowia; MZ): www.mz.gov.pl

Chief Sanitary Inspectorate (Główny Inspektorat Sanitarny; GIS): www.gis.gov.pl

National Institute of Public Health/National Institute of Hygiene (Narodowy Instytut Zdrowia Publicznego/Paristwowy Zaklad Higieny; NIZP-PZH): www.pzh.gov.pl

National Medicines Institute (Narodowy Instytut Leków; IL): http://www.il.waw.pl/english.html

Polish National Tuberculosis and Lung Disease Institute (Instytutu Gruźlicy i Chorób Płuc; IGICHP): www.igichp.edu.pl

Surveillance of communicable diseases

A total of 58 diseases and syndromes as well as hospital-acquired infections are by law

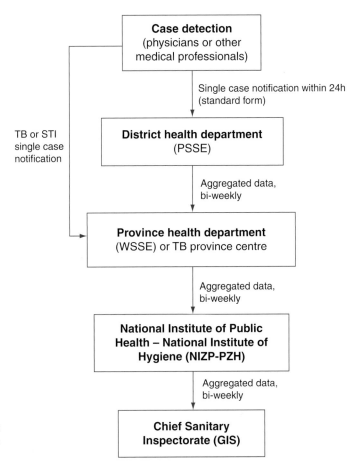

Fig. 5.25.1 Flow chart of statutory notification: Poland.

notifiable by physicians, some of them also by laboratories. For some of the diseases, specific case-based epidemiological information is collected. The information flow is hierarchical with first-level reporting of case data to the district Sanitary–Epidemiological Stations (PSSE). These pass on aggregated data to the Voivodeship (WSSE) level bi-weekly. The national level (NIZP-PZH) receives data from the second level, and it takes up to 14 days for data to reach the national level. Alert diseases are reported to national level in 24 hours (Figure 5.25.1).

Data from the national level is disseminated by the NIZP-PZH through a bi-weekly epidemiological bulletin, including tables of notified diseases and an annual epidemiological report (http://www.pzh.gov.pl/oldpage/epimeld/index_a.html).

Outbreak investigation and control

Control measures including contact tracing and outbreak investigation is generally the responsibility of the PSSE, with support at provincial and national level. The information is forwarded by the PSSE to the WSSE, which is responsible for outbreak detection and management at the provincial level. The WSSE reports to the NIZP-PZH and Chief Sanitary Inspectorate, which has national responsibility for outbreak control.

Childhood vaccination schedule

Updated data on the Polish childhood vaccination schedule are available from EU-VAC.NET (www.euvac.net). The national programme includes BCG, DTaP, DTwP, HepB, Hib, IPV, OPV and MMR (see List of abbreviations).

Updated data on vaccine coverage are available from the WHO Regional Office for Europe (http://data.euro.who.int/cisid/). Recent vaccine coverage rates: BCG (93.7%), DTP4 (95.6%), HepB3 (97.8%), HiB3 (98.8%), MCV2 (94.6%) and Polio3 (95.6%).

5.26 Portugal

Portugal (population 10,637,000) is a republic, administratively divided into 18 districts in mainland Portugal and two autonomous regions (Azores and Madeira). For health purposes, the mainland country is divided in 5 regional health administrations, and 74 primary healthcare centres groups, covering between 80,000 and 200,000 inhabitants.

Public health policy making is an important task for the Ministry of Health, while five Regional Health Administrations (mainland) and two Regional Health Directorates (Azores and Madeira) are in charge of implementing the policy and co-ordinating regional public health activities. National co-ordination of HIV/AIDS surveillance and prevention is a vertical programme directly under the Ministry of Health.

The General Directorate of Health (DGS) is under the Ministry of Health responsible for communicable disease prevention and control at the national level. It provides scientific advice, issues guidelines, organises the national surveillance, threat detection, training, preparedness and response, and communication about communicable diseases to the general public through its web portal.

The National Institute of Health 'Dr Ricardo Jorge' (INSA) is a state laboratory involved in microbiological surveillance and public health research. It acts under the Ministry of Health, and has as key areas of work food safety, infectious diseases, epidemiology, genetics, health promotion and chronic diseases and environmental health. It is also tasked with health research and produces scientific advice for public health policy and action. As a state laboratory it is responsible for co-ordinating quality assurance programmes.

In each Regional Health Administration (ARS) the public health department co-operates technically with DGS and ensures co-ordination between regional public health laboratory activities and INSA.

A network of local health authorities, consisting of public health doctors, is based in the primary healthcare centres groups. Among other tasks they are responsible for surveillance and control of communicable diseases.

National competent authorities for communicable disease control

Ministry of Health (Ministério da Saúde: www.min-saude.pt

Directorate General of Health (Direcção–Geral da Saúde; DGS), Disease Prevention and Control Department: www.dgs.pt

National Institute of Health 'Dr Ricardo Jorge' (Instituto Nacional de Saúde Dr Ricardo Jorge; INSA): www.insa.pt

Surveillance of communicable diseases

A total of 46 diseases are notifiable by law. Every physician identifying a case is responsible for reporting to the local health authority (Figure 5.26.1). DGS is responsible for the national surveillance, and is supported by INSA. Data dissemination is carried out by DGS, through periodic reports and yearly statistics on mandatory notifiable diseases which are published on the Internet (www.dgs.pt).

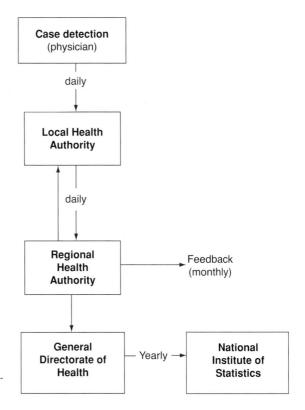

Fig. 5.26.1 Flow chart of statutory notification: Portugal.

Special bulletins are released when needed. In August 2009, new legislation has been published creating a national information system for surveillance and very soon it will be possible for clinicians and for laboratories to notify communicable diseases through a web platform.

cluding communicable disease outbreaks and food safety events) connects all levels of public health care.

Outbreak investigation and control

Control measures including contact tracing and outbreak investigation is generally the responsibility of the Public Health Service, primarily on local level with support from regional (ARS) and national level (DGS and INSA). A rapid alert and response system (Sistema de Alertas e Resposta Apropriada; SARA) for public health emergencies (in-

Childhood vaccination schedule

Updated data on the Portuguese childhood vaccination schedule are available from EU-VAC.NET (www.euvac.net). The national programme includes BCG, DTaP, dT, HepB, Hib, HPV, IPV, MenC and MMR (see List of abbreviations).

Updated data on vaccine coverage are available from the WHO Regional Office for Europe (http://data.euro.who.int/cisid/). Recent vaccine coverage rates: BCG (98%), DTP4 (95%), HepB3 (96%), HiB3 (96%), MCV2 (95%) and Polio3 (96%).

5.27 Romania

Romania (population 22,181,000) is a republic divided into 41 districts (*județe*) and the capital Bucharest with equal status, and further subdivided into 319 cities and 2686 municipalities. Each county is governed by a county council.

The national public health system is under the responsibility of the Ministry of Health, and in the area of communicable disease control the Ministry is responsible for initiation of legislative measures, implementation of surveillance systems, co-ordination of threat detection, preparedness and response, training, risk communication and international collaboration. This work is carried out by the Public Health and Communicable Diseases Surveillance and Control Department of the Public Health Authority within the Ministry through the co-ordination and supervision of a national network of communicable disease control and surveillance consisting of several national regional and district public health institutes and centres.

Under the Ministry of Health, the National Centre for Communicable Diseases Prevention and Control at the National Institute of Public Health Bucharest is integrating the parallel national surveillance systems and administrating the communicable diseases informational system, but it also monitors the national immunisation programmes, co-ordinates the national early warning and response system, and provides training.

The National Institute of Research and Development for Microbiology and Immunology Cantacuzino is an expert institute providing scientific support in the area of communicable disease control, including reference laboratory support, vaccine production and training.

National Institute for Infectious Diseases Prof. Dr. Matei. Bals is a tertiary care infectious disease unit providing care for HIV patients, but is also responsible for HIV surveillance and the national HIV prevention programmes. The Institute of Pneumology Marius Nasta has the same role for tuberculosis.

Four regional centres (Centrul Regional de Sanatate Publica; CRSP), subordinate to the National Institute of Public Health, have responsibilities for regional surveillance and control of communicable diseases, at local and regional level. The 42 district public health authorities (Direcții de sănătate public; DSP), in each district and the Bucharest Public Health Authority, have responsibility for control measures at district level, including implementation of the immunisation programmes and outbreak control.

National competent authorities for communicable disease control

Ministry of Health (Ministrul Sănătății): www.ms.ro

National Centre for Communicable Diseases Prevention and Control, National Institute of Public Health (Centrul pentru Prevenirea si Controlul Bolilor Transmisibile, Institutul National de Sanatate Publica Bucuresti; CPCBT-INSP): www.insp.gov.ro; http://www.insp.gov.ro/cpcbt

Institute of Pneumology Marius Nasta (Institutul de Pneumoftiziologie Marius Nasta), surveillance: www.marius-nasta.ro

National Institute for Infectious Diseases Prof. Dr. Matei Bals (Institutul National de Boli Infectioase Prof. Dr. Matei Bals), surveillance: www.mateibals.ro

National Institute of Research and Development for Microbiology and Immunology Cantacuzino (Institutul Cantacuzino), scientific advice, surveillance and response: www.cantacuzino.ro

Surveillance of communicable diseases

The Romanian surveillance system is regulated in the Communicable Disease Control and Surveillance Action Plan 2004. The reporting system covers 95 mandatory notifiable communicable diseases (suspect cases, confirmed cases, contacts and carriers) of

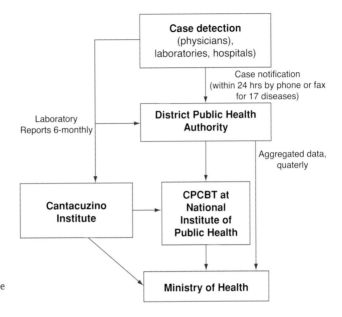

Fig. 5.27.1 Flow chart of case notification data: Romania.

which 17 are immediately notifiable (within 24 hours), while for the other 78 diseases there is a numerical reporting on a weekly, monthly, quarterly or annual basis. Physicians report to the DSPs, while all laboratories report aggregated information on the number of isolates and their antibiograms to the Cantacuzino Institute on a 6-monthly basis (Figure 5.27.1).

The DSPs report further to the Ministry of Health and to the CPCBT-ISPB on a quarterly basis. Data analysis is carried out at district, regional and national level. CPCBT-ISPB publishes weekly surveillance reports on its website.

There are separate systems for reporting on some diseases, for example HIV/AIDS, STI and tuberculosis.

Outbreak investigation and control

The DSPs have the main responsibility for controlling outbreaks in their district. Control measures may include mandatory treatment and hospitalisation. The CPCBT-ISPB holds the responsibility for co-ordination and control measures for outbreaks involving more than one district.

Childhood vaccination schedule

Updated data on the Romanian childhood vaccination schedule are available from EU-VAC.NET (www.euvac.net). The national programme includes BCG, DTaP, DtAP, HepB, IPV, MMR and R (see List of abbreviations).

Updated data on vaccine coverage are available from the WHO Regional Office for Europe (http://data.euro.who.int/cisid/). Recent vaccine coverage rates: BCG (99%), DTP4 (96.8%), HepB3 (95%), MCV2 (95%) and Polio3 (96.9%).

5.28 Slovakia

Slovakia (population 5,470,000) is a republic divided into 8 regions (*kraje*) and further subdivided into 79 districts (*okresy*). The

Ministry of Health has the overall responsibility for public health, including policy making, providing guidelines, health strategies, proposing legislation and co-ordinating preparedness, threat detection and response systems.

All the main activities in the area of communicable disease surveillance, prevention and control are carried out by the Public Health Authority of the Slovak Republic (PHA SR), an executive body under the Ministry of Health, and its network of 36 Regional Public Health Authorities (RPHA). PHA SR is headed by the Chief Hygienist of the Slovak Republic. This organisation is also responsible for the national child immunisation programme, food safety, environmental hygiene, health education, health statistics, as well as for other public health functions. Within PHA SR and selective RPHA are National Reference Centres, responsible for epidemiological and microbiological surveillance of specific infectious diseases. Surveillance is carried out closely together with the National Register of Communicable Diseases located in the Regional Public Health Authority in Banská Bystrica (RPHA BB).

Surveillance and control activities on tuberculosis are carried out by the National Institute for Tuberculosis, Lung Diseases and Thoracic Surgery in Vyšné Hágy which runs the national TB registry.

National competent authorities for communicable disease control

Ministry of Health of the Slovak Republic (Ministerstvo Zdravotníctva SR): www.health.gov.sk

Public Health Authority of the Slovak Republic (Úrad Verejného Zdravotníctva Slovenskej Republiky; PHA SR): http://www.uvzsr.sk/en/

National Institute for Tuberculosis, Lung Diseases and Thorax Surgery/National Register of Tuberculosis in Vyšné Hágy: http://www.hagy.sk/alias_admin/english/index.htm

Regional Public Health Authority in Banská Bystrica (RPHA BB): www.vzbb.sk

Surveillance of communicable diseases

A total of 64 diseases are mandatory notifiable by law. Physicians and laboratories report to the Regional Public Health Authority which passes the information on to the National Register of Communicable Diseases in RPHA BB. The national analysis of data is carried out together with the experts in PHA SR. The basis for the surveillance system is the national Epidemiological Information System (EPIS), and dissemination of data (mainly in Slovak language) is done through its portal, www.epis.sk (Figure 5.28.1).

Outbreak investigation and control

The physician reporting the patient is responsible for case management. Outbreak detection and control measures including contact tracing and outbreak investigation is generally the responsibility of the Regional Public Health Authorities with support from Public Health Authority of the PHA SR.

Childhood vaccination schedule

Updated data on the Slovakian childhood vaccination schedule are available from EUVAC.NET (www.euvac.net). The national programme includes BCG, DTaP, dT, HepB, Hib, IPV, MMR and PCV13 (see List of abbreviations).

Updated data on vaccine coverage are available from the WHO Regional Office for Europe (http://data.euro.who.int/cisid/). Recent vaccine coverage rates: BCG (97%), DTP4 (98.6%), HepB3 (99%), HiB3 (99%), MCV2 (99%) and Polio3 (99%).

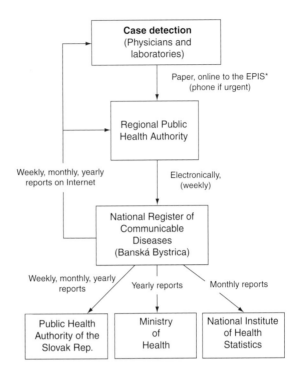

Fig. 5.28.1 Flow chart of statutory notifications: Slovakia.

* Epidemiological Infromation System

5.29 Slovenia

Slovenia (population 2,048,000) is a republic
divided into 12 regions and subdivided in 210
local municipalities, 11 of which have urban
status.

The Ministry of Health has the overriding
responsibility for the public health system:
public health policy, preparation of legislation and supervision of its implementation,
and overall monitoring of the public health
systems.

The National Institute of Public Health of
the Republic of Slovenia (IVZ) acts under the
Ministry of Health, and is a broad national
expert and reference institution. The IVZ co-
ordinates the activities of nine Regional Institutes of Public Health (RIPH). Within the IVZ,
the Centre for Communicable Diseases is responsible for epidemiological surveillance of

communicable diseases including healthcare-
associated infections. The centre is also involved in the preparation of proposals for legislation in the field of infectious diseases, and
in the implementation and evaluation of preventive and control measures. It issues recommendations and guidelines on all aspects of
communicable disease prevention and control and performs activities of a public health
microbiology laboratory. It is also involved in
research and training.

National competent authorities for communicable disease control

Ministry of Health: http://www.mz.gov.si/en/

National Institute of Public Health of the
Republic of Slovenia (Inštitut za varovanje
zdravja Republike Slovenije; IVZ): www.ivz.si

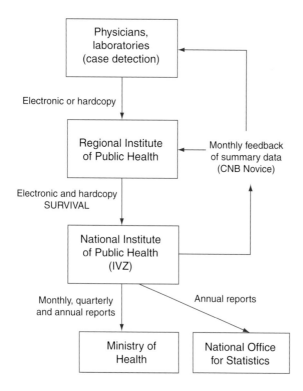

Fig. 5.29.1 Flow chart of statutory notification: Slovenia.

Surveillance of communicable diseases

The surveillance of communicable diseases is regulated by law, and the Ministry of Health is responsible for proposing changes in the legislation. Some 75 diseases are notifiable, and the diseases are grouped according to urgency of public health action. Group 1 disease must be reported by physicians within 6 hours of diagnosis to the RIPH and IVZ. Reporting is an obligation of both physicians and laboratories through a computerised reporting system (SURVIVAL) for the majority of infections and reconciliation of notifications and laboratory reports is undertaken at regional level. Specific surveillance systems have been developed for HIV and STIs. National healthcare-associated infections surveillance is under development.

National surveillance is co-ordinated by the Centre for Communicable Diseases at IVZ.

The Centre runs several national databases with reported data on communicable disease cases. There is a separate system for sexually transmitted infections and HIV (SPOSUR) with quarterly electronic reporting. Most of the results are disseminated through annual communicable disease surveillance reports and a monthly bulletin (CNB novice) available in Slovenian from the IVZ website (http://www.ivz.si/?ni=35).

Outbreak investigation and control

The responsibility for case management is held by the notifier. Outbreaks are detected at regional level by various information sources, including surveillance data and laboratory results. Reporting of suspected outbreaks to the IVZ is obligatory. Control measures such as contact tracing, clusters and outbreak investigation is under the responsibility of the RIPH (with the exception of HIV and STIs where it is the responsibility of the notifying physician) with support from IVZ.

Childhood vaccination schedule

Updated data on the Slovenian childhood vaccination schedule are available from EU-VAC.NET (www.euvac.net). The national programme includes BCG, DTaP, dTap, HepB, Hib, HPV, IPV, MMR and T (see List of abbreviations).

Updated data on vaccine coverage are available from the WHO Regional Office for Europe (http://data.euro.who.int/cisid/). Recent vaccine coverage rates: BCG (98%), DTP4 (83.8%), HepB3 (97%), HiB3 (96%), MCV2 (98%) and Polio3 (96%).

5.30 Spain

Spain (population 46,951,500) is a constitutional monarchy. The country is divided into 17 autonomous communities and 2 autonomous cities, subdivided into 52 provinces and further in municipalities. The autonomous communities have a large degree of autonomy with their own legislative assemblies, governments, supreme courts and public administrations. The public health services are organised regionally, and regional or local authorities are responsible for health protection, including surveillance and control of communicable diseases.

The Ministry of Health and Social Policy has the overall national responsibility to guarantee all inhabitants the right to health protection. Through its Directorate General of Public Health, the Ministry co-ordinates public health and is in charge of national health policy and initiation of appropriate legislation. The co-ordination of public health is carried out in the Inter-territorial Health Board, made up by national and regional Ministries

of Health, where the decisions are taken by consensus. At provincial (health area) level there are Provincial Health Units. At local level, the public health services are integrated within primary healthcare, and the main part of preventive medicine and health promotion is carried out by GPs and nurses.

There are several national expert institutions including the Institute of Health Carlos III (ISCIII), the Health Research Fund (with national centres covering research and service in epidemiology and microbiology), the National Plan on AIDS (in charge of co-ordinating research, information, prevention and treatment of AIDS) and the Spanish Food Safety Agency.

The ISCIII is the key national public health research and scientific support institute supporting and advising the Ministry of Health and Social Policy and the national healthcare system. The tasks include epidemiological surveillance, diagnostic and control of communicable diseases, the study of outbreaks and epidemics, and of other infectious or environmental health emergencies.

The Institute operates a number of special departments and agencies, including the National Epidemiology Centre (CNE), the National Centre for Tropical Medicine, the National Microbiology Centre and the National School of Public Health.

The CNE is responsible for managing the national surveillance and monitoring of both communicable and non-communicable diseases, as well as conducting research on health threats and providing training for experts in epidemiology and public health.

National competent authorities for communicable disease control

General Directorate of Public Health and Foreign Health (Dirección General de Salud Pública y Sanidad Exterior), Ministry of Health and Social Policy (Ministerio de Sanidad y Political Social): http://www.msc.es/en/home.htm

General Directorate of Public Health and Foreign Health, Ministry of Health and Social Policy (Dirección General de Salud Publica y Sanidad Exterior), Institute of Health Carlos III (Instituto de Salud Carlos III; ISCIII): www.isciii.es

National Centre of Epidemiology, Institute of Health Carlos III (Centro Nacional de Epidemiología, Instituto de Salud Carlos III): http://www.isciii.es/htdocs/centros/epidemiologia/epidemiologia_presentacion.jsp

Surveillance of communicable diseases

All physicians are required by law to notify 42 diseases or agents to the health authorities. The notifications follow a hierarchical system; physicians to provincial/area authorities to regional (autonomous community) authorities to the CNE to the Ministry of Health (Figure 5.30.1). The CNE manages surveillance at national level, and maintains the national epidemiological surveillance network (Red Nacional de Vigilancia Epidemiológica de España; RENAVE). The Ministry of Health and Social Policy gives direction to the system.

A non-statutory laboratory reporting system (Sistema de Información Microbiológica; SIM) compiles at the national level information provided by 53 clinical laboratories nationwide on 34 bacteria, viruses, fungi and intestinal parasites.

The CNE produces periodic reports on behalf of the Ministry of Health through a weekly epidemiological bulletin (*Boletín Epidemiológico Semanal*): http://www.isciii.es/jsps/centros/epidemiologia/boletinesSemanal.jsp

Outbreak investigation and control

Outbreak investigations as well as necessary control measures are carried out by the

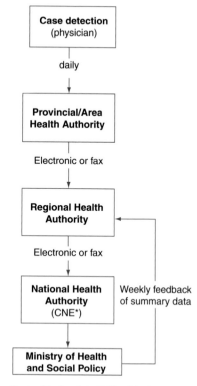

*CNE = Centro Nacional de Epidemiologia, Instituto de Salud "Carlos III"

Fig. 5.30.1 Flow chart of statutory notification: Spain.

health authorities at provincial or regional level with support from national level when necessary.

Childhood vaccination schedule

Updated data on the Spanish childhood vaccination schedule are available from EUVAC. NET (www.euvac.net). The national programme includes DTaP, dT, HepB, Hib, HPV, IPV, MenC, MMR and Var (see List of abbreviations).

Updated data on vaccine coverage are available from the WHO Regional Office for

Europe (http://data.euro.who.int/cisid/). Recent vaccine coverage rates: DTP4 (94.0%), HepB3 (95.5%), HiB3 (95.9%), MCV2 (90.1%) and Polio3 (95.9%).

5.31 Sweden

Sweden (population 9,074,000) is a constitutional monarchy, divided into 21 counties (*län*), and subdivided in 290 municipalities. Within each county there is a directly elected county council (*landsting*), responsible for healthcare and public health including communicable disease control at the county level. The role of the central government is to establish principles and guidelines for healthcare and public health, while its implementation is to a large degree decentralised.

The Ministry of Health and Social Affairs has the overall responsibility for policy and introduction of new legislation, but the main part of communicable disease control is carried out by the National Board of Health and Welfare (SoS) and the Swedish Institute for Infectious Disease Control.

The SoS has a co-ordinating responsibility for public health, and sets national standards, issuing guidelines, co-ordinating outbreak control and performing inspections. The SMI is the expert agency in charge of national surveillance of communicable diseases, reference microbiology functions, research and training. A national co-ordinating function for actions against antimicrobial resistance (STRAMA) is hosted by the SMI. The SMI also host the national Knowledge Centre for Microbiological Preparedness.

At the county level, the County Medical Officer for Communicable Disease Control (*smittskyddsläkaren*) has a far reaching responsibility for local surveillance and for prevention and control of communicable diseases, including healthcare-associated infections.

National competent authorities/bodies for communicable disease control

Ministry of Health and Social Affairs: http://www.sweden.gov.se/sb/d/2113

National Board of Health and Welfare (Socialstyrelsen; SoS): www.sos.se

Swedish Institute for Infectious Disease Control (Smittskyddsinstitutet; SMI): www.smi.se

Swedish Strategic Programme Against Antibiotic Resistance (STRAMA): http://en.strama.se/dyn/,84,,.html

Surveillance of communicable diseases

The surveillance of communicable disease is regulated in the Communicable Disease Act. Some 56 infections (including asymptomatic carriage) are notifiable within 24 hours, both by the physician and the diagnostic laboratory. Notifications are carried out in parallel to the County Medical Officer and to SMI through the electronic surveillance system, SmiNet (Figure 5.31.1). In this system, case notifications and laboratory reports are automatically merged using the unique personal identification number issued to all Swedish residents (HIV and STIs are notified coded without personal identification). The notifying physician is also obliged to enter relevant epidemiological information in each case notification.

At the county level, the surveillance information is used as a basis for direct public health action. At the national level, the information is analysed by the SMI for outbreak detection and following disease trends. Dissemination is carried out from SMI via a weekly electronic bulletin (*Epi-aktuellt*) and an annual surveillance report (both in Swedish). Monthly data are also available through the SMI website (http://www.smi.se/in-english/statistics/).

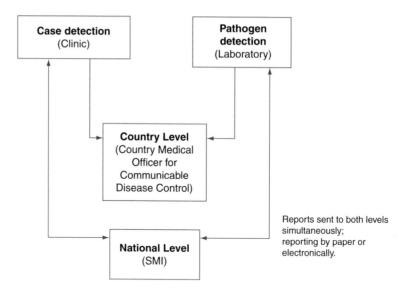

SMI = Swedish Institute for Infectious Disease Control Disease Control (Smittskyddsinstitutet)

Fig. 5.31.1 Flow chart of Statutory Notification: Sweden.

Outbreak investigation and control

The County Medical Officer is responsible for investigation, including contact tracing and control measures, assisted by the SMI when necessary. Depending on the kind of the outbreak the National Veterinary Institute (www.sva.se), the Swedish Board of Agriculture (www.sjv.se) and the National Food administration (www.slv.se) are also involved.

Childhood vaccination schedule

Updated data on the Swedish childhood vaccination schedule are available from EU-VAC.NET (www.euvac.net). The national programme includes BCG, DTaP, dTap, HepB, Hib, HPV, IPV, MMR and PCV7 (see List of abbreviations).

Updated data on vaccine coverage are available from the WHO Regional Office for Europe (http://data.euro.who.int/cisid/). Recent vaccine coverage rates: BCG (21.2%),

DTP4 (97.3%), HepB3 (22.5%), HiB3 (98.2%), MCV2 (94.9%) and Polio3 (98.4%).

5.32 Switzerland

Switzerland (population 7,623,000) is a confederation, consisting of 26 cantons, with a large degree of autonomy, and further subdivided into 2899 municipalities. Each canton has its own constitution, parliament, government and courts.

The confederation is limited to act in areas in which the constitution has granted it explicit powers, and health legislation is mainly a responsibility of the cantons. However, in the area of health protection, the federal constitution gives the confederation legislative powers in the area of combating transmissible diseases.

The responsibility for the control of infectious diseases lies with the 26 cantons, but under the Federal Authorities of the Swiss Confederation, the Federal Office of Public Health

(BAG) is the integrated centre of excellence for public health with a mandate to promote public health in the country. Its broad public health mandate covers surveillance and control of communicable diseases, including training, research and public campaigns, and it has a co-ordinating and supervisory function and issues national recommendations for surveillance and control.

The Division of Communicable Diseases in the BAG has separate functions for notification systems, epidemiological monitoring and assessment, strategies, principles and planning, vaccination programmes and control measures, prevention and promotion, as well as crisis management and international relations. The BAG is also responsible for national public health programmes, including the national HIV/AIDS programme and general child immunisation programmes, and is also tasked with legislation and oversight in the field of biological safety and consumer safety.

National competent authority for communicable disease control

Swiss Federal Office of Public Health (Bundesamt für Gesundheit; BAG): http://www.bag.admin.ch/index.html?lang=en

Surveillance of communicable diseases

The surveillance of communicable diseases is regulated by law (Epidemics Law of 18 December 1970 – now under revision). Some 35 diseases are notifiable. There are no financial incentives for notifying physicians. The majority of diseases are to be reported primarily by the laboratories to both the cantonal physician and the BAG (Figure 5.32.1). Statutory notification by physicians is restricted to diseases that may require prompt public health action in case of suspicion (e.g.

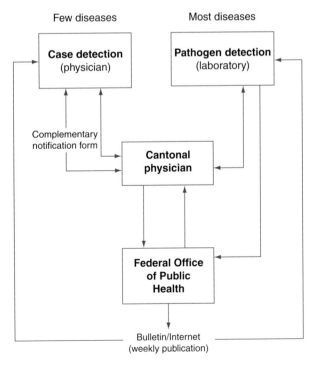

Fig. 5.32.1 Flow chart of statutory notification: Switzerland.

meningococcal disease) or for those where the diagnosis on clinical rather than laboratory grounds (e.g. AIDS).

An epidemiological bulletin (*Bulletin de l'Office Fédéral de la Santé Publique/ Bulletin des Bundesamtes für Gesundheit*) is published weekly by BAG (http://www.bag. admin.ch/dienste/publika/bulletin/d/index. htm) and surveillance data are also available on the Internet (http://www.bag.admin.ch/ infreporting).

Outbreak investigation and control

There is no national system for outbreak control in Switzerland. Outbreak management is the responsibility of the 26 cantons. The role of the BAG is mainly a coordinating one, and actions can only be taken by the BAG in exceptional situations.

Childhood vaccination schedule

Updated data on the Swiss childhood vaccination schedule are available from EUVAC.NET (www.euvac.net). The national programme includes BCG, DTaP, dT, HepB, Hib, HPV, IPV, MenC, MMR, PCV7 and Var (see List of abbreviations).

Updated data on vaccine coverage are available from the WHO Regional Office for Europe (http://data.euro.who.int/cisid/). Recent vaccine coverage rates: DTP4 (84%), HiB3 (93%), MCV2 (71%) and Polio3 (95%).

5.33 United Kingdom

The United Kingdom of Great Britain and Northern Ireland (population 61,792,000) is a constitutional monarchy that consists of four countries: England, Scotland, Wales and Northern Ireland. Health matters are devolved to the constituent nations and health protection arrangements therefore differ in each country.

England

The Department of Health in London has overall responsibility for health and healthcare and sets national policy for England. At local level, public health responsibilities are shared between the local NHS and Local Authorities, with the latter likely to take on more responsibility in the public health re-organisation planned for 2011. The Health Protection Agency (HPA) is the specialist agency that undertakes most specialised health protection functions through its local, regional and national teams and laboratories. At the time of writing, it is proposed that the HPA will be absorbed into a new service called Public Health England, which will become part of the Department of Health.

Scotland

The Scottish government is responsible for the development of health protection policy in Scotland and for NHSScotland and managing the performance of the latter. NHSScotland comprises 14 territorial NHS boards responsible for the planning and delivery of all health services in their area. These boards employ the local public health teams that undertake local health protection activities, supported by the relevant Local Authority environmental health teams. Health Protection Scotland (HPS) is the national centre for surveillance and investigation. It provides advice, support and information to health professionals, national and local government, the general public and other bodies that protect health. It commissions the national reference laboratories. For certain priorities, when requested by the government, it co-ordinates and assures the implementation of health protection policy. It leads the management of the health protection response when an incident affects more than one NHS board.

Wales

The Welsh Assembly government is responsible for health legislation and policy in Wales. Public Health Wales provides specialist health protection services, including the Communicable Disease Surveillance Centre, microbiology laboratories and local health protection teams that work with Local Authority environmental health departments and the NHS, which is organised into seven health boards.

Northern Ireland

The Department of Health, Social Services and Public Safety of the Northern Ireland Executive is responsible for health legislation and policy in Northern Ireland. The Public Health Agency provides a regional health protection service encompassing operational health protection response to both communicable and non communicable disease issues; surveillance; advice, information and support to healthcare professionals and related organisations, district councils and the general public.

National competent authorities for communicable disease control

The UK lead agencies for most international functions (e.g. links to WHO and ECDC), are the Department of Health (DH) and the Health Protection Agency (HPA), both based in England. However, within the UK, each nation has its own organisations that lead on communicable disease control issues within that country, for which they are not subordinate to DH/HPA.

England

Department of Health: www.dh.gov.uk
Health Protection Agency: www.hpa.org.uk

Scotland

Scottish Government Health Directorates: www.sehd.scot.nhs.uk
Health Protection Scotland: www.hps.scot.nhs.uk

Wales

Health and Social Care Department, Welsh Assembly Government: http://www.wales.gov.uk/topics/health/?lang=en
Public Health Wales: http://www.wales.nhs.uk/sitesplus/888/

Northern Ireland

Department of Health, Social Services and Public Safety, Northern Ireland Executive: www.dhsspsni.gov.uk
Public Health Agency: www.publichealth.hscni.net

Surveillance of communicable diseases

In England, notifications of communicable diseases are governed by the Health Protection (Notification) Regulations 2010, which makes it compulsory for medical practitioners to notify selected disease, infection or contamination in patients (http://www.legislation.gov.uk/uksi/2010/659/schedule/1/made) to the proper officer of the relevant Local Authority. In addition, diagnostic laboratories must notify selected causative agents found in human samples (http://www.legislation.gov.uk/uksi/2010/659/schedule/2/made) to the Health Protection Agency (or successor body).

Wales has similar arrangements to England, except that laboratory notifications are made to the proper officer of the Local Authority rather than the HPA. The list of notifiable diseases is slightly different in Scotland, where notification is to the local health board (http://www.legislation.gov.uk/asp/2008/5/contents), and in Northern Ireland, where notifications are to the DPH of the Public Health Agency (Figure 5.33.1).

(a)

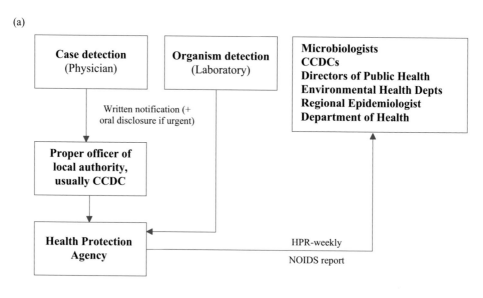

(b)

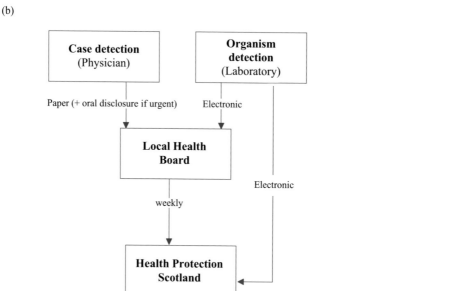

Fig. 5.33.1 Flow chart of statutory notifications: United Kingdom. (a) England; (b) Scotland; (c) Wales; and (d) Northern Ireland.

(c)

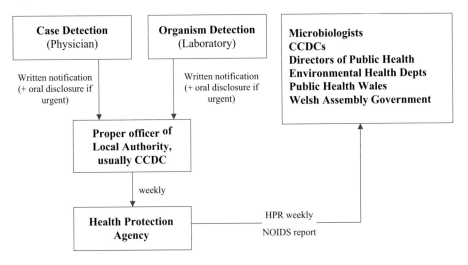

(d)

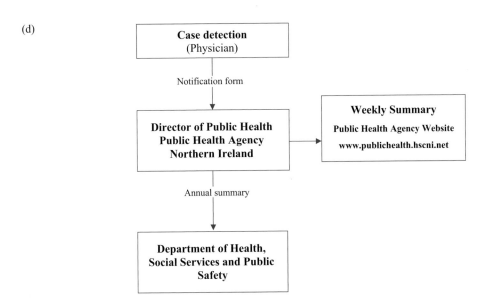

Fig. 5.33.1 (*Continued*)

Other sources of surveillance data used in the UK are discussed in Chapter 4.1.

Surveillance data are disseminated via the weekly Health Protection Report (http://www.hpa.org.uk/hpr/) for England and Wales and the HPS Weekly Report (http://www.hps.scot.nhs.uk/ewr/index.aspx) for Scotland. Other reports can be obtained from the relevant national agency website (see above).

Outbreak investigation and control

Outbreak investigation and management, including contact tracing, is generally undertaken by the local health protection unit (local public health department in Scotland) with support from local NHS, local authority, other relevant agencies (e.g. water company, Health and Safety Executive) and national health protection organisation as necessary.

Childhood vaccination schedule

Updated data on the UK childhood vaccination schedule are available from EUVAC.NET (www.euvac.net). The national programme is shown in Table 4.7.1.

Updated data on vaccine coverage are available from the WHO Regional Office for Europe (http://data.euro.who.int/cisid/). Recent vaccine coverage rates: DTP4 (81%), HiB3 (93%), MCV2 (79%) and Polio3 (93%).

Appendices

Appendix 1: Useful addresses and telephone numbers

European Union

European Centre for Disease Prevention and Control (ECDC)
Tomtebodavagen 11a, Solna, Sweden (Postal address: 171 83 Stockholm, Sweden)
Tel: (+46) 8586 01000

European Food Safety Authority (EFSA)
Largo N. Palli 5/A, 43121 Parma, Italy
Tel: (+39) 0521 036111

European Commission Directorate-General for Health and Consumers
B-1049, Brussels, Belgium
Tel: (+35) 243011

World Health Organization

WHO Regional Office for Europe (EURO)
Scherfigsvej 8, DK-2100 Copenhagen 0, Denmark
Tel: (+45) 3917 1717

WHO Headquarters
Avenue Appia 20, 1211 Geneva 27, Switzerland
Tel: (+41) 22791 2111

Health Protection Agency

Central Office, 151 Buckingham Palace Road, London, SW1W 9SZ
Tel: 0207 811 7000
Centre for Infections, 61 Colindale Avenue, London, NW9 5EQ
Tel: 0208 200 4400
Centre for Radiation, Chemical and Environmental Hazards, Chilton, Didcot, Oxon OX11 0RQ
Tel: 01235 831600
Centre for Emergency Preparedness and Response, Porton Down, Salisbury, Wiltshire SP4 0JG
Tel: 01980 612100

Health Protection Scotland (HPS)

Clifton House, Clifton Place, Glasgow, G3 7LN
Tel: 0141 300 1100

Public Health Wales Health Protection Division

Temple of Peace and Health, Cathays Park, Cardiff, CF10 3NW
Tel: 02920 402532

Public Health Agency (Northern Ireland)

Ormeau Avenue Unit, 18 Ormeau Avenue, Belfast BT2 8HS
Tel: 02890 311611

Departments of Health

England: Department of Health
Richmond House, 79 Whitehall, London SW1A 2NS
Tel: 0207 210 4850

Scotland: Scottish Government Health Directorate
St Andrew's House, Regent Road, Edinburgh EH1 3DG
Tel: 0131 556 8400

Wales: Welsh Assembly Government Department for Health and Social Services
Cathays Park, Cardiff CF10 3NQ
Tel: 02920 370011

Northern Ireland: Department of Health, Social Services and Public Safety,
Castle Buildings, Stormont, Belfast, BT4 3SJ
Tel: 02890 520500

Food Standards Agency

UK Headquarters: Aviation House, 125 Kingsway, London, WC2B 6NH
Tel: Switchboard 0207 276 8000; Emergencies only 0207 270 8960

Scotland: St Magnus House, 6th Floor, 25 Guild Street, Aberdeen, AB11 6NJ
Tel: 01224 285100

Communicable Disease Control and Health Protection Handbook, Third Edition. Jeremy Hawker, Norman Begg, Iain Blair, Ralf Reintjes, Julius Weinberg and Karl Ekdahl.
© 2012 Jeremy Hawker, Norman Begg, Iain Blair, Ralf Reintjes, Julius Weinberg and Karl Ekdahl.
Published 2012 by Blackwell Publishing Ltd.

Wales: 11th Floor, Southgate House, Wood Street, Cardiff, CF10 1EW
Tel: 02920 678999

Northern Ireland: 10c Clarendon Road, Belfast, BT1 3BG
Tel: 02890 417700

National Poisons Information Service (NPIS)
Tel: 0844 892 0111

National Travel Health Network and Centre (NaTHNaC)
Tel: 0845 602 6712

Advice Lines Available to General Public
NHS Direct: Tel: 0845 4647
National AIDS Helpline (now Sexual Health Line): Tel: 0800 567123
Hospital for Tropical Diseases Travellers Healthline: Tel: 0207 950 7799
Meningitis Trust: Tel: 0800 028 1828
Meningitis Research Foundation: Tel: 080 8800 3344

Appendix 2: Guidance documents and books

Please note that guidance documents are often updated and the documents given below are the most up-to-date at the time of writing. Checks for additional, more up-to-date or more local guidance can be made by accessing the appropriate national centre website (see Section 5 chapters) or by checking the list of websites at the end of this appendix.

Blood-borne viruses

UK Health Departments. AIDS/HIV Infected Health Care Workers: Guidance on the Management of Infected Health Care Workers and Patient Notification – A Consultation Paper. London: Department of Health, 2002. (Available at http://www.dh.gov.uk/assetRoot/04/01/85/96/04018596.pdf).

Expert Advisory Group on AIDS (EAGA). HIV Post-Exposure Prophylaxis: Guidance from the UK Chief Medical Officers' Expert Advisory Group on AIDS. London: Department of Health, 2008.

(Available at http://www.dh.gov.uk/en/Publicationsandstatistics/Publications/PublicationsPolicyAndGuidance/DH_088185?ssSourceSiteId=ab).

European Commission. *Recommendations for Post-Exposure Prophylaxis Against HIV Infection in Health Care workers in Europe.* Project number SI2.322294, March 2002. (Available at http://www.inmi.it/news/LineeGuida/RecommendationsHCW.htm).

Clinical Effectiveness Group (British Association for Sexual Health and HIV). UK guideline for the use of post-exposure prophylaxis for HIV following sexual exposure. *Int J STD AIDS* 2006, **17**: 81–92. (Available at http://www.bashh.org/documents/58/58.pdf).

European Commission. *Management of Non-occupational Post Exposure Prophylaxis to HIV: Sexual, Injecting Drug User or Other Exposures.* Project number 2000CVG4-022, April 2002. (Available at http://www.inmi.it/news/LineeGuida/ReccommendationsNONOCC.pdf).

Health Protection Agency. Standards for Local Surveillance and Follow Up of Hepatitis B and C. London: HPA, 2006. (Available at http://www.hpa.org.uk/web/HPAwebFile/HPAweb_C/1194947376936).

NHS Executive (England). *Hepatitis B Infected Health Care Workers: Guidance on Implementation of Health Service Circular 2000/020.* Leeds: NHS Executive, 2000. (Available at http://www.dh.gov.uk/assetRoot/04/05/75/38/04057538.pdf).

Ramsay ME. Guidance on the investigation and management of occupational exposure to hepatitis C. *Commun Dis Public Health* 1999, **2**: 258–262. (Available at http://www.hpa.org.uk/web/HPAwebFile/HPAweb_C/1194947393443).

Department of Health. *Hepatitis C Infected Health Care Workers*. London: Department of Health Publications, 2002. (Available at http://www.dh.gov.uk/assetRoot/04/05/95/44/04059544.pdf).

Gastrointestinal diseases

Working Group of former PHLS Advisory Committee on Gastrointestinal Infections. Preventing person-to-person spread following gastrointestinal infections: guidelines for public health physicians and environmental health officers. *Comm Dis Public Health* 2004, **7** (4): 362–384. (Available at http://www.hpa.org.uk/cdph/issues/CDPHVol7/no4/guidelines2_4_04.pdf).

Food Standards Agency (FSA). *Management of Outbreaks of Foodborne Illness in England and Wales*. London: FSA, 2008. (Available at http://www.food.gov.uk/multimedia/pdfs/outbreakmanagement.pdf).

Gastointestinal Programme Board VTEC working group (HQSD). *The VTEC Operational Manual*. London: HPA 2010. (Available at http://www.hpa.org.uk/web/HPAwebFile/HPAweb_C/1279889252950).

PHLS Viral Gastroenteritis Working Group. Managements of hospital outbreaks of gastro-enteritis due to small round structured viruses. *J Hosp Inf* 2000, **45**: 1–10. (Note: under revision in 2011: up-to-date guidelines on the management of norovirus outbreaks in hospitals and on cruise ships can be accessed at http://www.hpa.org.uk/webw/HPAweb&HPAwebStandard/HPAweb_C/1195733840182?p=1191942172932).

Hunter PR. Advice on the response from public and environmental health to the detection of cryptosporidial oocysts in treated drinking water. *Commun Dis Public Health* 2000, **3**: 24–27. (Available at http://www.hpa.org.uk/cdph/issues/CDPHvol3/No1/crypto.pdf).

Hepatitis A Guidelines Group. *Guidance for the Prevention and Control of Hepatitis A Infection*. HPA, 2009. (Available at http://www.hpa.org.uk/web/HPAwebFile/HPAweb_C/1259152095231).

Immunisation

Department of Health. *Immunisation against Infectious Diseases*. London: DH, 2007. (Available at http://www.dh.gov.uk/en/Publicationsandstatistics/Publications/PublicationsPolicyAndGuidance/DH_079917?CONTENT_ID=4097254&chk=isTfGX).

Royal College of Paediatrics and Child Health. *Immunisation of the Immunocompromised Child: Best Practice Statement February 2002*. (Available at http://www.rcpch.ac.uk/sites/default/files/asset_library/Publications/I/Immunocomp.pdf).

Imported infections and travel advice

World Health Organization. *International Travel and Health*. Geneva: WHO, 2010. (Available at http://www.who.int/ith/).

National Travel Health Network and Centre. *Health Information for Overseas Travel*. London: NaTHNaC, 2010. (ISBN 0-11-322329-3). (Available at http://www.nathnac.org/yellow_book/YBmainpage.htm).

Chiodini P, Hill D, Lea G, Walker E, Whitty C, Bannister B. *Guidelines for Malaria Prevention in Travellers from the United Kingdom 2007*. London: HPA, 2007. (Available at http://www.hpa.org.uk/Publications/InfectiousDiseases/TravelHealth/0701MalariapreventionfortravellersfromtheUK/).

Advisory Committee on Dangerous Pathogens. *Management and Control of Viral Haemorrhagic Fevers*. London: The Stationary Office, 1996. (ISBN: 0-11-321860-5). (Available at http://www.hpa.org.uk/Topics/InfectiousDiseases/InfectionsAZ/ViralHaemorrhagicFever/Guidelines/).

Bonnet JM, Begg NT. Control of diphtheria: guidance for consultants in communicable disease control. *Commun Dis Public Health* 1999, **2**: 242–249. (Available at http://www. hpa.org.uk/web/HPAwebFile/HPAweb_C/ 1194947407702).

Department of Health. *Memorandum on rabies: Prevention and Control.* London: Department of Health, 2000. (Available at http://www.dh.gov.uk/assetRoot/04/08/06/ 57/04080657.pdf).

Infection control and healthcare-acquired infections

Pratt RJ, Pellowe CM, Wilson JA, Loveday HP, Harper PJ, Jones SR, *et al.* epic2: National evidence-based guidelines for preventing healthcare-associated infections in NHS hospitals in England. *J Hosp Infect* 2007; **65** (Supplement 1): 1–59. (Available at http:// www.journalofhospitalinfection.com/issues/ contents?issue_key=S0195-6701(07)X6001-8).

Department of Health. *Infection Control Guidance for Care Homes.* London: Department of Health, 2006. (Available at http:// www.dh.gov.uk/prod_consum_dh/groups/ dh_digitalassets/@dh/@en/documents/ digitalasset/dh_4136384.pdf).

Coia E, Duckworth GJ, Edwards DI, Farrington M, Fry C, Humphreys H, *et al.* Guidelines for the control and prevention of methicillin-resistant *Staphylococcus aureus* (MRSA) in healthcare facilities. *J Hosp Infect* 2006, **66** (Supplement 1):1–44.

Nathwani D, Morgan M, Masterton RG, Cookson BD, French G, *et al.* on behalf of the British Society for Antimicrobial Chemotherapy Working Party on community-onset MRSA Infections. Guidelines for UK practice for the diagnosis and management of methicillin-resistant *Staphylococcus aureus* (MRSA) infections presenting in the community 2008. *J Antimicrob Chemother* 2008, **61**: 976–994.

Healing TD, Hoffman PN, Young SEJ. The infection hazards of human cadavers. *Commun Dis Rep CDR Rev* 1995; **5**: R61–68.

Meningitis and meningococcal infections

European Centre for Disease Prevention and Control. *Public Health Management of Sporadic Cases of Invasive Meningococcal Disease and their Contacts.* Stockholm: ECDC; 2010. (Available at http://ecdc.europa.eu/ en/publications/Publications/1010_GUI_ Meningococcal_guidance.pdf).

HPA Meningococcus Forum. *Guidelines for Public Health Management of Meningococcal Disease in the UK.* London: HPA, 2006. (Available at http://www.hpa.org.uk/web/ HPAwebFile/HPAweb_C/1194947389261).

Cartwright KAV, Begg NT, Rudd P. Use of vaccines and antibiotic prophylaxis in contacts and cases of *Haemophilus influenzae* type b (Hib) disease. *Commun Dis Rep CDR Rev* 1994, **4**: R16–17.

Tuberculosis

National Institute for Health and Clinical Excellence. Clinical Diagnosis and Management of Tuberculosis, and Measures for its Prevention and Control. National Institute for Health and Clinical Excellence (NICE) Tuberculosis Clinical Guideline. London: NICE, 2006. (Available at http://www.nice.org.uk/ CG033).

Influenza

European Centre for Disease Prevention and Control. *Interim Guidance: Public Health Use of Influenza Antivirals During Influenza Pandemics.* Stockholm: ECDC, 2009. (Available at http://ecdc.europa.eu/en/publications/ Publications/0907_GUI_Public_Health_use_ of_Influenza_Antivirals_during_Influenza_ Pandemic.pdf).

European Centre for Disease Prevention and Control. *Interim Guidance: Use of*

Specific Pandemic Influenza Vaccines During the H1N1 2009 Pandemic. Stockholm: ECDC, 2009. (Available at http://ecdc.europa.eu/en/publications/Publications/0908_GUI_Pandemic_Influenza_Vaccines_during_the_H1N1_2009_Pandemic.pdf).

Other infections

Lee JV, Joseph C. Guidelines for investigating single cases of Legionnaires' disease. *Commun Dis Public Health* 2002, **5**: 157–161. (Available at http://www.hpa.org.uk/cdph/issues/CDPHvol5/No2/guidelines1.pdf).

Health Protection Agency. *Guidelines for the Public Health Management of Pertussis*. London: HPA, 2010. (Available at http://www.hpa.org.uk/web/HPAwebFile/HPAweb_C/1287142671506).

Morgan-Capner P, Crowcroft NS. Guidelines on the management of and exposure to rash illness in pregnancy. *Commun Dis Public Health* 2002, **5**: 59–71. (Available at http://www.hpa.org.uk/cdph/issues/CDPHVol5/No1/rash_illness_guidelines.pdf).

Crowcroft NS, Roth CE, Cohen BJ, Miller E. Guidance for the control of parvovirus B19 infection in healthcare settings and the community. *J Public Health Med* 1999, **21**: 439–446.

Health Protection Agency. *Guidance for Managing STI Outbreaks and Incidents*. London: HPA, 2010. (Available at http://www.hpa.org.uk/web/HPAwebFile/HPAweb_C/1214553002033).

Health Protection Agency. *Initial Investigation and Management of Outbreaks and Incidents of Unusual Illness*. London: HPA, 2010. (Available at http://www.hpa.org.uk/web/HPAwebFile/HPAweb_C/1201265888951).

WHO. *Manual: The Public Health Management of Chemical Incidents*. Geneva:

WHO, 2009. (Available at http://www.who.int/environmental_health_emergencies/publications/Manual_Chemical_Incidents/en/index.html).

Health Protection Agency. *Guidance on Infection Control in Schools and Other Child Care Settings*. London: HPA, 2010. (Available at http://www.hpa.org.uk/web/HPAweb&HPAwebStandard/HPAweb_C/1203496946639).

Joint Formulary Committee. *British National Formulary*. London: British Medical Association, 2010.

Websites containing infectious disease guidelines

http://www.ecdc.europa.eu/en/publications/guidance/Pages/index.aspx

http://www.who.int/rpc/guidelines/en/index.html (plus some additional guidelines in disease sections of http://www.who.int/)

http://www2.evidence.nhs.uk/

http://www.library.nhs.uk/infections/

http://guidance.nice.org.uk/Topic/Infectious Diseases

http://www.neli.org.uk/IntegratedCRD.nsf/NeLI_Browse_Guidelines?OpenForm

http://www.hpa.org.uk/ (look in individual 'Topics A–Z')

http://www.escmid.org/escmid_library/medical_guidelines/escmid_guidelines/

http://www.idsociety.org/content.aspx?id=9088

http://www.cdc.gov/ncidod/guidelines/guidelines_topic.htm

Index

acetylsalicylic acid 152–3
actinomycetes 272–7
  see also fungi
acute chemical incidents
  see also chemicals
  management 336–9, 363–5
acute encephalitis 108, 287–90
  see also encephalitis
acute radiation incidents
  see also radiation incidents
  management 339–52
acute STIs 119–22
  see also sexual health and HIV infection services;
    sexually transmitted infections
adenovirus 30–3
Advice Line Available to General Public 422
Advisory Committee on Dangerous Pathogens
  247, 256
Afghanistan 191, 248, 326
aflatoxins 55, 281
African eye worm (loiasis) 266
Aga Khan Foundation 359–60
AIDS 46–52, 140–7, 313–17, 327, 356–60
  see also HIV
algae, shellfish poisoning 281
ambulances 337–9, 342–52, 370
ammonia 100, 128
amnesic shellfish poisoning 281
amoebic dysentery 39–40, 61–2, 270
  see also Entamoeba histolytica; protozoal diseases
Angola 248, 326
anthrax 62–5, 287–90, 349–52
  see also Bacillus anthracts
anti-helminthics 226
  anthrax 63–5
  sexually transmitted infections 120–2
  wound botulism 70
antimicrobial resistance 120, 172–6, 304–12, 367
  see also methicillin-resistant *Staphylococcus*
    aureus
antiretroviral therapy (ART), HIV 141–7
antitoxins, botulism 70–1
antivenoms 280
Arenaviridae 248–51, 278
ascariasis 260
aspergillosis 45–7, 55–6, 273, 306–10
  see also fungi
audits, clinical governance and audit 4, 15,
  353–6
Austria 372
Avian influenza 12–15, 148–9, 328–31
  see also influenza
azithromycin 87, 120, 224, 253

babesiosis 270, 272
  see also protozoal diseases
bacillary dysentery 215
  see also Shigella
Bacillus anthracts 62–5, 288–90, 349–52
  see also anthrax
Bacillus cereus 24–9, 65–7, 288–90
Bacillus licheniformis 67
Bacillus subtilis 22–9, 67
bacterial meningitis 19–22, 287–90
  see also meningococcal infection
bacterial vaginosis 40–4
Bartonella 241–4
  see also Rickettsia
bats 195, 247, 279
BCG 53, 230–7, 307–10, 319–21, 324, 327
bean sprouts, salmonella 55
bedbugs 280
bee stings 280
Belgium 4, 120, 142, 166, 189, 229–30, 373–4
Bell's palsy 137
bilharzia 269
Bill and Melinda Gates Foundation Global Health
  Program 360
biological incidents, deliberate release of
  biological/chemical/radiological agents
  12–15, 33, 62, 64–5, 67–71, 72–3, 188, 220–1,
  238–9, 291–8, 342–52, 363–5
bites 272, 280, 325–8
  see also stings; venoms
blastomycosis 273
  see also fungi
blogs, media relations and crisis communications
  353
blood flukes 269
blood-borne viral infections (BBV) 12–15, 47–52,
  56–7, 145–7, 302–4, 422–3
  see also hepatitis; HIV
  causes 47–52
  guidance documents and books 50–2, 302–4,
    321–2, 422–3
  individual measures against infections 3, 8–10,
    56–7, 325–8
boiled water 100–2
Bolivia 248–51
boosters, vaccines 106
Bordetella pertussis 253–5, 288–90
  see also whooping cough
Borrelia recurrentis 57, 196–7, 280
  see also relapsing fever
botulism 12–15, 55, 67–71, 280, 287–90, 349–52
  see also Clostridium botulinum
Bouchier report 101–2

Communicable Disease Control and Health Protection Handbook, Third Edition. Jeremy Hawker, Norman Begg,
Iain Blair, Ralf Reintjes, Julius Weinberg and Karl Ekdahl.
© 2012 Jeremy Hawker, Norman Begg, Iain Blair, Ralf Reintjes, Julius Weinberg and Karl Ekdahl.
Published 2012 by Blackwell Publishing Ltd.

Indexed by TERRY HALLIDAY

DATE DUE

			PRINTED IN U.S.A.